THE ETHICS OF
SURGICAL PRACTICE

THE ETHICS OF SURGICAL PRACTICE

Cases, Dilemmas, and Resolutions

James W. Jones

Laurence B. McCullough

Bruce W. Richman

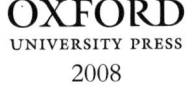

OXFORD
UNIVERSITY PRESS
2008

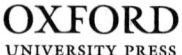

OXFORD
UNIVERSITY PRESS

Oxford University Press, Inc., publishes works that further
Oxford University's objective of excellence
in research, scholarship, and education.

Oxford   New York
Auckland   Cape Town   Dar es Salaam   Hong Kong   Karachi
Kuala Lumpur   Madrid   Melbourne   Mexico City   Nairobi
New Delhi   Shanghai   Taipei   Toronto

With offices in
Argentina   Austria   Brazil   Chile   Czech Republic   France   Greece
Guatemala   Hungary   Italy   Japan   Poland   Portugal   Singapore
South Korea   Switzerland   Thailand   Turkey   Ukraine   Vietnam

Published by Oxford University Press, Inc.
198 Madison Avenue, New York, New York 10016

www.oup.com

Oxford is a registered trademark of Oxford University Press

Library of Congress Cataloging-in-Publication Data
Jones, James W. (James Wilson), 1941–
The ethics of surgical practice : cases, dilemmas, and resolutions / James W. Jones,
Laurence B. McCullough, Bruce W. Richman.
p.   cm.
Includes bibliographical references.
ISBN 978-0-19-532108-1; 978-0-19-532109-8 (pbk.)
1. Surgeons—Professional ethics—Case studies.   I. McCullough, Laurence B.
II. Richman, Bruce W.
[DNLM: 1. Surgery—ethics—Case Reports.   2. Biomedical Research—ethics—
Case Reports.   3. Ethics, Medical—Case Reports.   4. Patient Rights—ethics—Case Reports.
WO 21 J77e 2008]
RD27.7.J66 2008
174.2'97—dc22   2007034983

9 8 7 6 5 4 3 2 1

Printed in the United States of America
on acid-free paper

This book is dedicated to Dr. Charles Dunlop, a beloved teacher of pathology at Tulane University, who never practiced clinical medicine but impressed a system of ethical values on generations of medical students. The following is a quote from Dr. Dunlop at a graduation address in 1966: "The affection and respect you will command from this day forward as doctors of medicine—these are not things of your own making. These things have been earned for you by the decency and humanity of countless generations of good men of all faiths over the past three thousands years. These men are dead and for the next few years you will hold in your own hands this magnificent heritage." Every physician would do well to accept this splendid challenge as guidance for their professional deportment.

· PREFACE ·

Probably no genre in all of literature is as little appreciated or as seldom read as the preface to a volume of nonfiction. Finding necessity to establish some context for the pages that follow, however, we shall commandeer the next few pages for that purpose, and make way for the body of a book we hope you will find both instructive and entertaining as you delve into the moral and intellectual processes of surgical ethics.

For many medical professionals, studying theoretical ethics is like reading a telephone book. Interest in medical ethics is directly proportional to one's immediate need to know, and you're not going to be interested in any of the undeniably valuable information in a phone book unless you have a specific question. Perhaps for surgeons, the study of gross anatomy would be a better example of the necessity to master material before its usefulness is fully apparent. We've tried to overcome the sense of artificiality with which even experienced practitioners study theoretical medical and surgical ethics by presenting a case-based course in practical ethics, an evaluation of ethical problems that are regularly encountered in the course of our work. We'll place you or people you're invited to observe in challenging ethical situations, ask you to make the best ethical choice, and discuss the strengths and weaknesses of the available options. Sometimes, as in actual surgical practice, no perfect answer will be available, and you'll be asked to make the best of the bargain by applying the ethical principles you've learned to select the most favorable course of action among those offered. We use this method to help you prepare yourself to handle ethical challenges when you encounter situations like these in the course of your independent practices, or be able in utterly different situations to extrapolate from these cases the principles of surgical ethics with which to resolve questions of good and bad action and good and bad character.

Our goal in this book is also to encourage the habits of preventive ethics. Ethical dilemmas are avoided by anticipating them. Anticipation is the key to success for students, stockbrokers, surgeons, and nearly everyone else. Anticipation in ethics is a skill developed by recognizing the conditions under which conflicting obligations arise and implementing standard choices and behaviors that help to obviate them. Ethical conflicts create an additional emotional burden for patients and families who are already trying to cope with the misery and anxiety routinely attendant to major illness. Ethical conflicts complicate the work of surgeons and clinical colleagues whose jobs are hard enough without them. We want to help you learn to avoid ethical conflict whenever you can, and learn to handle it adroitly when you can't.

The cases presented are edited versions of previously published papers in the "Surgical Ethics Challenges" section of the *Journal of Vascular Surgery*, which we initiated in 2001, and the "Ethics" series in *Surgery*, which we wrote from 2002 to 2005. You may have read condensed versions of some of the cases published in *Surgery News* or *Contemporary Surgery*. We have tried to make the fictional cases with which each study begins apply to a broad surgical audience, but many maintain vestiges of a vascular surgery orientation. Readers should be untroubled by this small slant, and understand that none of the cases is specialty-specific. Use each of them to explore how the ethical principles articulated will apply to your own surgical practice, in whatever subspecialty you study or work.

Surgical ethics is heavily context dependent, and we have attempted to provide all the information necessary to an informed choice without belaboring the issue. The informal style is intended to simulate discussions in the surgical lounge where colleagues might chat about such matters between cases. We also intend the style to promote teaching of surgical ethics to medical students, residents, and fellows, as curricular efforts in surgical ethics continue to develop and expand.

We have one disclaimer before we move on. As you read Chapter 2 on the subject of informed consent, you'll note that several cases involve Jehovah's Witnesses complying with their faith's interpretation of biblical passages. We want to make clear that we hold no special brief with this or any other religious denomination, as we hope the individual case discussions will confirm. We respect Jehovah's Witness members as having a deeply devoted faith that they are prepared to test with their lives. We utilized the Jehovah's Witnesses patients as exemplary of situations in which a surgeon may encounter a patient who exercises his autonomy by insistently withholding consent for treatment in the service of a value system that may be sharply at variance with the surgeon's instincts to preserve life whenever possible. No criticism of the beliefs or practices of Jehovah's Witnesses or any other faith community is intended or implied in these explorations of the principles of informed consent and patient autonomy.

We regard the ethical principles, rights, values, and virtues as humanitarian tools for discovering wisdom. Wisdom is one of the most desirable endpoints to be reached in life; it is our guide in deciding what to do next at every crossroad. We consider someone to be wise when we can count on him to reliably and sensibly suggest what difficult choice to make among contending imperatives. We hope that what you are about to read helps you to formulate wisdom in your medical practice.

Enjoy the rest of the book.

· ACKNOWLEDGMENTS ·

The case studies presented in this book are edited from versions that originally appeared in the *Journal of Vascular Surgery* and *Surgery*. They are republished here with permission.

Case 1: Jones JW, McCullough LB, Richman BW. Painted into a corner: unexpected complications in treating a Jehovah's Witness. *J Vasc Surg*. 2006; 44:435–438.

Case 2: Jones JW, McCullough LB. Refusal of life-saving treatment in the aged. *J Vasc Surg*. 2002; 35:1067.

Case 3: Jones JW, McCullough LB. Consent for an intraoperative video record. *J Vasc Surg*. 2001; 34:1133–1134.

Case 4: Jones JW, McCullough LB. Disclosure of intraoperative error. *Surgery*. 2002; 132:531–532.

Case 5: Jones JW, Richman BW, McCullough LB. The public's right to know? Surgical treatment of public figures. *J Vasc Surg*. 2002; 36:865–866.

Case 6: Jones JW, McCullough LB. Religiously based emergency treatment refusal. *J Vasc Surg*. 2001; 34:952.

Case 7: Jones JW, McCullough LB. Consent for residents to perform surgery. *J Vasc Surg*. 2002; 36:655–666.

Case 8: Jones JW, McCullough LB, Richman BW. Shifting sands of senility: canceled consent. *J Vasc Surg*. 2008 47: 87–89.

Case 9: Jones JW, McCullough LB, Richman BW. A surgeon's obligations to a Jehovah's Witness child. *Surgery*. 2003; 133:110–111.

Case 10: McCullough LB. Are ethics practical when externals impact your clinical judgment ? *J Vasc Surg*. 2007; 45:1282–1284.

Case 11: Jones JW, McCullough LB, Richman BW. What to tell patients harmed by other physicians. *J Vasc Surg*. 2003; 38:866–867.

Case 12: Jones JW, McCullough LB, Richman BW. The military physician's ethical response to evidence of torture. *Surgery*. 2004; 136:1090–1093.

Case 13: Jones JW, McCullough LB, Richman BW. Who should protect the public against bad doctors? *J Vasc Surg*. 2005; 41:907–910.

Case 14: Jones JW, McCullough LB, Richman BW. Management of disagreements between attending and consulting physicians. *J Vasc Surg*. 2003; 38:1137–1138.

Case 15: McCullough LB, Richman BW. Turf wars: the ethics of professional territorialism. *J Vasc Surg*. 2005; 42:587–589.

Case 16: Jones JW, Richman BW, McCullough LB. Professional self-regulation: eyewitness to incompetent surgery. *J Vasc Surg.* 2002; 36:1092–1093.

Case 17: Jones JW, McCullough LB, Richman BW. Ethics of operative scheduling: fiduciary patient responsibilities and more. *J Vasc Surg.* 2003; 38:204–205.

Case 18: Jones JW, McCullough LB, Richman BW. Do unto others: justice in surgical education. *Surgery.* 2003; 133:443–444.

Case 19: Jones JW, McCullough LB, Richman BW. The surgeon's obligations to the noncompliant patient. *J Vasc Surg.* 2003; 38:626–627.

Case 20: Jones JW, McCullough LB, Richman BW. Ethics of serving as a plaintiff's expert medical witness. *Surgery.* 2004; 136:100–102.

Case 21: Jones JW, McCullough LB, Richman BW. Standard of care: what does it really mean? *J Vasc Surg.* 2004; 40:1255–1257.

Case 22: Jones JW, McCullough LB. When does conventional surgical therapy become research? *J Vasc Surg.* 2002; 36:423–424.

Case 23: Jones JW, McCullough LB. A surgeon's obligations when performing new procedures. *J Vasc Surg.* 2002; 35:409–410.

Case 24: Jones JW, McCullough LB, Richman BW. The ethics of innovative surgical approaches for well-established procedures. *J Vasc Surg.* 2004; 40:199–201.

Case 25: Jones JW, McCullough LB, Richman BW. Ethics of surgical innovation to treat rare diseases. *J Vasc Surg.* 2004; 39:918–919.

Case 26: Jones JW, McCullough LB, Crigger NA, Richman BW. Ethics of introducing new operating room technology. *J Vasc Surg.* 2004; 39:482–483.

Case 27: Jones JW, McCullough LB, Richman BW. Ethics of patenting surgical procedures. *J Vasc Surg.* 2003; 37:235–236.

Case 28: Jones JW, McCullough LB, Richman BW. The ethics of sham surgery in research. *J Vasc Surg.* 2003; 37:482–483.

Case 29: Jones JW, McCullough LB. Stem cell research: Obligations when religious values conflict with professional values. *J Vasc Surg.* 2004; 40:589–591.

Case 30: Jones JW, McCullough LB, Richman BW. The ethics of odd ideas, good science, and academic freedom. *J Vasc Surg.* 2005; 41:1074–1076.

Case 31: Jones JW, McCullough LB, Richman BW. The ethics of bylines: will the real authors please stand up? *J Vasc Surg.* 2005; 42:816–818.

Case 32: Jones JW, McCullough LB, Richman BW. When the data won't get you there: the ethics of scientific error, and worse. *J Vasc Surg.* 2006; 43:1308–1310.

Case 33: Intentional overtreatment: the unmentionable conflict-of-interest. *J Vasc Surg.* 2007; 46:605–607.

Case 34: Jones JW, McCullough LB, Richman BW. Patient responsibilities, family responsibilities. *J Vasc Surg.* 2003; 37:698–699.

Case 35: McCullough LB, Richman BW, Jones JW. Nonmonetary conflicts of interest. *J Vasc Surg.* 2002; 36(6):1309–1310.

Case 36: Jones JW, McCullough LB. Ethics of over-scheduling: when enough becomes too much. *J Vasc Surg.* 2007; 45:635–636.

Case 37: Jones JW, McCullough LB, Richman BW. An impaired surgeon, a conflict of interest, and supervisory responsibility. *Surgery.* 2004; 135:449–451.

Case 38: Jones JW, McCullough LB. Surgeon-industry relationships: ethically responsible management of conflicts of interest. *J Vasc Surg.* 2002; 35:825–826.

Case 39: Jones JW, McCullough LB, Richman BW. Relationship funding of professional foundations: just another black sheep? *J Vasc Surg.* 2006; 44: 1126–1128.

Case 40: Jones JW, McCullough LB. When to refer to another surgeon. *J Vasc Surg.* 2002; 35:192.

Case 41: Jones JW, Richman BW, McCullough LB. HIV-infected surgeon: professional responsibility and self interest. *J Vasc Surg.* 2003; 37:914–915.

Case 42: Jones JW, McCullough LB, Richman BW. Ethical nuances of combining romance with clinical practice. *J Vasc Surg.* 2005; 41:174–175.

Case 43: Jones JW, McCullough LB, Richman BW. The ethics of operating on a family member. *J Vasc Surg.* 2005; 42:1033–1035.

Case 44: Jones JW, McCullough LB, Richman BW. Show me the money: the ethics of physicians' incomes. *J Vasc Surg.* 2005; 42:377–379.

Case 45: Jones JW, McCullough LB, Richman BW. Ethics of institutional marketing: role of physicians. *J Vasc Surg.* 2003; 38:409–410.

Case 46: Jones JW, McCullough LB, Richman BW. Ethics of boutique surgery. *J Vasc Surg.* 2004; 39:1354–1355.

Case 47: Jones JW, McCullough LB, Richman BW. Ethics and commercial insurance. *J Vasc Surg.* 2004; 39:692–693.

Case 48: Jones JW, McCullough LB, Richman BW. The ethics of clinical pathways and cost control. *J Vasc Surg.* 2003; 37:1341–1342.

Case 49: Jones JW, McCullough LB, Richman BW. Ethics of professional courtesy. *J Vasc Surg.* 2004; 39; 1140–1141.

Case 50: Jones JW, McCullough LB, Richman BW. The ethics of administrative credentialing. *J Vasc Surg.* 2005; 41:729–731.

Case 51: Jones JW, McCullough LB, Richman BW. Ethics of the new economic credentialing: conflicted leadership roles. *J Vasc Surg.* 2005; 41:365–367.

Case 52: Jones JW, McCullough LB, Richman BW. Whodunit? ghost surgery and ethical billing. *J Vasc Surg.* 2005; 42:1239–1241.

Case 53: Jones JW, McCullough LB, Richman BW. Other people's money: ethics, finances, and bad outcomes. *J Vasc Surg.* 2006; 43:863–865.

Case 54: Jones JW, McCullough LB, Richman BW. Consultation or corruption? The ethics of signing on to the medical-industrial complex. *J Vasc Surg.* 2006; 43:192–195.

Case 55: Jones JW, McCullough LB. Going public with amazing cases: fiat or fiasco? *J Vasc Surg*. 2007; 45:1084–1085.

Case 56: Jones JW, McCullough LB. Ethics of unprofessional behavior that disrupts: crossing the line. *J Vasc Surg*. 2007; 45:433–435.

Case 57: Jones JW, McCullough LB, Richman BW. My brother's keeper: uncompensated care for illegal immigrants. *J Vasc Surg*. 2006; 44:679–682.

Case 58: Jones JW, McCullough LB, Richman BW. From premiums to payouts: who's behind the malpractice crisis anyway? *J Vasc Surg*. 2006; 43:635–638.

Case 59: Jones JW, McCullough LB, Richman BW. A helping hand bitten: an ethical response to medical malpractice suits. *J Vasc Surg*. 2006; 43:422–425.

Case 60: Jones JW, McCullough LB. Caseload outcome credentialing: taking from the have-notes. *J Vasc Surg*. 2007; 45:214–216.

Case 61: Jones JW, McCullough LB. Fiduciary economization: your wealth or your health. *J Vasc Surg*. 2007; 45:858–860.

Case 62: Jones JW, McCullough LB. What to do when an international traveler's care goes south. J Vasc Surg. 2007; 46:1077–1079.

Case 63: Jones JW, McCullough LB. Futility and surgical intervention. *J Vasc Surg*. 2002; 35:1305.

Case 64: Jones JW, McCullough LB. Complying with advance directives in the operating room. *J Vasc Surg*. 2002; 36:199–200.

Case 65: Jones JW, McCullough LB. Abdominal aortic aneurysm in death row inmate. *J Vasc Surg*. 2002; 35:621–622.

Case 66: Jones JW, McCullough LB, Richman BW. Truth-telling about terminal diseases. *Surgery*. 2005; 137:380–382.

Case 67: Jones JW, McCullough LB. Arsenic and old lace: end-of-life care in the postoperative period. *Surgery*. 2002; 131:583–584.

Case 68: Jones JW, McCullough LB, Richman BW. Training on newly deceased patients. *Surgery*. 2004; 135: 108–109.

Case 69: Jones JW, McCullough LB, Richman BW. Advanced age, dementia, and an abdominal aneurysm: intervene? *J Vasc Surg*. 2003; 37:1132–1133.

Case 70: Jones JW, McCullough LB, Richman BW. Withdrawal of life-sustaining low-burden care. *J Vasc Surg*. 2005; 42:176–177.

Case 71: Jones JW, McCullough LB, Richman BW. Physician-assisted suicide: has it come of age? *Surgery*. 2005; 138:105–108.

· CONTENTS ·

6 The Ethics of Surgery as a Business • 192

7 Challenges to Medical Professionalism: Assaults from Within and Without • 247

THE ETHICS OF
SURGICAL PRACTICE

INTRODUCTION: A PRIMER ON SURGICAL ETHICS

Surgical Ethics: An Essential Component of Contemporary Surgical Practice

Ethics is now recognized as an essential supporting discipline in the practice of surgery.[1] Surgical ethics is the application of ethics to situations specific to surgical practice. We do not pretend that surgical ethics are of such specialized precision that they are completely unlike ethical situations and decisions found in other medical specialties. But surgery's mainstay is the operative experience, and that kind of work requires a unique frame of mind. Some of the ethical principles you'll read about in this book, such as avoidance of conflicts of interest, honesty with patients, and research integrity, can be easily extrapolated to any of the medical specialties. Other issues, such as suspension of do not resuscitate (DNR) orders, innovation versus controlled trials, ghost surgery, sham-controlled studies, and high-tech robotics, are largely specific to the surgeon's work, and their ethical implications must be individually considered. Best ethical practices are now an essential component of best surgical practices. As a result, rigorous ethical practices have become critical to the success of even the most technically skillful surgery.

The complexity of medical ethics has increased exponentially in the past half century for a number of reasons. Medical knowledge and technology, as in all scientific constructs, have outraced our understanding of when and how to make use of them. Dizzying reams of regulations constantly pour from the imaginations of well-meaning government agencies, legislatures, insurers, and professional organizations determined to improve our clinical practices, what and how we teach, what and how we investigate, and how and how much we get paid. The social context of patient relationships with physicians would hardly be recognized by a time-traveling surgeon who made the short trip from the mid-20th century. The basic ethical principles remain constant at their core, but as their context changes so do their applications. The era of "iron men sailing wooden ships" disappeared as MRIs, spiral CT scans, minimally invasive surgery, robotics, and the 80-hour workweek materialized.

Most surgical thinking takes the form of complex binary logic. Like a computer, the surgeon sees A or not-A. A patient lives or dies, bleeds or does not bleed, becomes infected or does not. Those who believe that their thought processes are more rich and nuanced than binary thinking seems to permit should be reminded that the critical decision processes we call clinical pathways are effectively binary algorithms. A completed surgical procedure is good or not good, as are judgments of nonprofessional performances. Ambivalence and polysemy are not well tolerated by surgeons. It is not coincidental that surgical board exams do not incorporate essay questions.

Against this mind-set, the study of medical and surgical ethics requires an ability to distinguish degrees of value or lack thereof. The best solution to an ethical question is often chosen from another solution that is not quite as good. But you must understand why the choice was made, and that skill development is the goal of this casebook. Contending imperatives are par for the course in situations requiring an ethical judgment. There is often more than one party in an ethical issue with a legitimate entitlement to have interests served. The ethical choice you make as a practicing surgeon will represent your best understanding of your moral responsibility in a given situation, but it also may mean that someone involved in the transaction is not getting all they want. And there should be no mistake—as the surgeon, you will be seen as the authority figure and ultimately be held responsible for how things turn out. This will be the case even when, despite your acknowledged expertise, you are not in control of the decision process, as we will discuss at length throughout this volume. In the cases presented here, the choice of available answers to the ethical dilemmas we present may twist and turn on degrees of reasonableness rather than be absolutely right. As in life, as in science, absolute truth's existence is denied because most truth is interpretive opinion. Even the perceived truths of religions change over time; disrespectful offspring are no longer stoned, witches are not hunted, and heretics need not fear being roasted. Amen.

The entry of ethical study into the rigorously scientific arena of surgery has been impeded by a belief that moral philosophy lacks the intellectual discipline and precision physicians rightly demand. The point is arguable. Like the application of grammar to language, ethics provides the structure that universalizes difficult moral decision making. But medical ethics is more than structural methodology; it incorporates principles, virtues, and values that predate medical science. The typical response to an event similar to one experienced in the past is to defend the actions previously taken and repeat them. One should never allow "clinical and ethical experiences" to mean making the same mistakes for 30 years. When practical ethics is mastered, as in the study of medicine, one can learn to avoid repetitive problems that attend trial-and-error learning.

Medical ethics is not an epiphenomenon to medical professionalism; it is the linchpin of professionalism. Medical ethics as moral philosophy examines reasons for behaviors, the correctness of behaviors, and evolves as reasoned reflection on clinical experience requires it to evolve. Medical ethics cannot be fully characterized as good professional manners, but it does promote them. A physician competent in medical ethics will be a better humanist, physician, and person, and will be confident that his or her moral choices are reflective of the highest professional ideals.

A Practical Method for Surgical Ethics: Achieving Discipline and Precision

Ethics has been understood for centuries in world intellectual traditions to be the disciplined study of morality.[1] Morality is a set of customary behaviors, governing how we act or don't act, as well as expectations of character that are regarded as proper for a particular culture at a particular time. The etymological root of the word moral meant customary. These expectations of right actions become our virtues and drive our values. Virtues are traits or habits of character that help us to routinely discern our obligations and direct us to fulfill them. Values are people's long-held standards and reflect what they feel is important; values drive our behaviors. Many are instilled in childhood, polished in early adulthood, and reorganized as ingrained professionalism. Ethical analysis is founded in a belief that current ideas of morality are always subject to re-examination and improvement, if only incrementally. Morality relies deeply on tradition, but uncritical acceptance of traditional morality can be a poor guide to ethically justified behavior: behavior for which we can give good reasons. If tradition were an indelible moral standard, exempt from examination, we would still be stoning and burning anyone who challenged us to learn and improve. Most people living in eras that endorsed those behaviors vigorously resisted any contemporary suggestions that their actions were wrong. Quite to the contrary, many of the people who most directly engaged in extreme forms of racial, social, and religious oppression considered themselves heroically moral for doing so. The consideration of ethics, in medicine, and in the culture at large, must be continuous, because our ideas of justice and fairness are always in need of critical assessment and improvement. Science, philosophy, and logic itself all deny the existence of an absolute truth beyond which inquiry is no longer necessary.

With the goal of improving morality, ethical study proposes to investigate what morality ought to be. Typically, this broad question is divided into two more concrete, manageable questions. First, what should our character be or not be? And, second, what should our conduct be or not be? The goal of studying ethics is to answer these questions in three steps, not unlike clinical medicine's processes. The first step in ethical evaluation is verification of the facts at issue. The second step is analysis, identifying and clarifying the meaning of concepts responsive to the two basic questions of character and conduct. Unclear concepts weaken the intellectual discipline of ethics, just as they weaken discourse in medical science, and almost always guarantee that conclusions will be imprecise and off-target. The third step is argumentation, the testing of ethical concepts against one another to reveal their relative strengths, flaws, and real-world durability. Ethical study does not accept unexamined assertions, what Plato's Socrates calls "mere opinion," even if those opinions originate from powerful authorities.

The intellectual authority of ethical argument depends not on the established eminence of the surgeon or philosopher who propounds it, but on the argument's ability to withstand assault by competing ideas and reach the status of ethical conclusion by maintaining its relevance and integrity. We've chosen the format of competition among intellectual formulations to demonstrate throughout this volume how ethical questions might be verified, refined, and argued in the context of daily surgical practice.

In popular discourse, it is sometimes said that in ethics there are no right or wrong answers. This is a mistake. There are well-reasoned and poorly reasoned and even unreasoned views about what morality should be, and with proper application one can differentiate between them. We intend to help you learn to do so.

Basic Concepts and Terms: Professional Virtues and Ethical Principles

The surgeon's responsibility to act as the patient's fiduciary is the ethical concept that guides how the surgeon thinks and behaves in virtually every clinical context. This concept especially means that the surgeon will consistently place the patient's health-related interests before his or her own interests, and that the patient may always rely on the surgeon to do so once a therapeutic relationship is established. The role of the surgeon as the patient's fiduciary demands that the surgeon provide vital care even when payment is not assured. It demands that care be provided even when the surgeon would rather be doing something else. It may even require the surgeon to provide treatment when doing so could place him or her at risk of personal injury. This concept has been confirmed in law as well as in ethical theory, and has survived the question of whether a duty exists for a surgeon to operate on an HIV-positive patient whose life-threatening disease may be communicated to the surgeon through a torn glove or an accidental nick at the operating table. Such a duty does exist. The surgeon must always make the protection and promotion of the patient's interests the primary consideration in the therapeutic encounter. Any and all elements of the surgeon's self-interest, however legitimate, must be considered secondary to the welfare of the patient. Most of everything else in the clinical application of surgical ethics derives from this principle.

Four professional virtues are essential to fulfilling fiduciary responsibility toward patients: integrity, compassion, self-effacement, and self-sacrifice. The fundamental professional virtue is integrity, indicating a moral wholeness with nothing of moral importance withheld. It requires surgeons to operate, conduct research, and teach in accordance with standards of intellectual and moral excellence. Intellectual excellence means that surgical judgment, decision making, technique, research, and education should reflect the most advanced state of medical knowledge and its technical application, requiring the surgeon to maintain educational currency in all elements of study affecting his or her work. A surgeon's medical education can never end if he or she is to serve patients with integrity throughout his or her career. Achieving and maintaining high levels of intellectual excellence, despite the obvious difficulty and inconveniences of always doing so while managing all facets of a demanding practice, are primary measures of the surgeon's professional integrity.

The professional virtue of compassion requires that the surgeon be alert to and prepared to respond to the pain, misery, and anxiety of patients and their families as they contend with significant illness and the sequelae of treatment. Although many surgeons place their greatest pride in their technical skills and breadth of knowledge, patients often evaluate their doctors by the degree to which they demonstrate understanding of the emotional blows accompanying their illnesses. Patients facing major surgery hate and fear the prospect of pain, disfigurement, disability, helplessness, threats to their self-esteem, interruptions or loss of their livelihoods, and disruptions in the accustomed patterns of their lives. They may or may not confide it to their surgeons, but they are afraid of death, dependency, and becoming a burden to those they love. In a revealing study of patients interacting with their surgeons during clinic visits, patients gave an average of 1.9 hints that they wanted to discuss their fears in more detail, and surgeons responded positively in only 38% of instances.[2] The best technical surgeons in the world will not have served their patients fully if they have not endeavored to help them through these uncertainties.

The professional virtue of self-effacement requires the surgeon to put aside personal preconceptions and be unaffected by them in the provision of equally excellent care to all who seek it. Certainly this is a virtue demanded nowadays of nearly all segments of our culture in their public capacities, but surgeons are nonetheless members of a tiny, elite subset of any social group. Surgeons are individually selected through an rigorous on-the-job trial of more than half a decade, challenging them to display superior intelligence, rare technical skills, emotional durability, human sensitivity, and an extraordinary capacity for hard work. Surgeons' power to heal and their authority within the doctor-patient relationship are remarkable, even when compared to other medical specialists. Unwavering self-confidence is an essential character element among men and women who invade living human bodies, rearrange the pieces, and put them back together better than before. These are traits that can easily inflate an ego and stimulate it to run away with itself. But the surgeon who displays a sense of personal superiority in dealing with patients will inevitably be considered ethically obtuse, and in relating poorly to patients he or she will necessarily provide them with suboptimal care. Self-effacement becomes another essential element of fiduciary responsibility because it sublimates the surgeon's personality to the needs of patients by containing the surgeon's pride of accomplishment.

The professional virtue of self-sacrifice is cited in acknowledgment of the extraordinary personal demands placed on the men and women who elect to work within the surgical profession. Lengthy and grueling training regimens, long hours away from family and private life, physically draining operations at the highest pitch of emotional intensity, and constant responsibility for the lives and deaths of others make surgery a very hard job indeed. The few who are capable of doing it must adopt a persistent ethical habit of self-abnegation. The great Duypuytren's personal historical footnote read, "Best among surgeons, least among men."

Like the virtues that describe the essential character traits, the principles of ethics provide the rules of how medical ethics works, its constitution. These principles are inviolate, except where they conflict. They are beneficence, respect for patient autonomy, nonmaleficence, and justice.[3] Beneficence instructs the surgeon to act in ways that are reliably expected to result in a greater balance of clinical goods over harms for the patient. Benevolence is an inclination; beneficence requires one to perform beneficial deeds. Respect for patient autonomy means that we will defer, without resort to coercion or deception, to the patient's wishes about whether to receive or refuse treatment, or to select among available treatment options. Nonmaleficence seems self-evident; it means that we will not intentionally harm a patient. But surgery harms before healing. Nonmaleficence in surgery entails carefully and accurately determining the risk/benefit ratio and operating only when it is favorable. Justice refers in this context to our role in ensuring that the availability of care will be fair and equitable. It would seem that these foundational principles ought to be absolute, but things can become more complicated when they intersect. The surgeon's respect for patient autonomy may sharply clash with an instinct toward beneficence when he or she struggles to stand by quietly while a patient makes a treatment choice the surgeon is quite certain will ultimately be contrary to the patient's health-related interests. The best that the surgeon might be able to do is to persuade the patient to listen once again to the surgeon's explanations and hope that the patient will finally see what the surgeon's greater knowledge and experience is trying to illuminate. But sometimes it doesn't turn out that way, and we will spend some time in the pages ahead discussing these kinds of complex situations.

The valuation of a surgeon's character and behavior ultimately becomes an evaluation of how good a surgeon is at performing the art and science of surgery. The evaluation of his or her actions reflects several levels of ethical obligation. The highest of these is an assessment of virtues, followed by consideration of principles, the issues of character and behavior we have briefly discussed. These are followed hierarchically by consideration of the surgeon's response to duties, and finally to contractual or legal obligations.

According to Cook, "the fundamental contract in surgery is an undertaking by one individual to cure another by operation, in the expectation of reward."[4] The passage characterizes in legalistic terminology the primacy of the immediate relationship between a surgeon and a patient, without the intercalations of third-party payers, government programs, referring physicians, support staff, or the institution in which the surgeon practices.

We can divide the concept of contractual obligations into four parts. The surgical contract is based in a reasonable certainty that the patient will get better, that the patient's health-related interests are paramount, that the surgeon will do the "best in his or her power" to effect clinical improvement, and, finally, that the "best in his or her power" will be sufficient to resolve the presenting problem. Whether sufficiency is reached remains a concern, with the accelerating rate of new untested technology coming into surgeons' hands.[5] All of these important elements are controlled by the surgeon, not the patient who must rely solely on the surgeon's knowledge, technical ability, and ethical integrity for a positive outcome. The surgeon will benefit financially regardless of how things turn out for the patient. This obvious inequity of power is why a strong and constantly refined commitment to ethical practice, important in all medical specialties, is literally vital to the surgical profession.

Duties are actions or prohibitions that must be generally obeyed to enable alliance of humans, but which may tend to be violated or ignored unless they are enforced by rules. It is the duty of auto drivers to stop at stoplights, for example. Miller and Brody have written that the physician's duties are to practice competently, to benefit and not disproportionately harm, to maintain fidelity in the therapeutic relationship, and to avoid misrepresenting the degree of his or her knowledge and skills.[6] Particularly with the overt entry of medicine into the competitive marketplace during the last two decades or so, complete with elaborate institutional advertising techniques that were once considered far out of medicine's ethical bounds, we must exercise particular care in keeping our practices within the limits of our individual competencies, to not encourage patients to accept untoward risks to further our personal goals, to not consider people who come to us as customers rather than as patients, and to not engage ourselves in the wiles of marketing by promising, or suggesting, more than we can reliably deliver. Violation of any or all of these constraints would constitute gross betrayals of our professional duties.

The Scope of Surgical Ethics

This brief first chapter is intended to serve as a general introduction, and its straightforward narrative format is atypical of the chapters that will follow. In the subsequent seven chapters, each of roughly equal length, we have organized illustrative case studies by their special relevance to major themes in the study of surgical ethics. The second chapter explores issues of informed consent in surgical practice, and some of the conflicts that a working surgeon might see arise in clinical practice. Our evaluations of the informed consent process will subsume such essential ethical components as physician honesty, patient autonomy, and the adequacy of disclosure. As with all the cases in the book, it is our intention to show you the ethical considerations that should shape and guide the informed consent process, so that you can find your way through ethical challenges you might encounter in your own practice, even if they're not identical to the ones you've read about here.

The third chapter concentrates on issues of professional self-regulation. The cases will be about your obligations to patients and to the profession when you encounter questionable behaviors among colleagues, when professional disagreements arise, and how your fiduciary responsibilities toward patients can sometimes feel strained by loyalties and responsibilities you feel toward the people with whom you work. Issues of professional integrity, collegiality, disclosure, and justice will be explored in the course of these discussions.

The fourth chapter is about ethical issues in surgical innovation and research. Many of the investigatory methods that advance the knowledge and methods of the surgical profession bear only slight resemblance to the well-controlled clinical trials common to other medical specialties. Individual innovation undoubtedly plays a bigger role in surgical research than it does in internal medicine, for example, creating all the more reason for the rigorous protection of patients' rights and safety. We'll explore the tensions that some of these issues create in surgical research, as well as how research results are most ethically handled.

Chapter 5 is about conflicts of interest and of commitment most often regarding conflicts between the surgeon's ethical obligations to his or her patient and the surgeon's own self-interest, but interests external to the surgeon can enter the equation as well. As you read this chapter, you may recognize conflicts not readily apparent. These issues get to the core of the surgeon's fiduciary responsibility toward patients, responsibilities toward family and colleagues, the qualified surgeon's entitlement to make a living, and how the surgeon can ethically balance his or her own legitimate interests with those of patients. The cases consider conflicts of interest involving money, involving personal convictions, and involving the convergence of personal and professional life. As might be anticipated in a profession dedicated to helping people who are at some form of disadvantage, confronting conflicted interests is a regular part of the surgeon's life.

Chapter 6 concentrates on ethical issues associated with how the surgeon handles the financial elements of practice. No surgeon wants to be mistaken for an automobile mechanic, but it is an inescapable fact that almost all of us exchange our highly skilled services for money, and for most of us surgery is a very lucrative profession. The cases in this section look at some of the issues involved in maintaining an ethical practice while attending to financial components that matter to us, that will continue to attract the best qualified of subsequent generations into the surgical professions, and ensure that we are able to continue our practices and remain available to the people who need us.

Chapter 7 addresses challenges to professionalism. These challenges concern the ethical concept of medicine as a profession and the physician as fiduciary of the patient, concepts that we explain in greater detail in the chapters that follow. Challenges to professionalism can arise from issues emerging from within or without medicine, such as uncompensated care, hospital credentialing practices, overscheduling in the OR, or publicity-seekers courting the lay press. Still other ethical entanglements can develop when our profession necessarily engages the interests and mores of the world at large, like the crisis in medical liability insurance, or how physicians should manage second careers that may not be guided by the principles of medical ethics.

Our final chapter confronts end-of-life issues, an inescapable decision point and often the most trying for every surgeon. The case studies explore the difficult moments when surgeons find that they can do no more, or that they should do no more. Sometimes the most ethical answer at what might appear to be one of those junctures is that more can and should be done, and we look at some circumstances in which those decisions should be made. Surgeons know better than most that every life ends, but no surgeon is inured to life ending for a patient in his or her care. Although everyone dies, death is still a complex and troubling ethical issue in the practice of surgery.

Conclusion

Ethics is an essential—literally vital—component of surgical practice, innovation, and research. Just as scientific reasoning in surgery requires adherence to the discipline of evidence-based reasoning, so ethics in surgery requires adherence to the discipline of using ethical concepts clearly and consistently and organizing appeals to those concepts into coherent arguments. The result is to create reliable ethical guides to the clinical judgment, scientific thinking, decision making, and behavior of surgeons. Ethics in surgery is thus not an "ivory tower" enterprise but a deliberately and intensely practical tool designed to improve patient care, innovation, and research. And the quality of the professional life of the surgeon.

References

1. McCullough LB, Jones JW, Brody BA. Principles and practice of surgical ethics. In: McCullough LB, Jones JW, Brody BA, eds. *Surgical Ethics*. New York: Oxford University Press, 1998:3–14.
2. Levinson W, Gorawara-Bhat R, Lamb J. A study of patient clues and physician responses in primary care and surgical settings. *JAMA*. 2000; 284:1021–1027.
3. Beauchamp T, Childress J. *Principles of Biomedical Ethics*. New York: Oxford University Press, 2001.
4. Cook J. The delegation of surgical responsibility. *J Med Ethics*. 1980; 6:68–70.
5. Jones JW. Regarding ethics of rapid surgical technological advancement. *Ann Thorac Surg*. 2000; 70:676–677.
6. Miller FG, Brody H. Professional integrity and physician-assisted death. *Hastings Cent Rep*. 1995; 25:8–17.

· 2 ·

Informed Consent
and Disclosure

We begin our inquiries into the conundrums of surgical ethics with a series of explorations into the process of informed consent. Informed consent is the practical beginning of the surgeon's clinical relationship with the patient and continues to be a vital influence throughout the episode of care. Informed consent is of further primary interest in any study of surgical ethics because it is a major manifestation of the bedrock ethical principle of respect for patient autonomy.[1,2]

Patient autonomy means that although the surgeon or other physician is knowledgeable on the subjects of disease, diagnosis, and healing by virtue of his or her training, skill, knowledge, and experience, it is the adult, competent patient who decides when it comes to determining what treatment is acceptable.[3] The physician is responsible for explaining in lay language the nature of the patient's disease, its untreated natural history, making a recommendation for the treatment deemed most appropriate to the patient's condition, and describing the relative risks and benefits of that treatment, the anticipated outcome, available alternative treatments, and the risks and benefits associated with each option. It is usually reassuring for the surgeon to provide some estimation of how the patient might expect the entire treatment experience to go. The physician cannot, however, require the patient to accept the treatment offered, no matter how certain the physician is that the patient will benefit from it, or how dire the clinical consequences should the patient reject it. Only the adult, competent patient can decide which of the available treatments to accept or reject. This decision is based on the thorough and accurate information provided by the physician before initiating treatment. A patient who agrees to a proffered treatment based on incomplete or inaccurate information provided by his or her physician has not been adequately informed, and therefore cannot be considered to have given informed consent.

In the United States, the legal obligations of the physician regarding informed consent were established in a series of court cases, starting in the second decade of the 20th century, that established the concept of simple consent and then the concept of informed consent.[4] Most of the legal and surgical ethics literature on informed consent assumes that the law, not ethics, shaped medical practice. Recent historical scholarship challenges this assumption.

The emerging, competing account is that physicians developed consent practices well before the 20th century. Surgeons led this major historical change. In the seventeenth century, British surgeons drew contracts with patients for surgical management of their ailments.[5] This was followed in the 18th century by the argument of the Scottish physician-ethicist John Gregory (1724–1773) that the patient has a right to speak in matters that concern life and health, and that the physician should take very seriously the expressed preferences of patients.[6] In the 19th century, the Brooklyn gynecologist, Alexander Skene (d. 1900), developed what 20th-century law and medical ethics would certainly recognize and endorse as informed consent practices for gynecologic surgery.[7] He offered his female patients surgical management when it was indicated and, if they refused, negotiated an alternative plan of care with them. This competing history of how physicians made decisions with patients supports the view that the common law of informed consent was influenced by emerging best ethical practices of informed consent. This view challenges the interpretation, common in the literature on informed consent, that the law invented the concept of informed consent and required medical practice to conform to it.

In 1914, the New York State Court of Appeals, in *Schloendorff v. The Society of The New York Hospital*, took the first step by articulating the concept of simple consent, that is, whether the patient says "yes" or "no" to medical intervention.[8] Judge Cardozo's conclusion is still quoted in the medical and bioethics literature: "Every human being of adult years and sound mind has the right to determine what shall be done with his body, and a surgeon who performs an operation without his patient's consent commits an assault for which he is liable in damages."[8]

Over the next half-century or so, the legal requirement of consent further evolved to include disclosure of information sufficient to enable patients to make informed decisions about whether to say "yes" or "no" to medical intervention, that is, whether to provide simple consent.[4] The physician's obligation to provide information adequate for the patient to make an informed decision added the concept of informed consent to that of simple consent, which was still required. Informed consent requires the physician to disclose an adequate amount of clinical information to the patient and then obtain his or her acceptance or refusal of offered or recommended clinical management. Standards that should guide the physician in fulfilling his or her disclosure obligation to the patient became central concerns of the courts.[4]

Two legal standards for the physician's disclosure obligation emerged. The *professional community standard*, now held in only a minority of the states, defines adequate disclosure in the context of what the relevantly trained and experienced physician tells patients.[4] The *reasonable person standard*, adopted by most states, goes further and requires the physician to disclose "material" information: what any patient in the patient's condition needs to know and the layperson of average sophistication should not be expected to know.[4] A rule of thumb for translating the reasonable person standard into clinical practice is for the physician to identify clinically salient information about the patient's condition and its management and then provide this information to the patient.[9]

The reasonable person has emerged as the ethical standard.[1,2] Using this standard, the physician should disclose to the patient the patient's diagnosis or condition, the medically reasonable alternatives to diagnose and manage the patient's condition, and the short-term and long-term benefits and risks of each alternative.

The main justification for the reasonable person becoming the preferred ethical standard is the history of systematic underdisclosure of information to patients when physicians successfully established that they met the professional community standard of disclosure.[4] Prominent examples that led courts, both state and federal, to reject the professional community standard in favor of the reasonable person standard included nondisclosure of the risks of cobalt radiation therapy[10] and nondisclosure of the risk of paralyzing injury from falls in the immediate postoperative period after a laminectomy.[11] The emergence of the reasonable person standard as the dominant legal and accepted ethical guideline acknowledged the professional community standard's tendency toward paternalism, with resultant failures to disclose clinically salient information to patients.[4]

The trust of patients in physicians plays an important role in the informed consent process. This investiture of trust was well documented by McKneally after interviewing a series of surgical patients about their decision processes.[12] Patients generally believe that members of the medical profession are not only honest and competent, but ethical as well. Fortunately for all of us, that trust is usually well placed.

Informed consent has become the "central dogma" of surgical ethics. Knowledge about the therapy originates with the surgeon, flows to the patient, and there becomes the basis for initiating therapy, never the other way around. The direction of this process is unlikely to change in the foreseeable future: ethical retroviruses don't exist. Provision of full disclosure to patients is joined irrefutably to the principles and pillars of professional integrity.[1] Providing truthful information upon which to base an unbiased decision demonstrates respect for the autonomy of another person, without which most of humanity's modern moral, religious, philosophical, legal, and cultural underpinnings would become invalid.

The present status of conventional informed consent is explicit; it is a necessary process of honest disclosure about a particular patient's medical treatment, starting when the surgeon agrees to evaluate the case and ending with the patient's discharge from the surgeon's care. It includes informing the patient of the surgeon's diagnosis and proposed surgical intervention, the goals of the intervention, the anticipated risks and benefits, available alternatives, including no treatment and its likely result, and the surgeon's record of personal experience in the performance of this particular operation. The patient should be informed postoperatively of any unanticipated intraoperative events, including physician errors, corrected or additional diagnoses, and complications affecting the pre-op prognosis.[2,13,14] The patient should receive frank and accurate progress reports, including news of any treatment-emergent abnormalities or recommendations for modifications in the plan of care.[15]

Some physicians find feelings of paternalism toward their patients hard to shake, and fear that patients might refuse essential treatment if they are exposed to detailed knowledge of the pain, complications, and long recovery a surgical procedure might involve. The informed consent process, as described here, is the antidote to these feelings of paternalism.

Anything well-intentioned can be overdone and become harmful, and the informed consent process is not immune to this paradox.[16] Patient autonomy bestows the right to decide which of the recommended therapies are permitted, not to dictate the therapy itself. Nor can the patient demand that the physician provide a therapy that the physician believes is dangerous or without therapeutic value.[17]

In the pages that follow, you will be presented with cases that examine various twists and turns that you may have already encountered or may expect to encounter in practice; most are from actual experiences.

The impulse toward acknowledging the patient's autonomy and easily submitting to the discipline of the informed consent process may not always come naturally. There are, however, ethical resolutions to these kinds of tenacious problems, resolutions that we believe will be sufficiently durable to forestall additional difficulties, and we invite you to explore them with us.

References

1. Beauchamp TL, Childress, JF. *Principles of Biomedical Ethics*. 5th ed. New York: Oxford University Press, 2001.
2. McCullough LB, Jones JW, Brody BA. Informed consent: Autonomous decision making of the surgical patient. In: McCullough LB, Jones JW, Brody BA, eds. *Surgical Ethics*. New York: Oxford University Press:15–37.
3. Engelhardt HT, Jr. *The Foundations of Bioethics*. New York: Oxford University Press, 1986.
4. Faden RR, Beauchamp TL. *A History and Theory of Informed Consent*. New York: Oxford University Press, 1986.
5. Wear A. Medical ethics in early modern England. In: Wear A, Geyer-Kordesch J, French P, eds. *Doctors and Ethics: The Earlier Historical Setting of Professional Ethics*. Amsterdam: Rodopi, 1993:98–130.
6. McCullough LB. *John Gregory's Invention of Professional Medical Ethics and the Profession of Medicine*. Dordrecht, The Netherlands: Kluwer Academic Publishers, 1998.
7. Powderly K. Patient consent and negotiation in the gynecological practice of Alexander J.C. Skene 1863–1900. *J Med Philos*. 2000; 25:12–27.
8. *Schloendorff v. The Society of The New York Hospital*, 211 N.Y. 125, 126, 105 N.E. 92, 93 (1914).
9. Wear S. *Informed Consent: Patient Autonomy and Clinician Beneficence within Health Care*. 2nd ed. Washington, DC: Georgetown University Press, 1998.
10. *Natanson v. Kline*, 186 Kan. 393, 350 P.2d 1093, 354 P.2d 670 (1960).
11. *Canterbury v. Spence*, 464 F.2d 772, 775 (D.C Cir. 1972).
12. McKneally MF, Martin DK. An entrustment model of consent for surgical treatment of life-threatening illness: perspective of patients requiring esophagectomy. J *Thorac Cardiovasc Surg*. 2000; 120:264–269.
13. Jones JW, McCullough LB, Richman BW. Informed consent: It's not just signing a form. *Thorac Surg Clin*. 2005; 15:451–460.

14. Jones JW, McCullough LB. Disclosure of intraoperative events. *Surgery*. 2002; 132: 531–532.

15. Jones JW, McCullough LB, Richman BW. Truth-telling about terminal diseases. *Surgery*. 2005; 137:380–382.

16. Jones JW, McCullough LB. Are ethics practical when externals impact your clinical judgment? *J Vasc Surg*. 2007; 45:1282–1284.

17. Brett AS, McCullough LB. When patients request specific interventions: Defining the limits of the physician's obligation. *N Engl J Med*. 1986; 315:1347–1351.

• CASE 1 •

Painted Into a Corner: Unexpected Complications in Treating a Jehovah's Witness

Prediction is very difficult, especially about the future.
Niels Bohr (1885–1962)

Although you are not often asked to treat members of the Jehovah's Witness denomination, you just accepted such a patient on referral from the radiology suite. He is among the most suitable candidates you've ever evaluated for endovascular repair of an infrarenal abdominal aneurysm. The patient was directed to you personally by a strongly supportive referring physician. You plan to treat the aneurysm with an endograft. During the informed consent process the patient tells you that he will not accept a blood transfusion under any circumstances. You clear your throat and ease past the possibility that conversion to an open procedure, and the associated increased need for transfusion, could become necessary intraoperatively. It has been quite a while since you've seen a patient with such straightforward anatomy have problems requiring conversion, and this patient has a cushiony hemoglobin of $> 16\,gm/dl$. Notwithstanding, the patient suddenly deteriorates during the procedure, forming an expanding retroperitoneal hematoma. His blood pressure becomes increasingly difficult to maintain as the operating room is being set up for open surgery. The patient's deep sedation makes discussion and an amended informed consent process impossible. You urgently discuss the situation with the patient's wife, who is not a Jehovah's Witness. She will sign permission for blood-transfusion therapy and strongly urges you to transfuse if necessary. What is your most ethical course?

(A) Assume that the patient did not fully appreciate that he could lose his life without a transfusion, and proceed to transfuse as clinically indicated.

(B) Since you did not specifically agree to withhold transfusion during an emergency open procedure, transfuse.

(C) Transfuse on the wife's authority.

(D) Transfuse and do not tell the patient.

(E) Do not violate the patient's autonomy by transfusing, even if it means the patient may die.

A number of new religious groups emerged in the United States during the latter half of the 19th and early 20th centuries. Distinguishing themselves from well-established Christian denominations, they based themselves upon novel scriptural interpretations and behavioral rituals as manifestations of what they believed to be superior righteousness and Biblical fidelity. The Pentecostal movement was begun by Charles Parham (1873–1929) in about 1901. Mary Baker Eddy (1821–1910) founded the Church of Christ Scientist in 1879. Charles Taze Russell (1873–1912) initiated the Jehovah's Witness movement in the 1870s. Scientology, not a Protestant denomination, was founded by L. Ron Hubbard (1911–1986) in 1952, who declared it a religion in 1960. To one degree or another, each of these new faiths considered modern medicine a rival contradictory to its principles, and they eschewed all or some of its practices. Christian Scientists typically reject all the ministrations of organized medicine. They correctly note that medicine began as a pantheistic pagan priesthood relying upon the graces of Apollo, Asclepius, Hygieia, Panaceia, and all other gods and goddesses believed to be sympathetic to healing. The original Hippocratic Oath confirms this contention. Having concluded that association with these ancient deities makes the medical profession anathema to Christianity, Christian Scientists reject medical interventions. They elect to seek health through prayer and rejection of the disease concept. Except in pediatric cases, their beliefs and practices are rarely considered ethically problematic, and they are seldom challenged. One published study showed that the longevity of Christian Scientists was significantly lower than the general population's.[1] Russell founded the Jehovah's Witnesses by disseminating what was then an unusual interpretation of Biblical Scripture. His first converts followed publication of his new magazine, "Herald of the Morning," which subsequently became "Zion's Watch Tower and Herald of Christ's Presence," and then "The Watchtower."[2] First known as "Russelites," the group developed a strong foundation of believers and able leadership by the time of Russell's death in 1916. Movement membership increased throughout the world in the 20th century, and it officially named itself the Jehovah's Witnesses in 1931. The Jehovah's Witnesses consider their practices and beliefs a return to original first century Christianity.[3] Like the earliest Christians whom they emulate, they take special pride in opposing to the utmost any form of authority that would separate them by force or persuasion from their beliefs and their literal interpretation of scripture.

Prohibition of blood transfusions was incorporated into the Jehovah's Witness dogma by its governing council, the Watchtower Society, in 1945. The basis for the doctrine is established by reference to three scriptural sources (Gen. 9:3, Lev. 17:14, and Acts 15:28–29) forbidding the consumption of sacrificial blood. The Watchtower Society annually issues wallet cards, effectively an advance directive (see Chapter 7), to the faithful explaining the risks (but not potential benefits) of transfused blood, require the member's signature, and admonish treating physicians against transfusion should the card holder be brought to care incapacitated and unable to speak for himself. The Watchtower Society threatens with "disfellowship," tantamount to excommunication from the faith, any Jehovah's Witness who accepts any transfused blood products other than those permitted by the Society. Compliance is almost universal among the faithful, who are steadfast in their refusal to be transfused with red blood cells that have been separated from their bodies. If the tubing remains connected to them, as in cardiopulmonary bypass or with use of erythrocyte retrieval and salvaging devices, they will usually accept reinfusions of the original autologous contents and postoperative drainage. The Watchtower Society does not prohibit acceptance of albumen or plasma, leaving this decision to each individual. Almost all Jehovah's Witnesses will accept treatment with erythropoietin, but they should be informed that the biological is suspended in human albumen.

By refusing to accept transfusion of erythrocytes, one of the pillars of surgical therapy, Jehovah's Witnesses impose a handicap on surgeons who accept them for major procedures.[4] These cases thrust physicians into the unusual position of agreeing to the possibility of allowing an otherwise salvageable mentally competent adult to die.

Seventy-nine and eighty-four percent of physicians responding to a pair of surveys reported that they had encountered at least one Jehovah's Witness patient needing urgent interventions like emergency surgery.[5,6] More than half these physicians reported having transfused the patients when they believed that blood was needed, whether or not there was a signed refusal statement. If a Jehovah's Witness patient was exsanguinating, more than half the physicians surveyed said they would transfuse against the patient's wishes, and 26% of them would not tell the patient what had been done.[7]

The informed consent process with a Jehovah's Witness patient may seem at first specific to this group and of little relevance to the care of the enormous majority of patients who do not subscribe to extraordinary religious beliefs that conflict with standard medical practice. On the contrary, informed consent actually encompasses the patient's right to an informed refusal to consent, including a refusal to accept life-sustaining care, for whatever reasons the patient finds the conditions of that care unacceptable. Physicians will easily accept a patient's refusal of open-ended life support in a persistent vegetative state without skeptically weighing the patient's value system against their own personally held beliefs. Almost certainly, physicians find it easier to cooperate with concepts of patient autonomy when treatment decisions closely reflect the values that they hold themselves and can therefore understand more readily. Seemingly alien value systems, including those based in extreme religious or supernatural beliefs, are more likely to be interpreted by physicians as mistaken, coerced, or suggestive of severe mental illness. As suggested by the recent surveys, many physicians will attempt to somehow circumvent the instructions of these patients, particularly when the patient's decisions may have irreversible consequences that the physician believes are contrary to the patient's best interests. For the Jehovah's Witness patient, the prospect of avoidable death in service to the religion's precepts, a tragic catastrophe in the view of most surgeons, would be of little importance when compared to righteous preparation for the eternal life to come. The apparently impossible reconciliation of two value systems at utter variance with one another, one supernatural and religiously based, one scientific and secularly based, becomes the substance of the surgeon's ethical paradox. What is ultimately more ethically valid, the patient's autonomy, even unto death, or the surgeon's obligation to preserve the patient's life and restore him to health?

Option (A) may in fact be your first instinctive response as a surgeon. Particularly when you are almost certain that with a routine procedure you can restore the patient to full function and a comfortable resumption of his daily life, it is practically impossible for a surgeon to imagine that a patient with an adequate understanding of the risks and benefits would surrender his life for a religious principle. In this case it would be you who is laboring under the misunderstanding, however. Jehovah's Witnesses are well-educated about the mortal risk associated with their refusal of transfusion, and their resistance almost always becomes more adamant in direct correlation to the immediacy of the danger and the intensity of arguments urging them to accept transfused blood. The advance directive they carry is reissued annually by their leadership, and members renew their fidelity to it annually with their signatures. You have no objective evidence for assuming that your patient has inadequately considered, or poorly understands, the consequences of his decision. You have in fact a great deal of evidence that his understanding is clear. Option (A) cannot be your ethical choice.

The failure to fully discuss the ramifications of converting to open surgery is an error entirely of your own making, and you cannot ethically proceed to use the mistake to justify forcing a sedated or anesthetized patient to undergo a procedure he would normally reject. Despite your abbreviated version of the informed consent process, the patient spontaneously made clear his refusal to accept transfusion. To justify disregarding his wishes on the basis of a linguistic trick is clearly unethical, and you cannot properly select option (B).

Option (C) exposes a serious weak point in modern medicine's application of the surrogate decision making principle. Surrogate decision making fails to reflect the patient's wishes accurately in 70% of important treatment issues.[8] Authorized surrogates (usually first degree relatives like spouses, parents, adult children, or siblings) are expected to conform to the ethical standard of substituted judgment: the surrogate should identify the patient's relevant values and beliefs and make a decision based on them. To the degree that they are known or can be determined, the patient's interests and wishes regarding his care have precedence over the surrogate's interests and wishes, should they diverge. This is also the legal standard of surrogate decision making in some jurisdictions. When those values and beliefs cannot be reliably identified, then the standard measure is the best interest of the patient. The surrogate is responsible for authorizing clinical management that will protect and promote the patient's health-related interests.[9] When it can be reliably established that the surrogate is failing to conform to the substituted judgment standard by incorrectly representing the patient's wishes, the surrogate's instructions are not binding.[10] When treating Jehovah's Witness patients, the durability of informed consent can be strengthened by completing the process in the presence of those designated as surrogate decision makers. All those who will participate in the decision-making process should be in agreement about transfusion therapy, or a written and signed statement should be obtained from the patient about the specific protocol to be followed should the need for blood products arise. This protects the patient's beliefs, and protects the surgeon from any subsequent suggestion of poor practice should an operation end disastrously because the patient withheld consent for life-saving transfusion therapy. It is clear that in this case the wife is advocating her own view rather than her husband's. Her authorization for transfusion is therefore not valid, and option (C) is not available.

Most surgeons understand their primary duty as the preservation of life, and can hardly imagine complicity in the willing surrender of life when a routine procedure will enable the successful completion of an operation and an almost certain restoration of the patient to full health. Most surgeons are furthermore intensely aware of working within a closely monitored profession, with our complication and death rates carefully tabulated and our competence judged by them. Few of us indeed will gladly see these figures inflated by the peculiar whims of our patients. After years and years of intellectual and technical training, and years more of experience, it may be difficult for surgeons to suppress the sense that we know what is best for our patients. The niceties of informed consent are fine until a patient codes in our OR, and then we will do things our way. These paternalistic instincts are at once both beneficent and self-serving, and they are not without virtue. They have nevertheless been trumped in the last century by common law and ethical theory that recognizes the surgeon as *an authority*, but places the patient *in authority* when decisions are made about his care.[11] The physician is not entitled to impose care upon an unwilling patient, or an unwanted procedure upon a patient seeking care. Though physicians have a duty to provide optimal, evidence-based care, they must do so while respecting the patient's autonomous decision about the care to be given. In a Jehovah's Witness's worldview, the surgeon who proceeds in this manner would imperil the patient's immortal soul. Though the preservation of life may be an absolute value to us as surgeons, life on earth may be a less absolute value to individuals with a fervent sense of a life hereafter, and it is not for us to insist that they are wrong. We are obligated to serve our patients, not dominate or determine their values for them. Option (D) is ethically inconsistent with the principles of patient autonomy to which our profession claims fidelity.

Though it may seem a bitter pill, option (E) is the surgeon's correct ethical choice. The surgeon should continue surgical management of this patient without transfusing him. Although a lower percentage of seriously ill patients survive surgery under the conditions imposed by the Jehovah's Witness faith, competent surgeons usually bring them through their operations satisfactorily, and even major surgical care should not be considered futile. Some surgeons decline to treat Jehovah's Witnesses because they find the constraints too confining and the risks too high. They are loath to surrender any of their therapeutic prerogatives, don't want to see their morbidity and mortality figures rise, and are unwilling to put themselves through the personal heartache of losing patients. Some others make a tiny subspecialty of treating Jehovah's Witnesses within their practices. Though they do not necessarily subscribe to the Jehovah's Witness faith, they make themselves fully conversant with its surgical prohibitions and allowances, study the special blood conservation and recycling techniques that can sometimes compensate for transfusion requirements, and readily agree to the faith's prescribed conditions for surgery. The Watchtower Society maintains an index of these surgeons and regularly refers members to them for care.

Though there are only 6.6 million members worldwide and about 1.5 million in the United States, Jehovah's Witnesses have precipitated one of the most vexing ethical conflicts in modern medicine. The dilemma posed by the Jehovah's Witnesses becomes fascinating not only as it impinges upon the critical care of these patients in and of themselves, but as the ethical problem they present is emblematic of the extreme assertion of patient autonomy against the medical profession's instinct for protective paternalism and dedication to preserving life to the extent of its scientific capacities. Patients come to physicians, to surgeons, because they need the knowledge and service that we can provide, and cannot do for themselves what we can do for them. Though it may sometimes seem that this dependence confers upon us broader entitlements, it does not. If we are fortunate enough to be able to extend or improve a life, the life nevertheless remains the patient's, to conduct according to his own lights.

References

1. Simpson WF. Comparative longevity in a college cohort of Christian Scientists. *JAMA*. 1989; 262:1657–1658.
2. Jehovah's Witnesses. Vol. 2006: Wikipedia, the free encyclopedia, 2006.
3. Pennsylvania WTBaTSo. *Jehovah's Witnesses—Who Are They? What Do They Believe?* Vol. 2006: Watch Tower Bible and Tract Society of Pennsylvania, 2006.
4. Jones JW, McCullough LB. Religiously-based treatment refusal. *J Vasc Surg*. 2001; 34:952.
5. Gouezec H, Ballay JL, Le Couls H, Malledant Y. Transfusion and Jehovah's witnesses. A review of medicosurgical attitudes in a University hospital in 1995. *Ann Fr Anesth Reanim*. 1996; 15:1121–1123.
6. Weinberger M, Tierney WM, Greene JY, Studdard PA. The development of physician norms in the United States: The treatment of Jehovah's Witness patients. *Soc Sci Med*. 1982; 16:1719–1723.
7. Vincent JL. Transfusion in the exsanguinating Jehovah's Witness patient—the attitude of intensive-care doctors. *Eur J Anaesthesiol*. 1991; 8:297–300.
8. Hare J, Pratt C, Nelson C. Agreement between patients and their self-selected surrogates on difficult medical decisions. *Arch Intern Med*. 1992; 152:1049–1054.

9. Buchanan A, Brock D. *Deciding for Others: The Ethics of Surrogate Decision Making.* New York: Cambridge University Press, 1989.

10. McCullough L, Jones J, Brody B. Informed consent: autonomous decision making of the surgical patient. In: McCullough LB, Jones JW, Brody BA, eds. *Surgical Ethics.* New York: Oxford University Press, 1998:14–37.

11. Engelhardt HT, Jr. *The Foundations of Bioethics.* New York: Oxford University Press, 1986.

• CASE 2 •

A Patient Refuses Consent for Life-Saving Surgery

The transition between life and death should be gentle in the winter of life.
Rudolph Matas, father of vascular surgery (1869–1957)

An 81-year-old widower with a dry gangrenous leg secondary to diabetes-related vascular insufficiency refuses amputation. A surgeon has explained the disease process and the prognosis with and without amputation, but the patient will not consent to the procedure. The surgeon's next step should be:

(A) Repeat the informed consent process with the next-of-kin present.
(B) Request a psychiatric consultation to determine the patient's competence.
(C) Discuss with the patient the reasons for his decision.
(D) Seek a court order to perform the amputation.
(E) Ask the patient to sign a medical release and treat him with antibiotics and morphine.

During the informed consent process, the physician will typically explain the diagnosis, the indications for treatment, and the risks and benefits associated with a recommended intervention. The patient's right to refuse the suggested treatment is implicit in the process. Patient consent can be neither commanded nor coerced by the physician, even when the consequences of nontreatment are known to be life-threatening. The patient can be reasonably asked (but not compelled) to explain his reasons for declining a recommended treatment. In acknowledgment of the patient's status as the "reasonable person"[1,2] for whom the surgeon has framed his explanations, and the patient's authority to make treatment decisions, the physician should try to fully understand the patient's thinking.

Our patient may explain that he believes the disability and disfigurement he associates with amputation of his leg would destroy the qualities of life he values, and ultimately outweigh any benefit he might receive in the form of extending his already long life. Perhaps he fears that, as his diabetic disease advances, this will be only the first of many painful and demoralizing treatment interventions, and he is content to conclude a full and satisfying life without additional suffering. He may reveal his concern that as a widower the amputation would render him unable to independently care for himself in his own home. Perhaps he envisions spending the remainder of his life in a bleak and joyless nursing home he cannot afford, or worries that his long-term care would exhaust the savings he looks forward to bequeathing his grandchildren. Or he may tearfully relate that since his wife died life has no meaning and he constantly ruminates about killing himself so that he can join her in heaven; permitting the gangrene to progress would relieve him of the fear and guilt of suicide. A patient might report that his dog told him his disease is punishment for a sinful life and that he deserves to die. Option (C), engaging the patient in further discussion about his reasons for refusing surgery, may reveal that he has clear and rational reasons for his choice. The conversation may also indicate that a psychiatric consultation is needed to determine whether the patient is delusional and in need of a guardian to make important medical decisions for him. We would suggest that it is the best first step to take among the available options.

Option (B) can follow if the surgeon finds that the patient's explanation suggests that an affective, psychotic, or organic brain disorder may be influencing the patient's judgment. Disagreeing with a physician's recommendation, or declining to extend a life of unremitting pain and disability, are not in themselves indications of mental illness. Some of our putative patient's possible explanations for refusing care reveal an appropriately apprehensive person with intact intellectual function, able to anticipate consequences and make realistic assessments of competing values. When evidence of conditions like major depression or delusional psychosis emerges during the consent process, however, psychiatry's role becomes clear.

Option (A), repeating the informed consent process with next-of-kin present, may be an ethical option after the surgeon has come to understand the patient's reasoning, but only with the patient's permission, and only if the intent is not to coerce the patient into accepting the surgeon's recommendation. The strong emotional influence of family can be intimidating, particularly to acutely ill and vulnerable patients. Furthermore, family sometimes benefit from a patient's demise, and potential conflicts of interest should be recognized when seeking alliance in their persuasive powers.

Option (D) presumes before further evaluation by the surgeon or a psychiatrist that the patient is incompetent to make rational treatment decisions. This disrespects the patient's integrity and violates the spirit of informed consent. A patient whose only choices are agreement or legal compulsion is not giving informed consent. Legal intervention may ultimately be sought if psychiatric evaluation suggests mental incompetence and there is no recognized surrogate decision maker. The court will typically appoint a guardian to make treatment decisions rather than directly approve the surgery itself.

Option (E) may be ethically permissible if the mentally intact patient ultimately refuses operative care. The surgeon should be afforded protection against later claims of poor practice by a detailed report of the patient's wishes and rationales in the medical record, and the patient should be made as comfortable as possible and provided with the medical treatment which offers the best, however slender, possibility of resolving the acute problem.

References

1. Faden RR, Beauchamp TL. *A History and Theory of Informed Consent. New York.* Oxford University Press, 1986.
2. McCullough LB, Jones JW, Brody BA. Informed consent: Autonomous decision making and the surgical patient. In McCullough LB, Jones JW, Brody BA, eds. *Surgical Ethics*. New York, Oxford University Press, 1998:15–37.

• CASE 3 •

Consent for an Intraoperative Video Recording

Those who cannot remember the past are condemned to repeat it.
George Santayana (1863–1952), *The Life of Reason*, Volume 1

You want to film a potentially landmark surgical procedure that will be performed for the first time anywhere, but you discover after anesthesia induction that no written consent for photography was obtained from the patient. There is a significant possibility of patient mortality with this procedure. The next of kin has refused permission to tape the operation. You discussed the videotaping with the patient the day before and received the patient's verbal permission, but no documents were signed and there were no witnesses to the discussion. What should you do?

(A) Record the operation and afterward get written permission from the patient to use the tape.

(B) Ask for permission to film from the hospital's ethics committee.

(C) Delay the procedure until you can obtain written permission from the patient.

(D) Continue with the operation without filming and film the next such procedure when the opportunity presents itself and all the written consents are in order.

(E) Have the hospital's legal counsel seek a court order permitting filming of the landmark event.

Videotaping without the patient's written informed consent is an invasion of privacy only if the patient can be identified and the tape is made available to others. In this case, the operative field and the scope of the camera will be limited to the area of the abdomen. Courts have imposed liability when patients' likenesses have been used, even for noncommercial purposes, if the patient has not consented. Section 160.103 of the U.S. Health Insurance Portability and Accountability Act of 1996 addresses the ethical implications of patient photographs by including them in the standards affecting individually identifiable health information. The Act also notes, however, that consent and privacy provisions do not apply when "full-face photographic images and any comparable images…are removed" (Section 164.514(b)(2)). Masking the eyes alone is not sufficient to insure complete patient anonymity. In a 1995 position paper, the International Committee of Medical Journal Editors determined that creation of an audiovisual record without any possibility of patient identification does not require consent. [1] This would apply in the present case, in which the operative field to be photographed does not include any facial characteristics. The Joint Commission on Accreditation of Healthcare

Organizations encourages its subscribers to obtain informed consent from patients for medical photography, specifying when appropriate that the material will be used for medical education. The Joint Commission also describes the ethical protocol that should be initiated when the photography has been performed prior to securing patient consent. In these cases, the film should be sequestered from use or release pending receipt of an appropriate consent. Under these circumstances, the surgeon may ethically videotape the operative procedure, secure the tape, and dispose of it should the patient postoperatively withdraw the verbal consent she provided prior to surgery. Furthermore, the surgeon may ethically and legally tape the operation with or without patient consent and use it for the education of other medical professionals and trainees if the patient's face or any other clearly identifying features do not appear.

Nonetheless, the fact that the issue was discussed with the family subsequent to anesthesia induction means that they must be offered consideration. The patient's prior verbal provision of informed consent for filming, although not written and signed, is sufficient to inform the surgeon of the patient's wishes, and alert him to the fact that the surrogate's decision does not accurately reflect them. Surrogate decisions that inaccurately represent the patient's wishes are not ethically binding on the surgeon, provided the surgeon has a basis for reasonable certainty that the surrogate is mistaken before acting contrary to the surrogate's instructions. Surrogate decision making fails to reflect the patient's wishes accurately in 70% of important treatment issues.[3] In this less critical decision, the surgeon knows that the surrogate's decision is contrary to the patient's verbally stated choice, and the surgeon is therefore not obligated to comply with the surrogate's instruction, even if the surrogate was otherwise entitled to control an anonymous filming.[4] Option (C), delaying the procedure until written permission to film can be obtained from the patient, could not justify exposing the patient to a second episode of anesthesia, and the right of the patient to be protected from unnecessary risk must prevail over the contribution to medical science the tape might provide.

Option (D), continuing the operation without taping and making plans to videotape the next such opportunity is a cautious but not entirely ethically acceptable option because it abandons the surgeon's responsibility to advance medical knowledge, a fundamental professional duty.[2] Because this procedure is considered a potentially unprecedented advance in operative care, the video record may be valuable to the future treatment of patients with similar conditions, and the lost opportunity to create such a record could be a significant scientific sacrifice.

Anesthesia has been induced and the operative team has assembled. The ethics committee cannot realistically be convened in time to help resolve the impasse with the family. This eliminates option (B) from consideration. Besides the impracticality of timing, there is no emergent patient care issue upon which to legitimately seek legal override of the family's refusal to grant permission, and option (E) is thus eliminated from among our choices.

Most importantly, the patient has agreed to the videotaping of the procedure after receiving suitable explanations from the operating surgeon. She has given consent, lacking only the signature that documents it. The patient's signature documents agreement; it does not by itself constitute the consent process. Option (A), recording the procedure with no identifying patient features and sequestering the tape until she is able to provide signed consent postoperatively, meets the patient's expressed wishes and legally meets the surgeon's scientific and educational needs. It is the best available ethical option.

References

1. Editors ICoMJ. Protection of patients' rights to privacy. Vol. 311. *Br Med J*. 1995; 1272.
2. Joint Commission Perspectives. 2000; 20:6.
3. Hare J, Pratt C, Nelson C. Agreement between patients and their self-selected surrogates on difficult medical decisions. *Arch Intern Med*. 1992; 152,1049–1054.
4. McCullough LB , Jones JW, Brody BA. Informed consent: Autonomous decision making of the surgical patients. In: McCullough LB, Jones JW, Brody BA, ed. *Surgical Ethics*. New York: Oxford University Press, 1998:15–37.

• CASE 4 •

Disclosure of Intraoperative Error

"What is truth?" said jesting Pilate; and would not stay for
an answer.
Francis Bacon (1561–1626), *Essays*, "Of Truth"

During an urgent colon resection for diverticular bleeding in an 86-year-old man, a medical student assistant applied too much pressure with a retractor, creating a four-centimeter tear in the area of the splenic hilum. The repair was complex but completed satisfactorily, and the spleen was salvaged. The patient's elderly wife has been very upset by her husband's sudden illness. Their grown children are due in town in a few hours. What is the most ethical form of postoperative disclosure?

(A) Do not disclose the intraoperative error because there will probably be no lasting consequences and disclosure might needlessly upset the patient's wife further.

(B) Provide a detailed description of the tear to the patient's wife immediately after surgery.

(C) Wait until the children arrive before giving the wife a detailed description of the error.

(D) Immediately disclose to the patient's wife only that the operation involved unforeseen complications, but that the surgery was successful.

(E) Await the patient's recovery from anesthesia and the children's arrival, and then disclose to the family and patient only that the bypass involved unforeseen complications, but that surgery was successful.

No surgeon wants to be sued, lose patients' confidence, or undergo the humiliation of admitting errors; all are among the distinct dangers of full disclosure. But the spirit of informed consent has ethically and legally replaced paternalism in surgery. Informed consent does not stop with the agreement to accept treatment. Mutual decision making by the physician and patient (or family, when the patient agrees or cannot participate) about treatment throughout the course of an illness is grounded in respect for the patient's right to autonomy. The renowned ethical philosopher Immanuel Kant's (1724–1804) belief that although deception must be avoided, truth may be revealed selectively is inappropriate to the physician–patient relationship. The physician must help the patient to understand both what is planned preoperatively and how treatment is proceeding. The extent of disclosure is generally based on the physician's provision of information that should influence diagnosis, treatment planning, and outcomes. This includes knowledge that the average layperson cannot be expected to have, but needs to know in order to participate meaningfully in treatment decisions and planning their future. The character of such information should satisfy what is known in both law and ethics as the "reasonable person" standard.[1,2] The physician is not expected to give the patient a "mini medical education," or even everything that is known about iatrogenic splenic tears, but the patient should be told about the risks of complications involved in the proposed treatment, and the actual outcome of his treatment. Patients should also be specifically informed if trainees will participate in their treatment, what they will do, and how they will be supervised.[2]

The reasonable person standard must guide the surgeon in the process of mutual decision making before surgery, and postoperatively as well. A 4 cm tear of the spleen, even when repaired successfully, may cause such clinically significant complications as subsequent bleeding and abscess. The surgeon's postoperative care will therefore include additional evaluation procedures and response to these and other potential complications. This is part of the clinically relevant information that properly shapes the surgeon's judgment and, consistent with the reasonable person standard, it should be shared with the patient or his surrogate in the early postoperative period.

Option (B) would be ethically acceptable only if there were not going to be family available soon to support the already distraught wife. Options (D) and (E) risk underdisclosure, because details of the complications, and how they could affect the postoperative course, are not explained. Moreover, underdisclosure may be even more anxiety-provoking for the family and patient, mobilizing fears that the complications were worse than they really were.

Option (A) involves nondisclosure. It is inconsistent with the reasonable person standard, and therefore ethically unacceptable. Indeed, the reasonable person standard as the benchmark of the informed consent process emerged in specific response to a particularly notorious case of physicians electing not to disclose unpleasant information that patients actually needed when selecting therapy: the severe complications of cobalt radiation therapy in treating breast cancer.[1]

Option (C) is the best ethical choice. Assuming that the patient has not prohibited his wife's involvement in the decision-making process, she should be informed about the complication, its management, and its clinical implications. Given her fragile emotional condition, the impending arrival of her adult children, and the necessity for timely but not urgent notification of the surgical error, a proper concern for all involved suggests waiting until her children are there to support her. When the patient can again function as the primary decision maker in his care, he should be informed in a similarly detailed way about the complications. He should also be told that the manner in which the spleen was handled caused the tear, and that responsibility for the student's error resides fully with the supervising surgeon.

References

1. McCullough LB, Jones JW, Brody BA. Informed consent: Autonomous decision making of the surgical patient. In: McCullough LB, Jones JW, Brody BA, eds. *Surgical Ethics*. New York: Oxford University Press, 1998:15–37.
2. Faden R, Beauchamp T. *A History and Theory of Informed Consent*. New York: Oxford University Press, 1986.
3. *Natanson V. Kline:* 186 Kan. 393, 404, 350 P.2d 1093,1104, 1960.

• CASE 5 •

The Public's Right to Know? Surgical Treatment of Public Figures

Fama volat (The rumour has wings)
Virgil (70–19 BC), Aeneid

The governor of your state has had a three-vessel coronary bypass graft at your center. Three weeks later he is returned unconscious to the hospital after suffering a right hemiparetic stroke while catching up on paperwork in his office. An emergency arteriogram reveals embolus to the left internal carotid artery at the bifurcation. As you leave the operating room following an emergency carotid endarterectomy with embolectomy, you are met by the hospital's public information officer and the governor's top political aide. They inform you that the press corps is assembled in the auditorium and expects you to provide them with a detailed description of the governor's condition and prognosis. You should respond by:

(A) Acknowledging the press's right to know about a public official and providing an immediate and complete report on the governor's presenting symptoms, the operation performed, his current condition, and his prognosis.

(B) Requesting advice from the political aide about how the governor would like the situation presented.

(C) Insisting that a report to the press await authorization from the governor or his next-of-kin.

(D) Refusing to meet the press.

(E) Relying upon the public information officer to direct you in implementing the hospital's disclosure policy on treatment of public figures.

Many of us have been involved in or observed the frenzy of activity generated by hospitalization of a celebrity or prominent public official, particularly when emergency treatment for a life-threatening condition is involved. The convergence of news media places extraordinary demands upon the hospital, and the institution's staff and management naturally want to be favorably represented by these highly influential opinion-makers. Representatives of the press will often assert the public's right to know important information about high-ranking government officials or entertainment figures who experience medical crises, cite the press freedoms guaranteed by our Constitution, and insist upon your full cooperation in describing the patient's condition and medical care. Nevertheless, neither the public nor the press have a statutory entitlement that outweighs a patient's right to confidentiality in seeking or receiving medical care, and patients do not relinquish that right when they become public figures.[1] The American College of Surgeons' *Statement on Principles* requires that "the surgeon should maintain the confidentiality of information from and about the patient, except as such information must be communicated for the patient's proper care or as is required by law."[2] The United States Constitution's guarantee of a free press imposes an obligation upon government to refrain from interfering with the gathering and dissemination of information; it does not require individuals or nongovernmental institutions, such as physicians or hospitals, to satisfy the demands of journalists.[3] The "public's right to know" is an artificial concept promoted by the press, not a constitutional or moral right. Option (A) is inconsistent with your ethical obligation to insure confidentiality in the doctor-patient relationship.

Option (B), accepting guidance from the governor's aide about the manner and degree of information to be disclosed about the governor's condition, is unacceptable because the aide has no authority as next-of-kin or legal surrogate to speak for the governor in personal matters. Although the political adviser may speak with great authority and in the expectation that you and other members of the hospital staff will respond obediently to his directives, his opinions and desire to control the flow of information are irrelevant to your professional relationship with your patient.

Option (D), refusing to meet with the assembled press, is certain to project an unnecessary attitude of arrogance and hostility that will poorly serve the fine hospital in which you practice, and which values the community's good will. Your refusal will also insure that some other member of the hospital staff, one who does not share your special fiduciary relationship with the patient, will be sent to the press room and probably discuss the governor's condition and your case management in a manner neither you nor your patient is likely to approve of. You may visit the press room and advise the assembled journalists that until your awake and alert patient, his next-of-kin, or legally designated surrogate authorizes you to release medical information, you are prevented by rules of confidentiality from doing so. You may apologize for any inconvenience to the group, ask that they respect the patient's right to privacy in his medical care, and assure them that appropriate information will be made available at such time as the patient's permission is received.

Option (E), permitting the hospital's public relations officer to interpret the hospital's disclosure policy and direct your actions, surrenders your fiduciary role. Maintaining confidentiality in the physician–patient relationship is your responsibility, and it should not be ceded to a nonprofessional whose primary goals may not entirely reflect your ethical values. Even assuming no unethical or misguided motives in the public relation's officer's recommendations, you as the attending physician should not permit yourself to be governed by support staff who do not share your responsibilities.

Option (C), declining to disclose sensitive medical information about your well-known patient until he or an appropriate surrogate authorizes such disclosures, insures that the physician–patient privilege is protected. Although your patient is an important political figure upon whom the public depends for the complete and efficient operation of state government, the physician's relationship with him is identical to that of a patient who does not reside in the public arena. Famous patients are entitled to all the consideration the medical profession affords private citizens, including personal respect and confidentiality. Even when, and if, the patient, spouse, or legal surrogate authorizes public release of medical information, the patient maintains the authority to control how and how much material will be made publicly available. The patient, not the physician, not the hospital, and not the press, is the owner of his medical information, and only he and his designated surrogates should decide upon the form and content of its disclosure.

References

1. Marshall MF, Smith CD. Confidentiality. In: McCullough LB, Jones, JW, Brody BA, eds. *Surgical Ethics*. New York: Oxford University Press, 1998: 38–56.
2. American College of Surgeons. Statement on Principles. Chicago, ACS, 1989.
3. Medical Ethics Advisor. October, 1995:126–127.

• CASE 6 •

Religiously Based Emergency Treatment Refusal

In all affairs it's a healthy thing now and then to hang a question mark on the things you have long taken for granted.
Bertrand Russell (1872–1970)

You are the only vascular surgeon within 70 miles when a devout 55-year-old, otherwise healthy male patient presents in your ER, hypotensive and unconscious, with a rupturing abdominal aortic aneurysm. You recall that several months ago this same patient was referred to you for an elective procedure and he described to you his faith as a Jehovah's Witness and the denomination's refusal to accept transfused blood. You explained to him at that time, and to other such patients throughout your career, that you did not operate on Jehovah's Witnesses because of this restriction upon your ability to administer a basic life saving procedure should the need arise. The patient's wife does not subscribe to the Jehovah's Witness faith. She asks you to perform emergency surgery, with blood transfusions if necessary, but not to tell the patient if blood is given.

(A) Transfer the patient to another competent surgeon at the nearest available center.

(B) Treat the patient according to the wife's wishes.

(C) Treat the patient doing everything possible to avoid transfusion, but transfuse the patient if survival depends upon it, and tell him when he recovers.

(D) Treat the patient and allow an anesthesiologist who is willing to comply with the wife's request to be responsible for transfusion therapy.

(E) Treat the patient and comply with his prior refusal of blood transfusion, regardless of associated risk.

In one survey, 79% of physician respondents had encountered a Jehovah's Witness patient needing emergency surgery.[1] More than half these physicians reported having transfused the patients when they believed that blood was needed, whether or not there was a signed refusal statement. Notwithstanding, the strongest ethical argument can be made for (E).

With no other vascular surgeon immediately available, option (A) is not feasible in an emergency situation. The patient would not survive a transfer of more than 70 miles. Surgeons are committed to serving each patient's best interests as defined by the patient. In a nonemergency situation, an alternative surgeon willing to work under these conditions could be called in. Without recourse to an adequately trained and experienced colleague, however, a surgeon is obligated to treat an emergent patient regardless of the circumstances. Refusing to treat a dying patient when therapy is possible is clearly unethical.

(C) is a close second best answer and could not be summarily dismissed, but it places the surgeon's values above the values of the patient. You cannot ethically pretend that you don't recall your earlier meeting with the patient or otherwise don't understand the operative restrictions imposed by his faith. It is likewise unethical to deceive the patient option (B), even to comply with the wishes of the next-of-kin.[2] Normally, treatment is guided by the family's wishes, but this standard is not binding when it is clear that the surrogate decision maker is not faithfully representing the patient's desires. You are the attending surgeon responsible for the patient's care, and cannot knowingly sponsor an equivalent deception by a surrogate physician option (D). The competent patient is entitled to treatment consistent with his or her value system, even if it increases risk and is inconsistent with the surgeon's own beliefs. An argument could be made that the surgeon is relieved of the obligation to treat because this course of action is futile, defined as the reliable expectation that clinical intervention will not have the intended therapeutic effect. Although a lower percentage of seriously ill patients survive surgery under the conditions imposed by the Jehovah's Witness faith, competent surgeons usually bring them through their operations satisfactorily, and surgical care should not be considered futile. [3]

References

1. Gouezec H, Ballay JL, Le Couls H, Malledant Y. [Transfusion and Jehovah's witnesses. A review of medicosurgical attitudes in a University hospital in 1995]. *Ann Fr Anesth Reanim.* 1996; 15:1121–1123.
2. McCullough LB, Jones JW, Brody BA. Informed consent: Autonomous decision making of the surgical patient. In: McCullough LB, Jones JW, Brody BA, eds. *Surgical Ethics.* New York: Oxford University Press, 1998:15–37.
3. Baker CE, Kelly GD, Perkins GD. Perioperative care of a Jehovah's Witness with a leaking abdominal aortic aneurysm. *Br J Anaesth.* 1998; 81:256–259.

• CASE 7 •

Consent for Residents to Perform Surgery

To study the phenomena of disease is to sail an uncharted sea, while to study books without patients is not to go to sea at all.
Sir William Osler (1849–1919)

A senior member of the Board of Trustees at your University Hospital has asked to see you in consultation. After studying his diagnostic workup, you will recommend that he undergo a laparoscopic distal gastrectomy. As usual, a surgical resident will be assigned to perform the procedure under your supervision. The operation will count as an index case for the resident's board credit. Which of the following should you tell the patient during the informed consent process?

(A) That surgery is a team effort and you are the captain of the team.
(B) That a supervised resident will perform and be credited for the procedure.
(C) That you will be performing the surgery with the involvement of a trainee.
(D) That your morbidity and mortality rates for performing this procedure with assisting residents are excellent compared to national averages.
(E) That you appreciate his special status in the hospital and will not impose upon his busy schedule by describing procedural details he is surely familiar with.

The medical profession has an ethical and social obligation to educate physicians and surgeons to meet the needs of future generations of patients. The compelling need to train our successors was articulated by the author of the Hippocratic Oath in the fifth century BCE, and was probably well established long before that. Our responsibility to prepare students, residents, and fellows to practice independently and competently requires that we provide them with opportunities to assume graduated responsibility for the assessment and care of patients, while insuring that the patients we entrust to trainees are treated safely and effectively.

The first teaching hospitals in America were modeled on the British infirmaries and funded from public and private sources. These hospitals provided free care to the poor, and were seen by academic physicians as training sites where a presumed sense of reciprocity would obligate indigent patients to willingly serve as teaching material in exchange for their care.[1] This assumption is now considered incompatible with the process of informed consent, which is understood to include the patient's awareness and agreement that trainees may participate in his care.

The AMA Council on Ethical and Judicial Affairs has established a clear position on the relationship between patients and trainees on clinical rotations:

Patients should be informed of the identity and training status of individuals involved in their care, and all healthcare professionals share the responsibility for properly identifying themselves.[2]

As we've noted earlier, the prevailing ethical measure for disclosure in the informed consent process is referred to as "the reasonable person standard."[3,4] This guideline effectively obligates the physician to provide the information that any reasonable person in the patient's circumstances would need to know, and that the layperson of average sophistication cannot be expected to know, in order to make an informed decision about pertinent treatment options. Patients need to know about the nature of their surgical procedure, who will perform it, and the benefits and risks of the operation.

Option (A), substituting reassuring homilies for specific information, deprives the patient of information he needs under the reasonable person standard and diminishes his ability to make an informed decision about whether to proceed with the operation you are planning. In this case, such an approach evades discussion of the resident's actual role and is essentially misleading.

Option (C), informing the patient that you will be the primary surgeon, and that the resident will be only vaguely "involved" in some implied inessential capacity, clearly misrepresents both the resident's function and your own. Although this characterization of the surgical resident's work in the OR remains the standard of disclosure in many teaching hospitals, it does not meet the reasonable person measure, which assumes that the information provided the patient will be neither untrue nor designed to be misunderstood. Before the patient can accept the role of teaching subject, he must be made aware that he has been offered the part.

Option (D) is not an adequately complete disclosure of operative conditions. Although pertinent morbidity and mortality rates are important in the surgical consent process, your own outcome data are not the salient statistic in this case. Even with close supervision, a resident's work at the operating table can add an increment of risk to surgical care. Infra-renal aneurysmectomies, for example, run an average of 75 minutes longer when performed by surgical residents[5]. Citing your own outcome data when you will not be the primary surgeon obfuscates the resident's relative inexperience, and deceives the patient by guiding his attention away from a key risk element to which he might reasonably object.

Option (E), assuming that your patient's association with the hospital obviates the need to explain procedural elements of the operation to him, can actually deprive him of his entitlement to informed consent. Even when the sign over the door reads, "University Hospital," the layperson of average sophistication should not be expected to intuit that an incompletely trained but supervised surgeon will be performing his operation. And even though this patient sits on the hospital's governing board, we should not presume that he is closely familiar with the structures and practices of surgical training. It has long been acknowledged in medical practice that VIP status guarantees that a patient will receive substandard care; show this patient the respect that you give every patient, and remember that the well-honed standard practices of the informed consent process ensure that all patients receive the information they need to make critical decisions.

Option (B), explaining that a surgical resident will perform the key elements of his operation under your direct supervision, provides the patient with an accurate account of what is planned, assures him that a senior surgeon will be present to offer guidance and control risk, and establishes that this is a regular and fully transparent method of clinical care and surgical training. The patient so-informed will have an opportunity to explore his questions, including any misgivings, with you and assess his choices in the manner typical of reasonable people.

References

1. Bard S. A discourse upon the duties of a physician. In: Bard S, *Two Discourses Dealing with Medical Education in Early New York*. New York: Columbia University Press, 1921.
2. Council on Ethical and Judicial Affairs, American Medical Association. Medical students' involvement in patient care. *J Clin Ethics*. 2001,12:111–115.
3. Faden RR, Beauchamp TL. *A History and Theory of Informed Consent*. New York: Oxford University Press, 1986.
4. McCullough LB, Jones, JW, Brody BA. Informed consent: autonomous decision making. In: McCullough LB, Jones JW, Brody BA, eds. *Surgical Ethics*. New York: Oxford University Press, 1998:15–37.
5. Bridges M, Diamond DL. The financial impact of teaching surgical residents in the operating room. *Am J Surg*. 1999,177:28–32.

• CASE 8 •

The Shifting Sands of Senility: Canceled Consent

Time often puts more wrinkles on the mind than on the face.
Anonymous

Mrs. G. Arbled, an 88-year-old woman with mild Alzheimer's disease was well informed and gave consent for a colectomy last evening. She has now arrived in the OR holding area, is very agitated, and unalterably refuses surgery. A psychiatric consultant declared her competent during a lucid period a month ago. She has had a comprehensive workup, bowel prep, a large-bore IV placed, and insertion of an arterial line. Her operative indication is an obstructing colon cancer. She appears mentally competent during lucid periods and there is a cousin who refuses participation. The most ethical course of management is:

(A) Give her IV sedation until she calms down and proceed with the operation.
(B) Return her to her room, negotiate a "Ulysses contract," and operate as soon as possible.
(C) Return her to her room and sign off the case.
(D) Consult another psychiatrist to reevaluate her mental competence to refuse essential care.
(E) Restrain her, roll her into the OR, and ask the anesthesiologist to provide "crash induction."

One of the most stable, well-understood concepts in medical and surgical ethics is that a competent adult patient has the right to accept or reject medical or surgical intervention, even when therapy is necessary to preserve the patient's health or life.[1,2] The strength of this right, whether its exercise should be respected and implemented, is based in an assumption that the patient's decision-making capacity is intact and directed toward serving the patient's best interest as the patient understands his or her interests. When a patient's cognitive, decision-making capacity is significantly impaired, the right to refuse diminishes proportionately. Patients whose organic brain syndromes have significantly affected their perceptual and intellectual processes cannot reliably be said to exercise a right to make their own health care decisions; they are entitled to surrogate decision makers to protect their right to treatment and life that their errors in judgment would otherwise threaten.[2] Surrogate decision makers can be assigned by the patient in a durable power of attorney for health care or, in the absence of such an advance directive, according to applicable law, but part or all of the decision making process often falls to the surgeon.

Because the relative in this case refused to participate, a surrogate decision maker is unavailable. Surrogates for assistance with older patients' medical decisions are not without ethical conflicts. Surrogates supposedly are expected to reflect accurately the patient's wishes, but that is not always the case; it ranges from a high concurrence of 81%[3] to 66%[4] in terminal illness. Surrogates regularly attending church were less likely to reflect the views of those they represented.[4] The difference in therapy is almost always more treatment than the patient would choose. [5]

This patient does not have the advantage of surrogate representation which is not unusual in modern times; 21% of patients admitted to one ICU lacked both decision-making capacity and a surrogate decision maker.[6] Without a court-appointed guardian, the matter should be handled by the surgeon when the patient is not capable. Surgeons should appreciate that failures in communication with patients can sometimes result in refusal of surgical management.[7,8] Patients, especially the elderly, have a variety of frightening experiences and fears of infirmity as frailty relentlessly dominates. When refusal of needed medical care occurs, surgeons should review basic information, including especially risks and benefits, about the proposed operation with their patients, reiterating and remaining alert to a special need for clarity of information and the likelihood of patient misunderstanding.[2] Exploring the feelings of such patients, especially the issues behind the issues, can often provide the understanding necessary to resolve the patient's misapprehension.

Finally, it is well understood in medical and surgical ethics that a patient's refusal of indicated surgery, including urgently indicated surgery as in this case, is not, by itself, evidence of significantly diminished decision-making capacity. At the same time, a patient's refusal of indicated surgery should prompt the conscientious surgeon to question whether the patient's decision-making capacity is intact.[8,9]

When patients refuse indicated surgery that can be safely postponed, the surgery should be postponed. The clinical situation described here can be only briefly postponed. Although the patient had appeared to understand the elements of the informed consent process and seemed otherwise intellectually intact when she signed the consent agreement last evening, she now refuses. The abrupt change of mind without a change in operative conditions suggests that the patient may not be reasoning well this morning. Preoperative medications, exposure to the unaccustomed hustle of the perioperative area, and the discomfort of the insertion of IVs and monitoring apparatus produces anxiety in everyone. Simply taking the patient to surgery without first reevaluating her present circumstances and her decision-making capacity is inconsistent with the intent of informed consent, and is disrespectful to the patient. Option (E) is therefore not ethically viable. Option (A) is coercive, in that the patient's decision-making capacity after administration of a psychoactive drug is clearly impaired, and cessation of her protests cannot be ethically interpreted as informed or even legal consent. Option (C) abrogates the surgeon's obligation to evaluate this patient's refusal and constitutes abandonment.

This patient has a history of a mild dementia with fluctuating periods of lucidity during which she is competent to make her own decisions, and periods of confusion with markedly diminished intellectual function. This has been verified by a previous psychiatry consult. The most likely explanation of her refusal of surgery is that she is in an exacerbated period of dementia. Arriving at the operating room without adequate sedation can be very stressful to an elderly patient with diminished cognitive reserves. In her stable periods she is competent to make decisions. Thus, temporarily postponing surgery and waiting for the patient to regain decision-making capacity respects her autonomy without putting her at clinically unacceptable risk. When she recovers capacity, the informed consent process should be repeated and the patient should be informed that, as a result of her dementia and the nature of preoperative interventions, she refused surgery, but did so while in a condition of diminished decision-making capacity. She should be asked whether she again consents to surgery. If she does and there is no clinical evidence of significantly diminished decision-making capacity, she should then be given the opportunity to accept a plan in which subsequent refusal that is judged to be symptomatic of her dementia will not be considered representative of her reasoned decision. This form of advance directive has been called a "Ulysses contract,"[9,10] and it can be ethically used to ensure that episodes of acute anxiety associated with the preoperative period do not cause the patient to deprive herself of necessary care. In this case, the intensity of the patient's preoperative anxiety has kindled her previously stable organic brain syndrome and affected her reasoning capacity. With this preventive ethics strategy in place, surgery can be performed with complete confidence that the patient has competently authorized it. Option (B) is therefore the ethically justified response to this patient's refusal of surgery. Should the patient not regain intellectual capacity in a sufficiently brief period to permit timely surgical resolution of her intestinal disease, a psychiatric consultation option (D) becomes the clinically and ethically necessary alternative to arrange temporary guardianship and authorization for essential medical care.

The scenario presented does not address true emergency circumstances wherein minutes or at most an hour or less might be decisive. Other measures in the true emergency depend on context but could include getting an emergency psychiatry consult in the operating room to save time. We use the "true emergency" designation because of the practice of some surgeons to designate emergency freely for the surgeon's convenience. This form of deception solely for convenience is patently unethical.

References

1. Jones JW, McCullough LB, Richman BW. Informed consent: it's not just signing a form. *Thorac Surg Clin* 2005; 15:451–460, v.
2. McCullough L, Jones J, Brody B. Informed Consent: Autonomous Decision Making of the Surgical Patient. In: McCullough L, Jones J, Brody B, eds. *Surgical Ethics*. New York: Oxford University Press, 1998.

3. Sulmasy DP, Haller K, Terry PB. More talk, less paper: predicting the accuracy of substituted judgments. *Am J Med* 1994; 96:432–438.

4. Sulmasy DP, Terry PB, Weisman CS, Miller DJ, Stallings RY, Vettese MA, et al. The accuracy of substituted judgments in patients with terminal diagnoses. *Ann Intern Med* 1998; 128:621–629.

5. Li LL, Cheong KY, Yaw LK, Liu EH. The accuracy of surrogate decisions in intensive care scenarios. *Anaesth Intensive Care* 2007; 35:46–51.

6. White DB, Curtis JR, Lo B, Luce JM. Decisions to limit life-sustaining treatment for critically ill patients who lack both decision-making capacity and surrogate decision-makers. *Crit Care Med* 2006; 34:2053–2059.

7. Appelbaum PS, Roth LH. Patients who refuse treatment in medical hospitals. *JAMA* 1983; 250:1296–1301.

8. Connelly JE, Campbell C. Patients who refuse treatment in medical offices. *Arch Intern Med* 1987; 147:1829–1833.

9. Faden R, Beachamp T. *A History and Theory of Informed Consent*. New York: Oxford University Press, 1986.

10. Buchanan A, Brock D. Deciding for Others: *The Ethics of Surrogate Decision Making*. New York: Cambridge University Press, 1989.

· CASE 9 ·

A Surgeon's Obligation to a Jehovah's Witness Child

*It were better for him that a millstone were hanged about his neck, and he
cast into the sea, than that he should offend one of these little ones.*
Luke 17:2

An 11-year-old boy is seen at 2 AM in the emergency room of a rural medical center with a classic case of appendicitis. The child has a hemoglobin of
9 grams/dl and a white count of 24,000 with 95% bands. You evaluate and
schedule the child for urgent operative intervention based upon signs and
symptoms of impending rupture. As the parents are reviewing routine preoperative authorizations, they reveal that they are Jehovah's Witnesses and will not
give permission for allogenic transfusions. There are no other surgeons in your
area who will operate on a Jehovah's Witness's child. What should you do?

(A) Refuse to treat the child without permission to transfuse.
(B) Refuse to treat the child without permission to transfuse and request
emergency judicial intervention.
(C) Accept the patient for surgery and explain to the parents that if administration of blood products becomes necessary to prevent the patient's
death, they will be given.
(D) Treat the child, and if complications occur deal with the problem at
that time.
(E) Refer the case to another equally competent surgeon who is willing to
accept the stipulations imposed by the parents' religious beliefs.

Jehovah's Witnesses are among the few religious denominations that can
expect to test their religious beliefs with their lives. By refusing transfusion of
blood products, Jehovah's Witnesses show fortitude that frequently confronts
the beneficent characteristics of the medical profession.

The physician's fiduciary relationship with the patient is primary. This
means that the physician is committed to protecting and promoting the health-
related interests of the patient. This duty sometimes has to include protecting
patients from their own poor judgment about medical care, or the bad medical
decisions made for them by surrogates.

It is well recognized in medical ethics that competent adults have the right
to refuse medical care, even care necessary to save their lives.[1,2] Pointing out
that the decision is inconsistent with good health and asking the patient to
reconsider are compatible with respect for the patient's right to refuse. Ultimately, however, the decision of the competent, conscious, and sober adult
patient is determinative.[1,2]

Confusion can arise about the physician's moral responsibilities to pediatric patients when the focus is on the right of parents to decide, as their minor child's duly constituted surrogates, appears to conflict with their fiduciary obligation to protect and promote the life and health of their child. The primary moral relationship between a parent and his or her child is the latter, that is, one of obligation and not rights. Parents are expected to protect their children as their primary concern, an obligation that is encouraged and enforced by laws addressing child abuse and neglect, schooling, vaccinations, and labor. Although the transmission of moral, cultural, and religious values from parent to child is societally sanctioned, this parental responsibility is acknowledged as secondary to the responsibility to insure the physical safety of the child.

The parental obligation to protect and promote their child's health-related interests is fundamental, because life and health are necessary conditions for independent development of human values. Minor children are not thought to be capable of informed consent, and so are not accorded in medical ethics or law the decision-making authority of adults.[3] This presumed authority devolves on their behalf to the responsible parents on the assumption that the parents will act as advocates of the child's health. If parents elect a course which promotes their own interests to the detriment of the child's health, however, other authority may supervene. The Committee on Bioethics of the American Academy of Pediatrics has summarized the ethics of parental responsibility in health care:

> Although physicians should seek parental permission in most cases, they must focus on the goal of providing appropriate care and be prepared to seek legal intervention when parental refusal places the patient at clear and substantial risk.[3]

In this case, the child is anemic but still a candidate for safe induction of anesthesia. The proposed appendectomy carries a low risk for significant intraoperative blood loss requiring transfusion. Such subsequent complications as intraoperative abscess with prolonged catabolic depletion could nevertheless create an eventual need for allogenic blood products. The surgeon should explain to the parents the potential surgical complications of appendectomy, then explain the complications that could necessitate administration of blood products to maintain the child's life and health. The parents should be asked to consent to surgery with the knowledge that you will administer blood products for life-saving purposes.

If the parents refuse the surgery on those terms, the American Academy of Pediatrics' criteria for legal intervention becomes applicable. Without surgery, it is probable that the child's appendix will rupture, precipitating peritonitis and other life-threatening complications. It is not reasonable to expect the child's appendicitis to resolve spontaneously without surgery. With respect to blood products, the child's condition intraoperatively, but most likely postoperatively, could become life-threatening, and administration of blood products may become necessary to prevent death.

The surgeon should explain this clinical and ethical reasoning to the parents and ask them to reconsider. Should they continue to refuse and assert religious grounds for doing so, the surgeon should urgently initiate proceedings to obtain a court order for surgery and/or blood products. Parents do not have the right to refuse life-saving treatment for minor children in American common law.[4]

The American Academy of Pediatrics recommends that in cases of "serious conflict, physicians and families should seek consultative assistance and only in rare circumstances look to judicial determinations."[3] Option (C) is thus the best approach, supported by *urgent* ethics consultation to help persuade the parents. A court order should be sought if these efforts fail. Option (A), simply refusing to treat the child, fails to distinguish between the need for surgery, which is plain, and the need for blood products, which at this point is unlikely but must be planned for. Option (B) neglects to explain the potential need for blood products to the child's parents, an explanation that is obligatory as an essential component of the informed consent process. Option (D) is not entirely unacceptable, but fails to inform the parents of the surgeon's intent to honor his or her fiduciary responsibility to his or her patient and disregard their religious prohibitions if a life-threatening event requiring blood transfusion occurs. Option (E) is not acceptable because, with no other surgeon nearby who is willing to do the case, transfer of the patient out of the area would increase the risk of a catastrophic rupture which would surely threaten the patient's survival. Furthermore, the ethical issues in this case are not operator dependent; all surgeons should be prepared to address them prospectively and effectively.

References

1. Faden R, Beauchamp T. *A History and Theory of Informed Consent*. New York: Oxford University Press, 1986.
2. McCullough LB, Jones JW, Brody BA. Informed consent: Autonomous decision making of the surgical patient. In: McCullough LB, Jones JW, Brody BA, eds. *Surgical Ethics*. New York: Oxford University Press, 1998, pp 15–37.
3. Committee on Bioethics, American Academy of Pediatrics. Informed consent, parental permission, and assent in pediatric practice. *Pediatrics*. 1995; 95:314–317.
4. Kennedy L. Blood transfusion. In: Reich W, ed. *Encyclopedia of Bioethics*. New York: Macmillan, 1995:289–293.

• CASE 10 •

Are Ethics Practical When Externals Impact Your Clinical Judgment?

Every man is a damn fool for at least five minutes every day. Wisdom consists in not exceeding that limit.
Elbert Hubbard (1856–1915)

You were somewhat flattered when the foremost donor to the hospital where you practice consulted you 6 months ago for an infrarenal aneurysm. He is 85 years of age and has enjoyed fully his leisurely lifestyle. In the interim he has pledged to fund a much needed hospital children's wing. The aneurysm measured 4 cm then. When he came in for a 6 months' checkup, the same equipment measured no change in the size of the aneurysm. Both the patient and his wife insist that their lives have been constantly tormented by the knowledge that he has a "weak spot that could suddenly rupture and kill him". Your citations of data and scientific evidence, appeals to reason, and attempts to reassure do nothing to calm the couple's fears or reverse their insistence that you operate on the aneurysm without further delay. In consideration of the gentleman's VIP status, and at the urging of hospital executives, you agreed to repair the aneurysm. The hospital administrator and chief-of-staff have called you to register their support. The preoperative workup revealed no imposing data causing you to reconsider operating. The patient's children and influential friends have flown in from around the country to be attentive. But you continue to be troubled about the unfavorable risk/benefit ratio. What should you do?

(A) Do the procedure. You agreed.
(B) Get called out of town for a family emergency and have one of the equally experienced colleagues who encouraged you to operate do the procedure.
(C) Do the procedure. A generation of patients will benefit from the new hospital wing.
(D) Do the procedure. The opportunity to relieve the emotional distress of the elderly couple tilts the ordinarily unfavorable risk/benefit ratio back to an acceptable level.
(E) Don't do the procedure. Your integrity depends on objectively practicing evidence-based medicine.

In a modern medical environment, high-profile physicians encounter all kinds of external pressures. Political pressures about what to do or say, demands on time and energy, and VIP patients with special claims or requests make an elite practice "interesting." In contrast to the interesting cases of medical students, to experienced surgeons the designation "interesting" usually euphemistically means an association with sphincter tetany. In this case, the interesting portion is ethical not medical.

Major vascular surgery saw miraculous advances in the last half of the twentieth century, but complex procedures can still be attended by horrific complications. It is therefore crucial that each operation's ratio of risks to benefits weigh heavily toward the beneficial. The surgeon's beneficence-based obligation to protect the health and life of the patient is otherwise violated, and professional integrity does not permit such violations. Externalities, such as the hospital's quite legitimate self-interest in securing funding for its expansion, are irrelevant to this integrity-based ethical requirement.

Maintenance of professional integrity and the protection of patients from clinically unnecessary and, especially, unnecessary and potentially harmful interventions, provide the basis of the culture's vital trust in physicians. Patients who are considering major operations have a great deal of trust, frequently unreasonable, in what their surgeon can do and what their clinical outcome will be.[1] The physician is and should remain someone worthy of the intellectual trust that he or she will practice medicine to scientific evidence-based standards, and the moral trust that he or she will consistently sublimate self-interest, or the interest of his organization, however legitimate in other contexts, to insure the primacy of the patient's health-related interests.

Because subspecialty surgeons are conclusive referral specialists, they are less likely to receive a patient's requests for tests or procedures, but the era of patients' participation in their medical care is clearly upon us. Kravitz noted that one third of patients requested specific tests or procedures, and 9.6% of physicians complied.[2] Another study determined that when physicians were confronted with requests for unindicated MRIs, 8% ordered the expensive tests, 22% stated they would order them in the near future, and 53% ducked the issue with a needless referral to a neurologist. It sometimes appears that government, patient advocates, insurers, national medical organizations, and an increasing number of ethicists have hopped on the autonomy bandwagon to insist that not only should patients be accurately informed and participate in decision making about their treatment, but should be entitled to dictate their therapy. The pharmaceutical industry recognizes the emergence of "power to the patient" by peppering the airways with enticements pressuring physicians to prescribe life-enhancing supplementary drugs that do not treat diseases. They legitimize these advertisements by providing an encapsulated medical education, including contraindications and side effects in rapid undertones or microscopic print, which patients generally ignore or even find desirable. What impotent layman, when warned about erections lasting 4 hours, would not confuse satyriasis (good) with priapism (bad) unless specifically advised that his penis could thrombose and require amputation? Talk about polysemous advertising. Over a decade ago, Pellegrino warned that enthusiasm for patients' rights could be harmful to their health. He wrote that,

In the last 25 years, patient autonomy has displaced physician beneficence as a dominant principle in medical ethics. This has enhanced the moral right of patients to refuse unwanted treatment and to participate in clinical decisions. But now, in some cases, patient autonomy is being absolutized. The right to refuse is becoming a right to demand treatment. The result is danger to the moral and professional integrity of physicians. A reassessment of the mutual moral obligations of physicians and patients to respect each other's autonomy is in order.[3]

That reassessment has involved distinguishing between negative and positive rights. A negative right is the right to be left alone. Negative rights shape the informed consent process. Once the physician has presented the adult, competent adult patient (and all adults are presumed to be competent) with the medically reasonable alternatives for the clinical management of the patient's condition, the patient has the right to select one of them or the right to reject some or all. Positive rights differ. A positive right includes the right to identify for oneself what clinical management is reasonable and then request it. Because they place no or little demand on the resources of others, negative rights have no or only modest limits. By contrast, positive rights do place demands on the resources of others. Positive rights always come with limits. The ethics of positive rights concern what those limits are, not whether they exist in the first place.[4] The distinction between positive and negative rights may be lost on some patients. Physicians, however, should never lose sight of the distinction, lest they prefer to abandon professional integrity and become mere technicians of medical knowledge and its clinical application.

In this context, it is crucial to appreciate that when one grants patients the right to direct their own therapy, it must be recognized that a patient's values may directly conflict with the physician's values.[5] Evidence-based medicine cannot be understood completely, much less mastered to proficiency, by a highly intelligent layperson querying the Internet. Explaining concepts of disease and therapy to such a patient using advanced scientific terminology would be equivalent to showing card tricks to a dog. Beneficence-based judgment is the linchpin of surgical therapy; without it deficits accrue that technical skills cannot overcome. When the patient's extended autonomy modifies the surgeon's best judgment it creates the paradox of something good becoming bad. Surgical judgment must thus be mindful of when respect for autonomy has gone too far and trodden beneficence must reassert itself. That point is reached when the patient asserts positive rights to a therapy for which there is no adequate evidence base and a substantial risk of harm. Performing such a procedure violates beneficence-based obligations to the patient and thereby professional integrity. The devout Jehovah's Witness patient may exercise his autonomy by refusing transfusion therapy, even unto death, but he or she is not entitled to demand a clinically unindicated operation that is likely to be harmful.[6]

Recommendations for treating abdominal aneurysms are current and devised by competent and experienced investigators who have evaluated large bodies of evidence before reaching reasoned conclusions.[7] The size of our patient's aneurysm is below the authoritatively recommended threshold for surgical repair. Combined with his advanced age and reliable follow-up evidence of disease stability, there is ample foundation for you as the surgeon to rethink your decision to operate. The recommendation of the Joint Vascular Council's subcommittee includes consideration of the patient's preference in the decision to operate or monitor, but one may assume the patient's positive rights apply to borderline cases and do not trump unfavorable risk-benefit ratios.

Excellence in the practice of evidence-based medicine requires a continuous readjustment of decisions as data input changes. Rethinking decisions becomes absurd unless there is a willingness to alter previous conclusions. Changing the decision to operate will be embarrassing for the surgeon and inconvenient for the patient and his family. But is doing an operation for the wrong reason less important? One would suspect that the ego strength of our surgeon will suffice; the ego appears the most regenerable part of the human psyche. Option (A), proceeding with the operation, cannot be considered ethically correct.

If recruiting another willing surgeon to take over a Jehovah's Witness case is ethically acceptable, why not equally so this case? As the responsible surgeon, you cannot disregard the fact that by making arrangements for the procedure you will still be responsible for an unindicated procedure being done.[8] Should you refuse and the patient seek another surgeon himself, you would not be at fault. Option (B) has some entertainment value, but it has no legitimate virtues. It must be rejected.

Option (C) has no legitimate place in the decision making process here, representing as it does a transparent failure of professional integrity. Option (D) is insufficient to validate the operation and should be replaced by a careful explanation of the relative risks, a recommendation against surgical intervention at this time, and psychological reassurance of closer follow-up. The same is true for option (A).

The remaining choice is option (E), canceling the procedure. It is the ethically correct decision. It is sometimes difficult indeed to disregard worldly importance, including the risk of losing a badly needed new hospital wing or irritating one's administrative superiors, in reaching clinical decisions, but bad judgment, whether arising from insufficient knowledge or irrelevant enticements, pollutes all the same.

References

1. McKneally MF, Martin DK. An entrustment model of consent for surgical treatment of life-threatening illness: Perspective of patients requiring esophagectomy. *J Thorac Cardiovasc Surg*. 2000; 120:264–269.
2. Kravitz RL, Bell RA, Azari R, Krupat E, Kelly-Reif S, Thom D. Request fulfillment in office practice: Antecedents and relationship to outcomes. *Med Care*. 2002; 40: 38–51.

3. Pellegrino ED. Patient autonomy and the physician's ethics. *Ann R Coll Physicians Surg Can.* 1994; 27:171–173.

4. Minkoff H, Powderly KR, Chervenak F, McCullough LB. Ethical dimensions of elective primary cesarean delivery. *Obstet Gynecol.* 2004; 103:387–392.

5. Blustein J. Doing what the patient orders: Maintaining integrity in the doctor-patient relationship. *Bioethics.* 1993; 7:290–314.

6. Brett AS, McCullough LB. When patients request specific interventions: Defining the limits of the physician's obligation. *N Engl J Med.* 1986; 315:1347–1351.

7. Brewster DC, Cronenwett JL, Hallett JW, Jr., Johnston KW, Krupski WC, Matsumura JS. Guidelines for the treatment of abdominal aortic aneurysms: Report of a subcommittee of the Joint Council of the American Association for Vascular Surgery and Society for Vascular Surgery. *J Vasc Surg.* 2003; 37:1106–1117.

8. Jones JW, McCullough LB. Religiously-based treatment refusal. *J Vasc Surg.* 2001; 34:952.

· 3 ·

PROFESSIONAL SELF-REGULATION

Self-regulation within surgery, either individually or as a collective effort of the profession, is among the most demanding elements of medical leadership and independent practice. It is typically a process of internal oversight and restraint that is emblematic of the dedication to professionalism observed by surgeons.

Self-regulation in surgery reflects a key component of the ethical concept of fiduciary responsibility for patient care: accountability for the scientific and clinical quality of that care. The English philosopher of science and medicine, Francis Bacon (1561–1626), was among the first to call for scientific improvement of medicine, noting with scorn how physicians' clinical judgment was more often a function of personal bias and self-interest than it was of scientific rigor. Bacon, as part of a broader proposal that helped birth the Enlightenment, called for the replacement of knowledge grounded in tradition and authority by knowledge based on "experience," probably the first expression of the concept of evidence-based medicine.[1]

Bacon's ideas began to have real influence on medicine and medical education at the medical school of the University of Edinburgh at the end of the 18th century. There, the physician-ethicist John Gregory (1724–1773) called explicitly for physicians to adopt the intellectual virtue of candor, which requires physicians to accept the scientific discipline of being open to new, evidence-based information and to making evidence-based improvements in clinical practice. Gregory was skeptical, however, about whether physicians could be counted on to put candor into regular clinical practice, displacing the powerful allures of individual self-interest in wealth, prestige, and power. He recommended the creation of a group of "learned gentlemen," laypersons of wealth and leisure who would have time to learn medical science. Physicians, Gregory proposed, would then routinely submit their theories and practices to what, in effect, was an external review board.[1,2]

Then and now, surgeons, including those in group and academic practices, have historically and proudly functioned with a large degree of autonomy. They command their operating rooms and wards as the last word on the major patient care decisions made there. Unsolicited advice about one's practice is seldom well-met. Once an application is submitted, hospital privileges without limitations are expected, privilege renewal is considered a right, and withdrawal or reduction of privileges an unspeakable, often legally actionable, affront.

Skepticism may be politely, if pointedly, expressed about a particular case's management within the closed confines of a divisional morbidity/mortality conference, where problematic outcomes are analyzed for errors in judgment, knowledge, or technique, but criticism is expected to remain muted and to stop there, with future adjustments in case management left to the discretion of the individual surgeon. Still, the fact that surgery is the only medical specialty that consistently incorporates such critical reviews in its regular schedule of activities confirms the profession's intention to systematically regulate itself.

In fact, self-regulation among surgeons occurs in many contexts and at various intensities. The individual practitioner who asks that another surgeon in his or her specialty be consulted when a patient is seen with a complex condition that he or she cannot responsibly treat because of inexperience is exercising self-regulation at ground level. The division chief or department chair who travels to observe a new applicant's technique in the applicant's operating room before approving a new hire is exercising self-regulation on behalf of the supervisor's own group and the profession at large. The state medical boards that review complaints from patients and other physicians in some of the most troubling claims of sexual abuse, drug abuse, and poor practice are trying indirectly to exercise professional self-regulation. Committees of our national professional societies codify the technical and ethical standards of their specialties and effectively establish standards that serve as important internal regulators of our behavior as surgeons.

Despite so many types and levels of self-regulation functioning to ensure that the surgical profession conducts itself ethically and to high standards of technical and intellectual competence, imposition on a surgeon's authority and autonomy is still exercised only with the greatest reluctance and restraint. A surgeon with only a little experience with a complex disorder may disregard the fact that a world-class expert in treating the condition is available a few miles away and elect to cavalierly do the case himself without much certainty of how things will turn out for the patient. Such a surgeon has allowed self-regard to overcome self-regulatory standards. One close friend may choose not to criticize another friend in a morbidity/mortality conference, despite knowing that the friend handled the case poorly. A state medical board may find that its membership simply doesn't have the specialty knowledge necessary to conclude that a surgeon is incompetent and should not be allowed to practice. A professional organization's committees may be slow or tentative in reaching and publishing conclusions about right behavior. No one will argue that precipitous leaps to negative conclusions, or a persistently suspicious and accusatory posture, is good for surgeons or their patients, but a profession-wide tacit decision to see no evil is also wrong.

There is a claimant and growing need for rigorous self-regulation within the surgical profession to protect our patients, ourselves, and our position as ethical doctors. Professional integrity, as Gregory argued with remarkable foresight, requires processes of accountability within which protection of patients, physicians, and the profession can be routinely accomplished. The cases described in the pages ahead will suggest how this balance can be achieved.

References

1. McCullough LB. *John Gregory and the Invention of Professional Medical Ethics and the Profession of Medicine.* Dordrecht, The Netherlands: Kluwer Academic Publishers, 1998.
2. Gregory J. *Lectures on the Duties and Qualifications of a Physician.* London: W. Strahan and T. Cadell, 1772. In: McCullough LB, ed. *John Gregory's Writings on Medical Ethics and Philosophy of Medicine.* Dordrecht, The Netherlands: Kluwer Academic Publishers, 1998:161–245.
3. Percival T. *Medical Ethics, or a Code of Institutes and Precepts, Adapted to the Professional Conduct of Physicians and Surgeons.* London: Johnson and Bickerstaff, 1803.

· CASE 11 ·

What To Tell Patients Harmed By Other Physicians

He is a folyshe phisition that cannot cure his patientes disease, unless he caste him in another syckenes.
Sir Thomas More (1478–1535), *Utopia*

A 60-year-old obese diabetic woman with a history of CABG underwent a successful right femoro-distal nonreversed vein graft salvage procedure 6 years ago. She has done well since, and has been compliant with an antiplatelet medication regimen. She had a laparoscopic cholecystectomy performed yesterday at another local hospital. Her antiplatelet drugs were held and the anesthesiologist tried to start a femoral arterial line on the grafted side. She was transferred to your care at the university medical center that afternoon with a painful avascular right leg. While operating, you find that the badly damaged proximal graft has thrombosed and you are unable to reestablish blood flow to the leg. The rest of the observable graft remains pristine. An amputation is going to be required, and the family wants to know what happened. You should:

(A) Advise them that you believe the other physician's care resulted in the catastrophe.

(B) Tell them that the graft was worn out and probably would have failed soon.

(C) Tell them nothing.

(D) Respond fully to the family after discussing his case management with the surgeon who performed the cholecystectomy.

(E) Notify the patient, their family, the chief of surgery at the other hospital, and the state medical board.

In an era of medical specialization, complications of one physician's therapy often must be managed by another. Nonsurgical specialties regularly refer major anatomical complications to surgeons, and, correspondingly, surgeons often depend on nephrologists, neurologists, cardiologists, gastroenterologists, radiologists, pulmonologists, and others to help resolve postoperative complications. In the practice of technologically advanced medicine, cooperation among specialties is essential to resolution of complex complications associated with another physician's clinical management. In such an environment, a tangled maze of informed consent, self-protection, abundant opinions about what should have been done, guild mentalities, and multiple simultaneous patient-physician relationships can create an atmosphere rife with conflict. What should a consultant physician reveal about another physician's clinical errors and their sometimes terrible consequences?

The Council on Ethical and Judicial Affairs (CEJA) of the American Medical Association recommends full disclosure when medical errors injure patients:

> Patients have a right to know their past and present medical status and to be free of any mistaken beliefs concerning their conditions. Situations occasionally occur in which a patient suffers from the physician's mistake or judgment. In these situations, the physician is ethically required to inform the patient of all the facts necessary to insure understanding of what has occurred. Only through full disclosure is a patient able to make informed decisions regarding future medical care.[1]

The goal of full disclosure is for the patient to understand the nature and basis of her surgeon's clinical judgment about her condition and the plan to address it. As Brody puts it, disclosure of information by the physician in the informed consent should be "transparent."[2] The informed consent process obligates the physician to explain to the patient or family the nature of her condition, the medically reasonable and available therapies, and the benefits and risks associated with each option, including nonintervention.[3,4] Discussion of this patient's condition should include an account of its etiology. If medical/surgical management was among the causes of the current ailment, then the patient and family should be so-advised, but transparency in this case is best achieved by first consulting the patient's previous surgeon to determine what he or she believes occurred and why.

As the surgical specialist who has been asked to resolve the complication and explain it to the family, you should determine whether the lamentable outcome followed the first surgeon's medically reasonable treatment or was the result of a departure from the accepted standard of care. "Medically reasonable" means that a properly implemented method of treatment can be reliably expected to produce more clinical benefit than harm to the patient. Medically reasonable care is beneficence-based, in the formal terms of bioethics.[5] "Reliably expected" means that the general surgeon and anesthesiologist had some evidentiary basis, beyond his or her opinion, for a belief that the treatment they gave and the methodology used would benefit the patient. When established treatment methods are available, a departure from the standard of care violates both evidence-based and beneficence-based obligations to the patient, precisely because no physician could reasonably expect the treatment to produce clinical benefit.

The availability of evidence can of course broaden or narrow the range of reasonable treatments for a given condition. In this case, therefore, the central ethical test revolves around the question of whether preoperative discontinuation of anti-platelet therapy and placement of the femoral line on the same side as the graft were medically reasonable. Judgments on these matters shape the remaining ethical questions about how the case management should be explained to the patient and her family.

Briefly discontinuing the anti-platelet medication before surgery very slightly increases the risk to graft patency, but most physicians would agree that this should be done to control intraoperative blood loss. A femoral arterial line at the site of an arterial graft is problematic. Was an arterial line even necessary? If so, why was it not sited in a less vulnerable extremity? You determined that damage from the attempted femoral line caused the graft failure, and will probably result in loss of the limb. Was the offending procedure justifiable?

This case has the earmarks of a serious error in judgment, but surgical judgment is heavily context dependent. What, when, and how well an individual intervention is made have everything to do with its result. Exploration of such contexts is typically the subject of inquiry in divisional D&C conferences, and they provide a structured arena for open discussion and criticism within an institution's surgical department. In this case, however, your practice is located in a separate tertiary care hospital, so combined case analysis in a D&C conference is not likely to happen. You should nevertheless make an effort to contact the other physician to discuss your concerns and hear his sense of the context in which events occurred before reaching a conclusion about the reasonableness of his thoughts and actions. You are ethically bound to notify and educate him to prevent similar future problems. You could invite him to join you in meeting with the family to discuss how the case was handled, but you are the patient's current moral agent and as such bear responsibility for truth telling. Option (D) would therefore be our first choice in responding to the family's request.

Option (A) is precipitous, and deprives the other physician of an opportunity to explain his reasoning and intent. Option (B) is intentionally misleading, and violates the patient's unqualified right not to be deceived.[6] Option (C) is similarly indefensible, because it denies the patient her right to the truth about her care, the ethical underpinning of the concept of informed consent. Option (E) is premature, excessive, and because of the responses it is certain to provoke may place you and/or the other surgeon in an unfairly embarrassing position.

The medical fraternity has historically protected itself against disclosure of its errors and poor judgment, and to the extent that the habit persists, it is to the detriment of our professional integrity. CEJA's guidance is a significant corrective to this regrettable tradition.

References

1. Counsel on Ethical and Judicial Affairs, American Medical Association. *Code of Medical Ethics*, section 8.12. Chicago, IL: American Medical Association, 1998.
2. Brody H. Transparency: Informed consent in primary care. *Hastings Cent Rep.* 1989; 19:5–9.
3. Faden RR, Beauchamp TL. *A History and Theory of Informed Consent.* New York: Oxford University Press, 1986.

4. McCullough LB, Jones JW, Brody BA. Informed consent: Autonomous decision-making of the surgical patient. In: McCullough LB, Jones JW, Brody BA, eds. *Surgical Ethics*. New York: Oxford University Press, 1998:15–37.

5. McCullough LB, Jones JW, Brody BA. Principles and practice of surgical ethics. In: McCullough LB, Jones JW, Brody BA, eds. *Surgical Ethics*. New York: Oxford University Press, 1998:3–14.

6. Halevy A, Baldwin JC. Poor surgical risks. In: McCullough LB, Jones JW, Brody BA, eds. *Surgical Ethics*. New York: Oxford University Press, 1998:153–170.

• CASE 12 •

The Military Physician's Ethical Response to Evidence of Torture

. . . a savage who delights to torture his enemies . . . knows no decency, and is haunted by the grossest superstitions.
Charles Darwin (1809–1882), *Descent of Man*, 1871

A surgeon with whom you developed a close friendship during residency is visiting while on leave from military duty in the Middle East. Over cocktails in your home, he reveals that he has been deeply troubled because the kinds of injuries he has treated among enemy prisoners have repeatedly suggested intentional and severe physical abuse by their captors, his fellow military personnel. He has a strong sense of patriotism and has planned to make his career in the military, aspiring to general officer status after having quickly advanced to the rank of Lieutenant Colonel. He has written comprehensive medical records and made copies of them, but cannot decide how he should proceed. What should he do?

(A) Wait until he has achieved a policy-making rank before revealing his concerns.

(B) Notify the news media.

(C) Remain silent. His findings will probably be denied or ignored, considered betrayal of fellow soldiers, and cause retributive ruin of his military career.

(D) Accept the decision of the civilian and military chain of command that prisoner abuse is necessary to save lives and achieve political goals, and help to implement the program.

(E) Submit the information to military superiors immediately.

A substantial proportion of American surgeons have served for some part of their careers in the nation's military. Surgeons in particular are especially valued in an organization that is designed specifically to inflict severe physical trauma on an enemy and expects to receive its most devastating manifestations in return. Professionally dedicated to preservation rather than destruction of life, military physicians are exempted from combat and other aggressive action. The military physician is a health care professional and a professional soldier. The two roles can generate an obvious potential for conflicting obligations.[1] The combat surgeon is responsible for resolving the physiologic consequences of serious injury; the combat soldier beside whom he serves is trained and ordered to inflict it. Both military physician and soldier are bound by the Uniform Code of Military Justice, which dictates that "a lawful command or order" is required to obligate obedience (USUCMJ, subchapter X, 889, article 90). Orders which violate laws are not legally binding.

Systematically injuring or causing pain to other people is so antithetical to the traditions of medicine that it would seem unnecessary to formalize prohibitions against physicians' participation. Nonetheless, the medical profession, through collusion or actual participation, has established a notable record of involvement in torture throughout modern world history. The role of Nazi physicians has been well-established. A survey of Iraqi physicians showed that most had been exposed to torture as part of their medical practices.[2] 50% of Iraqi physicians interviewed had implemented government-directed punishment by performing nontherapeutic surgical mutilations. Physicians in Turkey falṣified records and otherwise disguised the activities of government agents who tortured prisoners and subsequently brought to them for care. Many of them reported that they did not consider beatings of prisoners to be torture.[3] Forty-nine percent of Mexican physicians employed in federal prisons have forensic evidence of detainees being tortured, and 69% have had prisoners complain to them of abuse by civil and military authorities.[4]

There is a wealth of authoritative literature available to guide our military colleague in his present dilemma. Though frequently invoked in both criticism and defense of U.S. government policies since the tragic events of September 11, 2001, the 1949 Geneva Convention Relative to the Treatment of Prisoners of War has been most often misquoted. It has been used recently in a way unintended by its framers for the determination of whether prisoners can be tortured or subjected to any of the torments that have been variously euphemized. The document does not address conditions for imprisonment of guerrillas, terrorists, and other paramilitary personnel.

The Geneva Convention states specifically that proper and timely medical care must be provided, if possible by one of the enemy's own medical officers, and supervised by a commission comprised of physicians representing both sides of the conflict. Seriously injured prisoners who are unable to resume combat are to be released, POWs are to have contact with the outside world, be paid for their labors, and even given creature comforts such as tobacco. Most importantly, they are to be humanely treated at all times:

> Any unlawful act or omission by the Detaining Power causing death or seriously endangering the health of a prisoner of war in its custody is prohibited, and will be regarded as a serious breach of the present Convention.... Prisoners of war must at all times be protected, particularly against acts of violence or intimidation, and against insults and public curiosity.[5]

These moral obligations, agreed upon by most nations following WW II, were intended to prevent in future armed conflicts the kind of oppressive and punitive treatment afforded neutralized captured combatants during that just-ended war and too many others. The enormity and horror of world events since the turn of the millennium have nevertheless created a question in the minds of some about whether the unethical actions of terrorists, particularly large-scale attacks upon civilians and brutal execution of captives, have exempted them from the moral world of mankind. It has also been asked whether independent terrorist groups not representing any organized national authority subscribing to the Geneva Conventions are entitled to its protections after provoking an armed response. Neither the Geneva documents nor the United States Uniform Code of Military Justice addresses such distinctions, and it must therefore be assumed that none were intended. Regardless of the provocations for war, the weapons or tactics chosen by the enemy, or the authority represented by the combatants, the Uniform Code is written to apply to prisoners, not just people meeting criteria as prisoners of war, and grants the same legal status to enemy captives as to members of the U.S. military incarcerated for violations. And it prescribes that, "Any person subject to this chapter who is guilty of cruelty toward, or oppression or maltreatment of, any person subject to his orders shall be punished as a court-martial may direct."[6]

Medical officers assigned to military prisons have moral obligations beyond those of the line soldier; the incarcerated are their patients, not just prisoners. The United Nations has resolved (111th plenary meeting passed resolution 37/194) that:

> It is a gross contravention of medical ethics, as well as an offence under applicable international instruments, for health personnel, particularly physicians, to engage, actively or passively, in acts which constitute participation in, complicity in, incitement to, or attempts to commit torture or other cruel, inhuman, or degrading treatment or punishment.

The World Medical Association's 1997 Declaration of Hamburg urged physicians worldwide to resist pressure to participate in torture and mistreatment of prisoners.[7] It is clear that the full weight of international and professional moral authority opposes option (C), remaining silent. Stated eloquently by Edmund Burke, "The only thing necessary for the triumph of evil is for good men to do nothing."

The justification is support of political goals, without regard to law or ethical ideals. Military groups have always valued their insularity and their prerogatives. The history of hostility and retaliation afforded whistleblowers by the military establishment cannot realistically be denied, and your friend must confront the likelihood that by properly rejecting option (C) he will be denied advancement and his career goals may be dashed. Whether he can happily spend the remainder of his professional career in an organization which would respond accordingly to his deepest ethical sensibilities is a question he must address secondarily.

Informing the news media of his suspicions as a first response could constitute an injustice to the brave and self-sacrificing officers and enlisted men and women, many of whom will have become his personal friends and close colleagues, and with whom he serves under the most stressful conditions. Although the regularity with which he has seen what appear to be torture-related injuries strongly suggests implementation of a standard policy, and therefore command influence, the mistreatment could conceivably be confined to a few low-level jailers. As a military officer, your friend is obligated to assume his leadership's honor and integrity and afford them the first opportunity to investigate and resolve the injustice within the parameters specified by military law, and before publishing potentially harmful and demoralizing unsubstantiated allegations. Option (B) would therefore not be an ethically justified initial action.

Maintaining silence until achieving his career goal of general rank, and the career protections it would afford, countenances the continued abuse of prisoners, deferring its revelation for at least the decade required for a lieutenant colonel to be promoted to brigadier. It does so in order to advance the physician's self-interest, without regard to the interim consequences such timid procrastination holds for others. It is hypocritical because postponement constitutes complicity, the passive participation in illegal acts which the United Nations condemns, while securing his career within an organization which he cannot sufficiently respect or trust to give fair hearing to his ethical concerns as a lower-ranking officer. The question again arises of whether lifetime dedication to a group that behaves antithetically to law and one's own morality is the career ideal he once believed it to be. He must be able to trust that his superiors will hear his concerns without prejudice or retaliation, or reconsider the integrity of his career goals. Option (A) cannot be ethically supported.

Military personnel are given the strongest encouragement to honor the chain of command and respond to orders. Though sworn to defend a democratic ideal, the organization within which they function is distinctly not democratic, and decisions are not subjected to group approval. Nevertheless, the Nuremberg trials confirmed the responsibility of every soldier to obey only orders that are legally issued. Your friend has not been ordered to countenance war crimes, and he cannot be ordered to suspend his conscience and his consciousness. The proper practice of medicine requires high intellect, astute judgment, and ethical discernment. Most of the people who survive the extraordinary rigors of our profession's selection and training processes to become physicians, and then surgeons, have shown that they are up to these demands. Unquestioning obedience to all authority despite terrible evidence of ethical error, hypocrisy, or illegality is wholly inconsistent with the physician's essential role as an independent critical intellect. Expressing group allegiance by actively participating in torture, either by using the surgeon's special skills to inflict pain and disfigurement or by maintaining secrecy on behalf of others who do, violates each of the military and international laws just cited, and all established ethical principles of medicine. Option (D) is not the correct choice.

The professional responsibilities of military physicians include preventive ethics. In this context, that means an obligation to prevent torture of prisoners in the first place and to report it promptly to forestall its continuation and repetition. Bloche, who served as a human rights investigator, has written that the more involvement physicians have in prisoner advocacy, the less torture and loss of life will occur.[9] Military physicians share with their civilian counterparts the obligation to act as their patients' fiduciary by placing the patients' health-related interests before their own. Option (E) may put this maxim to a hard test, requiring courage and significant personal sacrifice, but it is the only ethically consistent action available in these difficult circumstances.

References

1. Howe E. Ethical issues regarding mixed agency of military physicians. *Soc Sci Med.* 1986; 23:803–815.
2. Reis C, Ahmed A T, Amowitz L L, Kushner A L, Elahi M, Iacopino V. Physician participation in human rights abuses in southern Iraq. *JAMA.* 2004; 291:1480–1486.
3. Iacopino, V, Heisler M, Pishevar S, Kirschner R H. Physician complicity in misrepresentation and omission of evidence of torture in postdetention medical examinations in Turkey. *JAMA.* 1996; 276:396–402.
4. Heisler M, Moreno A, DeMonner S, Keller A, Iacopino V. Assessment of torture and ill treatment of detainees in Mexico: Attitudes and experiences of forensic physicians. *JAMA.* 2003; 289:2135–2143.
5. Geneva Convention relative to the Treatment of Prisoners of War in Diplomatic Conference for the Establishment of International Conventions for the Protection of Victims of War. 1949.
6. Military Forces, U.S.A., Title 10, Subtitle A, Part II, Chapter 47, Uniform Code of Military Justice.
7. World Medical Association. Consent for an Intraoperative Video Record Declaration of Hamburg in Support for Medical Doctors Refusing to Participate in, or to Condone, the Use of Torture or Other Forms of Cruel, Inhuman, or Degrading Treatment. 1997.
8. U.S. Department of the Army, Field Manual 34–52, Washington DC, 9/28/92.
9. Bloche, M, Physician, turn thyself in. *New York Times.* June 10, 2004.

• CASE 13 •

Who Should Protect the Public Against Bad Doctors?

Out, you impostors!
Quack salving, cheating mountebanks! your skill
Is to make sound men sick, and sick men kill.
Philip Massinger (1583–1640) and Thomas Dekker (1572–1632)
(1620; *The Virgin-Martyr*, act IV, sc. 1)

Not long ago, the board of medical examiners in one of our largest states revoked the medical license of a surgeon and fined him $845,000 for habitually poor practice. The surgeon began his career by failing his specialty certification exams three times, but eventually became the highest paid physician in the state's workers' compensation program, earning $3.3 million from the agency in 2002. He lived ostentatiously in a multimillion dollar home and owned a jet plane. He first came to the notice of the state board in 1985, when he was arrested after 30 grams of cocaine were found in his car during a traffic stop. He was convicted and placed on probation by the medical board for "intemperate use of drugs." In 1995, administrative law judges recommended that his license be revoked, but the board of medical examiners again voted for probation. During these two decades, the surgeon was a respondent in more than 60 malpractice suits, had a peer review board find that he performed 29 unnecessary operations—two of which resulted in the deaths of patients—and was the subject of 125 complaints filed with the state board. Described as charming, with an excellent bedside manner, he routinely prescribed patients large doses of narcotics and regularly convinced them to let him reoperate, "often the same procedure in the same spot," when his procedures failed to correct the original complaint.[1] It took more than 20 years of chronic and dangerous malpractice and many cries for help from his patients and other doctors before this physician was stopped. Who was ethically responsible for protecting the public from him?

(A) The state medical board.
(B) Hospital-based peer review.
(C) The malpractice tort system.
(D) Specialty certification boards.
(E) His specialty's professional society.

Is the case we have described so rare and isolated that only its oddity is worth notice, perhaps just a mention in some tabloid on sale at supermarket checkout aisles? Similar cases of chronic, poor, and dangerous practice, proceeding virtually without impediment, have been the subjects of exposés in national news magazines and network television features.

Virtually all measurable human activity, particularly medical practice, can be displayed in Gaussian distribution on a bell-shaped curve. In scientific theory, variations of more than two standard deviations from the mean determine significance, confirming a performance level that is either better or worse than that of the composite group. We recognize and reward those at the higher end of the profession by referring the most difficult cases to them, seeking their opinions, electing them to prestigious medical societies, and lining their office walls with awards. If some doctors are the best, there will inevitably be some who are among the worst, people who never mastered the craft, accumulated the knowledge, or accepted the enormous ethical responsibilities that properly go with the job.

According to the National Practitioner Data Bank,[2] only 5% of physicians are responsible for 33% of all the malpractice awards paid in the United States. Physicians who sustain more malpractice awards were also the subjects of more adverse administrative actions by hospitals and professional organizations than were doctors with fewer payable liability verdicts and settlements,[2] indicating a convergence of dissatisfaction and disapprobation between the medical and legal professions.

Weycker analyzed the malpractice history of 8,700 physicians in Michigan and found that a past history of patient lawsuits strongly predicted future mal-practice suits,[3] which is precisely why an individual's malpractice insurance premiums are raised as lawsuits accumulate. These kinds of data confirm that habitually bad physicians are abroad in the land, routinely practicing unsound medicine on vulnerable and unsuspecting patients. Our rogue surgeon is not *sui generis*.

The Englishman Dr. Thomas Percival (1740–1804) argued that an essential component of the development of medicine as a profession should be the physician's acceptance of the healer's training and role as a social contract. Percival advocated removal from the profession of those who are unwilling or unable to work in a fiduciary capacity:

> Let both the Physician and Surgeon never forget that their professions are public trusts, properly rendered lucrative whilst they fulfill them, but which they are bound by honour and probity to relinquish as soon as they find themselves unequal to their adequate and faithful execution.[4]

The implication for self-regulation within the profession is clear: to maintain the profession as a public trust, physicians have an obligation to monitor the quality of their own and colleagues' performance. The medical profession is a moral community with an ethical obligation to keep its members from harming the larger society within which it functions.

With the advent of medical licensure in the 19th century, the medical profession accepted an explicit social contract which codified its ancient implicit bond.[5] In exchange for a monopoly over medical services, graduates of accredited schools of allopathic and osteopathic medicine, the only people eligible for full medical licensure in the United States, have made assurance that the profession will regulate itself consistent with the public interest. The surgeon whose poor and predatory practices were winked at or who was permitted to slide through the cracks for 20 years, and the statistical certainty of others much like him, makes it clear that the medical profession has been insufficiently successful in honoring this contract.

State medical boards are the only legally authorized organizations for stopping incompetent doctors from continuing to practice medicine. In fact, the number of physicians disciplined by medical boards is a fraction of one percent of those licensed to practice.[6,7] The magnitude of the problem faced by state medical boards is much greater than the average physician may estimate. About 115,000 physicians are licensed in the state of California. The California Medical Board receives 10,000 complaints against its physicians each year.[7] Of these, it investigates 2,000 and prosecutes 500, resulting in about 250 annual disciplinary actions. Only about one fifth of those disciplined have their licenses revoked or suspended, as our surgeon eventually did. State medical boards, composed mostly of physicians, primarily serve to monitor qualifications for granting privileges and generally perform well in that capacity. In their disciplinary roles, however, they actually focus and act upon physicians' substance abuse, improper prescriptions, and sex with patients far more than upon demonstrable malpractice. These charges are much less defensible, and require no specific medical specialty expertise.

Almost no state boards have physician representatives from every one of the twenty-four practice groups comprising the American Board of Medical Specialties (ABMS), and they are therefore severely limited in the level of expertise they can bring to bear in overseeing the quality of care within their jurisdictions. With invariably small apportionments from their states' budgets, the boards have neither the manpower nor the mandates to systematically protect the public against incompetent or ill-intentioned practitioners.

For all the money and quality assurance hoopla associated with hospital-based specialty-specific peer review, it really has minimal effect on the ability of careless or incapable doctors to practice bad medicine. Good social skills among colleagues will usually be enough to get an errant practitioner out of a jam at his hospital, particularly because no institution really wants to go through the ordeal of removing a professional staff member anyway. Most physicians have witnessed the abundant benefit of liberally bestowed doubt go to colleagues who have been the subjects of internal investigations.

Not too long ago, one of us sat among the dissenting membership of a hospital committee reviewing the records of a surgeon who had three consecutive cases of transplanted kidneys donated by living relatives fail acutely, an occurrence many thousands of times in excess of chance. The investigating committee dismissed an independent expert's highly critical review because the consultant was deemed unnecessarily harsh. The transplant surgeon was not even censured. Fewer than 4% of the complaints made to state medical boards are the result of hospital peer review.[7] The societal goals of malpractice litigation are compensation of those wrongfully injured, identification and discipline of bad doctors, and consequent improvements in the quality of medical care within a community. The malpractice tort process does little to accomplish any of these goals.[5] In a study of correlations between negligent injuries and malpractice claims, Localio concluded that, "Medical malpractice litigation infrequently compensates patients injured by medical negligence and rarely identifies and holds providers accountable for substandard care."[8] Within this extraordinarily large study population, only 1.5% of patients who sustained negligent injuries brought suit, and in 86% of the cases that were filed there was no medical fault. Studdert's group studied 14,700 medical records, confirmed these findings, and reported that 77% of malpractice actions filed were evaluated as unrelated to actual medical malpractice.[9] The association between negligent injury and a court's finding for the plaintiff was no better correlated.[10] Awards to the plaintiff were granted in 46% of cases in which injuries were not caused by medical negligence, a rate not significantly different from the 45% of patients who did not receive awards after actually being harmed by malpractice. Awards were granted in 42% of cases with no serious injury. In a study of 8,000 cases with iatrogenic injuries, defense attorneys considered 62% defensible, but 21% of plaintiffs in this subgroup still received payments.[11] Furthermore, in jury trials, no relation was found between severity of injury and the awards. A comprehensive epidemiologic evaluation of the malpractice problem concluded that "substantial improvements in negligent care will not lead to a large reduction in claims rates."[12]

Specialty boards are responsible for determining the adequacy of candidates' qualifications for certification as specialists. Most first-time candidates for certification by the 24 member boards that ABMS coordinates are relatively young, recent graduates of approved residencies or fellowships who are just beginning their careers as independent practitioners. In many specialties, veteran practitioners must now seek recertification periodically throughout their careers. The Board's stated mission is to provide assurance to the public that a physician specialist certified by a Member Board of the ABMS has successfully completed an approved educational program and evaluation process, which includes an examination designed to assess the knowledge, skills, and experience required to provide quality patient care in that specialty. Widely believed to be predictive of a diplomate's competence in the specialty, medical board certification has been associated with reduced risk for subsequent sanction by a state medical board.[6,7]

Paradoxically, indicators of superior medical knowledge such as specialty board certification, election to medical honor societies, and high professional prestige have been associated with a higher incidence of malpractice lawsuits.[13, 14] The antinomy of this relationship has several possible explanations, primarily because the two subgroups are not identical. Those who failed to obtain board certification compose a small proportion of uncertified practitioners lacking necessary training credentials, a deficiency likely to reveal itself in their clinical practices. And just a few of the most flagrant offenders with repeated violations are punished by Medical Boards; better qualified practitioners are better able to avoid the multiple offenses that lead to disciplinary actions. Perhaps, superior practitioners have a higher incidence of malpractice suits because they are typically referred the most complex cases with the highest risk for failure. At any rate, the paradox reinforces the need for a better malpractice tort system.

Specialty medical boards do not represent themselves as guarantors that the knowledge and experience level they are certifying will screen for future bad doctors. The process of certification renewal for seasoned practitioners is typically limited to validation of adequate case experience and successful reexamination of a knowledge base. Application for recertification is not treated as an occasion for career evaluation by peers. The suspicion that multiple failures to pass specialty board examinations, as our surgeon experienced, predicts poorer quality practice is intuitively inescapable, but unproven, chiefly because it has not been studied.

The mission statements of the leading professional medical organizations implicitly commit them to protecting the public from substandard physicians. The American Medical Association promises that, "The AMA's envisioned future is to be an essential part of the professional life of every physician and an essential force for progress in improving the nation's health." The American College of Surgeons assures us that it is "dedicated to improving the care of the surgical patient and to safeguarding standards of care in an optimal and ethical practice environment." Both statements confirm that improving patient care is the organizations' paramount goal.

No representatives of organized medicine are better qualified to identify bad doctors and make authoritative corrective recommendations to state medical boards than the professional specialty societies. Certainly, no organized element of the medical profession has made a bolder public avowal of its intention to globally improve patient care. Nevertheless, the sage physician–ethicist Edmund Pellegrino has been deeply critical of our learned societies' failures to thus far do very much about these pledges:

> Physicians must now choose more definitively than ever whether their professional associations will assert the primacy of ethical commitment or shed any pretense of being moral enterprises and, instead, allow economic considerations to dominate their policies. The time is propitious for the medical profession to act responsibly to reaffirm the ethical commitment that grounds physicians' authenticity. Only then can physicians justify the claim to the moral integrity that patients expect.[15]

The present dilemma provides an opportunity for professional medical associations to shift the balance from self-interest to the interests of patients, thereby regaining public support and influence. Judging from recent trends, it is an opportunity that may not come again.

So the correct response to our multiple-choice question is (A), (B), (C), (D), and (E), "all of the above." Every one of the groups and processes cited has somehow assured the public that it will pursue quality in clinical medicine, sought and gained the public's confidence that it is doing so, and has thereby established its own ethical responsibility for insuring that bad practitioners cannot flourish. Each has had some success, but all have at least partly failed, and each can do much better.

As a matter of practical application, the leading professional specialty associations should lead by maintaining and strengthening medicine as a public trust. They can do this by following Dr. Pellegrino's advice and adopting a proactive, rather than a merely rhetorical, stance in the systematic improvement of medical care. They can do a great deal by directing some of their considerable expertise to the eradication of chronic medical malpractice. By appointing and offering the services of committees in each of the 24 medical specialties to each of the 50 state boards of medical examiners, the professional societies can arm the boards with the specialized knowledge and manpower they need to properly investigate and fairly judge physicians suspected of habitual poor practice. The state boards must agree to accept the assistance of the professional societies. They will make the necessary records available to the consulting committees appointed by the societies to provide them with authoritative opinions in allegations of persistent poor practice. The consulting committees will give the records their confidential expert study and submit their recommendations to the boards for such legal redress as might be indicated. The professional specialty societies lack the legal authority to take corrective action when chronic malpractice is discovered. The state medical boards lack the manpower and the specialized expertise to fairly and completely investigate each such allegation. Working together, the professional associations and the state boards can compensate for one another's disadvantages and fulfill their mutual goals of protecting the public by insuring the integrity of the medical profession.

References

1. Hopper L. Slapped with $845,000 fine, oft-sued surgeon loses license. *Houston Chronicle*. February 5, 2005:1,15.
2. National Practitioners Data Bank Annual Report. 2002, U.S. Department of Health and Human Services: Washington DC.
3. Weycker DA, Jensen GA, Medical malpractice among physicians: Who will be sued and who will pay? *Health Care Manag Sci*. 2000; 3:269–277.
4. Percival T. *Medical Ethics, or a Code of Institutes and Precepts, Adapted to the Professional Conduct of Physicians and Surgeons*. London: Johnson and Bickerstaff, 1803.
5. Jones JW, McCullough LB, Richman BW. Ethics of serving as a plaintiff's expert medical witness. *Surgery*. 2004; 136:100–102.
6. Clay SW, Conatser RR. Characteristics of physicians disciplined by the State Medical Board of Ohio. *J Am Osteopath Assoc*. 2003; 103:81–88.

7. Morrison J, Wickersham P. Physicians disciplined by a state medical board. *JAMA.* 1998; 279:1889–1893.

8. Localio AR, Lawthers AG, Brennan TA, Laird NM, Hebert LE, Peterson LM, et al. Relation between malpractice claims and adverse events due to negligence: Results of the Harvard Medical Practice Study III. *N Engl J Med.* 1991; 325:245–251.

9. Studdert DM, Thomas EJ, Burstin HR, Zbar BI, Orav EJ, Brennan TA. Negligent care and malpractice claiming behavior in Utah and Colorado. *Med Care.* 2000; 38:250–260.

10. Brennan TA, Sox CM, Burstin HR. Relation between negligent adverse events and the outcomes of medical-malpractice litigation. *N Engl J Med.* 1996; 335: 1963–1967.

11. Taragin MI, Willett LR, Wilczek AP, Trout R, Carson JL. The influence of standard of care and severity of injury on the resolution of medical malpractice claims. *Ann Intern Med.* 1992; 117:780–784.

12. Mello MM, Hemenway D. Medical malpractice as an epidemiological problem. *Soc Sci Med.* 2004; 59:39–46.

13. Ely JW, Dawson JD, Young PR, Doebbeling BN, Goerdt CJ, Elder NC et al. Malpractice claims against family physicians. Are the best doctors sued more? *J Fam Pract.* 1999; 48:23–30.

14. Sloan FA, Mergenhagen PM, Burfield WB, Bovbjerg RR, Hassan M. Medical malpractice experience of physicians: Predictable or haphazard? *JAMA.* 1989; 262: 3291–3297.

15. Pellegrino E, Relman A. Professional medical associations: Ethical and practical guidelines. *JAMA.* 1999; 282:984–986.

• CASE 14 •

Disagreements Between Attending and Consultant Physicians

*I have opinions of my own—strong opinions—but I don't always
agree with them.*

George H. W. Bush, 41st President of the United States

You disagree with a referring internist who has recommended that a mutual friend receive a carotid angioplasty. You suggest a standard carotid endarterectomy. The patient has a 99% stenosis from a complex plaque of the left internal carotid artery, with recent onset TIAs. The internist is the attending physician, and is well-known for a progressive attitude toward innovative treatment. The patient has asked that the internist seek your consultation. The carotid angioplasty procedure has been very recently introduced at your institution. Your recommendation for surgery has been dismissed by the attending, who is the senior partner in the medical group that provides your largest referral base. You should:

(A) Inform the patient and his family of your opinion.
(B) Consult another surgeon and do not relate the impasse.
(C) Make your recommendation to the internist in writing and inform him that you are withdrawing from the case immediately.
(D) Negotiate with the internist on how to present both alternatives to the patient.
(E) Place an anonymous note on the patient's food tray.

Disputes between physicians and surgeons about how best to manage patients' problems have remained a staple of the medical as well as the ethics literature for centuries. At one time, surgery was not included in the curriculum of medical education. Surgeons had their own guilds and colleges, and were neither licensed nor certified in the same manner as physicians. The Hippocratic Oath itself admonished physicians to refrain from surgery, and the two professions saw themselves as competitors rather than colleagues. Neither group was fully committed by present-day standards to the concept of the care-giver as fiduciary, protecting and promoting the best interests of the patient. Without shared professional knowledge and training, consultation and collaboration were rare, disputes frequent, and vitriol and even violence routinely characterized the interactions of physicians and surgeons.

Early physician-ethicists such as John Gregory in Scotland and Thomas Percival in England lamented the often hostile relationship and called on both surgeons and physicians to base clinical judgment and practice as much as possible on scientific evidence and use their knowledge and skills primarily for the benefit of patients rather than for financial or other personal gain.[1,2]

Percival encouraged cooperation between physicians and surgeons in their care of hospitalized patients,[3] arguing that both professions based their work in common ethical principles.

The surgeon should discuss with the attending internist all of the reasonable options for managing their patient's disease. The surgeon should explain to the internist why he believes surgical management is significantly more likely than medical care to successfully establish control of the abnormality. He should include in his consultation report the clinical risk factors, published data, and, respectfully, any concerns about the adequacy of available facilities or professional experience. Jecker and Allen write that a major ethical consideration in preventing and managing disputes is "maintaining high standards of competence in order to promote the patient's interests."[4]

Option (A), independently advising the patient and his family of your opinion when differing from the attending physician, places upon them the difficult burden of making a major medical decision that even his doctors seem unable to reach. The patient's personal request notwithstanding, the internist has engaged you to advise him, and as the attending physician it is he who should receive your evaluation and recommendation. He should likewise be afforded an opportunity to probe more deeply and perhaps debate still other alternatives with you. The patient's entitlement to information upon which to base his consent for treatment can be defeated rather than promoted by raw data from contending specialists. Although this patient has requested your involvement, the attending physician is his choice to manage his care. The role of the consultant is to assist the attending physician in formulating a plan of care.

Option (B) avoids the dispute, but in a manner that is disrespectful to the attending internist, and places a second surgeon at risk for being drawn into a dispute without his knowledge or consent. You deepen that risk by withholding the complete history of the case. Furthermore, the privilege of engaging consultants is exclusively the attending's, upon whom you are practicing a second deception by surreptitiously seeking additional support with which to defeat his conclusions.

Option (C) is an expression of personal pique unbecoming a medical professional and certain to disrupt any future relationship you might envision with this internist and his practice group. Although you are neither obligated nor entitled to send him a falsely flattering report to insure future referrals at this patient's expense, you do owe him collegial courtesy. This course is clearly intended to provide you with liability coverage in the event that the carotid angioplasty promoted by the internist is tried and fails; in that respect, such a consultation report would be accurately viewed as accusatory and hostile toward the attending physician. Furthermore, your sudden withdrawal from the case immediately after submitting your statement abrogates your responsibility as a consultant by making you unavailable for further discussion, clarification, or exploration of other options. In the codes of ethics formulated by the American colonial medical societies, members were fined if they engaged in fisticuffs during meetings, and expelled if they engaged in duels to resolve scientific disputes. The display of stubborn petulance described in option (C) is consistent with the censured behavior of a rowdier age.

Option (E) is childish behavior thoroughly contrary to your professional role. It will generate massive anxiety in the patient by encouraging complete mistrust in the profession to which he has entrusted his life, without even identifying the medical and scientific authority behind whatever information or recommendation the note contains. Like option (C), this method places the surgeon's egotistical interest in having the last word in the position of primacy. Communication of this sort serves neither your professional nor your personal relationship with this patient.

The primary focus of the surgeon's concern should be on protecting and promoting the patient's health by fulfilling the consultant's role in all its aspects. The internist is responsible for presenting the patient with all of the medically reasonable alternatives for managing his disease. Your colleague's ability to fulfill this obligation will be strengthened if you provide him with your complete, evidence-based evaluation of the relative clinical values of carotid endarterectomy and carotid angioplasty, for this patient and under the presently available conditions. Your evaluation of treatment options can and should include the observation that risk may be increased when even the most skilled interventionist is in the early stages of learning to implement a new procedure. Having pointed this consideration out to your colleague, it then becomes his responsibility as the attending to convey it to the patient. He may choose to seek your further advice about how best to do so, and it is important for this reason that you maintain your availability. Should you suspect that the internist is insisting upon angioplasty in an overabundance of financial self-interest, you should temper that concern with an awareness that selection of a surgical procedure could be similarly construed as an expression of yours.[5] Mutually respectful, informed, and patient-centered cooperation is the most desirable course, clinically and ethically, making option (D) your best choice.

References

1. Gregory J. *Lectures on the Duties and Qualifications of a Physician*. London: W. Strahan and T. Cadell, 1772. In: McCullough LB, ed. *John Gregory's Writings on Medical Ethics and Philosophy of Medicine*. Dordrecht, the Netherlands: Kluwer Academic Publishers, 1998:161–245.
2. McCullough LB. *John Gregory and the Invention of Professional Medical Ethics and the Profession of Medicine*. Dordrecht, the Netherlands: Kluwer Academic Publishers, 1998.
3. Percival T. *Medical Ethics, or a Code of Institutes and Precepts, Adapted to the Professional Conduct of Physicians and Surgeons*. London: Johnson and Bickerstaff, 1803.
4. Jecker NS, Allen MD. Surgery and other medical specialties. In: McCullough LB, Jones JW, Brody BA. *Surgical Ethics*. New York: Oxford University Press, 1998:280–301.

• CASE 15 •

Turf Wars: The Ethics of Professional Territorialism

Let each man pass his days in that wherein his skill is greatest.
Sextus Propertius (50–16 BCE), *Elegies*

A 300-bed general hospital in a mid-sized city has a busy cardiac catheterization laboratory, with 12 invasive cardiologists and over 4,000 annual procedures. An invasive radiology suite, the only one in town, is staffed by a single invasive radiologist and two vascular surgeons. They perform about 150 diagnostic angiograms and endovascular procedures each year, about half of which are generated by consultation requests from the cardiologists. The invasive radiology team has worked together for the last 5 years, since an endovascular fellowship-trained vascular surgeon joined the staff. The invasive radiologist helped to develop an endovascular team and mentored the more senior vascular surgeon until he could accumulate the requisite number of procedures to become credentialed. The program's finances and work schedule have been arranged to the satisfaction of all three participants. Until recently, whenever cardiologists found evidence of vascular occlusive disease during catheterizations, they changed host arteries; if symptoms and signs indicated a need for therapy, they referred patients to the invasive radiology clinic. Lately, the cardiologists have begun to perform terminal angiograms on all their patients to detect injuries. They have requested clinical privileges to perform peripheral endovascular procedures as well as traditional cardiac work. The hospital administrator is afraid that the cardiologists may become disenchanted with the hospital if their request is denied. The invasive radiology staff are concerned that their caseload will become insufficient to maintain quality if they must divide it with the cardiologists. You are the hospital chief of staff and must decide whether to grant the cardiologists privileges which have thus far been reserved to the endovascular team. What should you do?

(A) Grant all cardiologists full privileges in endovascular procedures.
(B) Maintain privileges in their current alignment.
(C) Grant endovascular privileges to the most productive cardiologists.
(D) Close the invasive radiology suite.
(E) Assign an ad hoc committee to study the situation.

The power of self-interest, including legitimate self-interest in expanding one's fund of knowledge, clinical skills, and ability to make a living, can sometimes distract physicians from their fiduciary roles and responsibilities. The distorting influence of self-interest can increase with the development of new technologies that straddle traditional specialty boundaries or eliminate the need for a particular discipline's bread-and-butter therapies. Radiotherapy took treatment of hyperthyroidism away from surgeons and made it a radiologist's disease. Discovery of the gastric bacteria, *Heliobacter pylori*, and development of medications that protected the gastric mucosa, effectively ended surgical treatment of nonmalignant gastric diseases, some of general surgery's bread and butter procedures until medical management proved superior. The still-growing sophistication of various endoscopes has eliminated whole fields of disease that once required open surgery. From time to time, these disruptions of territorial boundaries constitute improvements in patient care, with reductions in infection, pain, inpatient days, and recovery time. Usually the motivation for the incursions is less grand, but almost always they've provoked some mighty tiffs among physicians, and they lay at the bottom of some of the oldest and most persistent ethical problems in the history of medicine. Dr. John Gregory did the first extensive ethical analysis of doctors' therapeutic boundary disputes in 18th-century Edinburgh. He correctly concluded that physicians should avoid them because they had nothing to do with responsible patient care and everything to do with pique, turf, and money.

Twenty-four distinct medical specialties were recognized in the last century as a sufficient body of medical knowledge was accumulated to justify a division of labor and concentrations of study. The prescribed areas of specialization were severally defined, by anatomy (e.g., thoracic or neurological surgery), by organ systems (urology, gastroenterology), or sometimes by individual organs (cardiology, dermatology). Pathological systems, like infectious diseases, or necessary skill sets (radiology, pathology, nuclear medicine) determined some other specialty classifications. Sub-specialties emerged from the ever-growing body of knowledge and procedural skills developed within the parent specialties, and cardio-electro-physiologists, congenital heart surgeons, hepatologists, and pediatric psychiatrists now thrive. None of the specialties has been as fragmented as internal medicine and general surgery, with what seems like dozens of sub-specialists doing the work the parent specialties used to do and chipping away at their traditional caseload. And some of the old established specialties have themselves made grand forays into territory that once was exclusively claimed by another. Otolaryngologists have gradually become the preeminent head and neck specialists, and now contend with plastic surgeons for cosmetic work. The invasion of cardiology upon ground once exclusively held by thoracic surgeons is legend. When multiple specialties work in the same anatomical territory it typically stimulates physician conflict, especially if one discipline begins to be consulted most often for a particular abnormality and goes on to develop superior expertise, more exposure for its residents, better research opportunities, and more luxurious incomes.

About 40 years ago, angiograms were done unenthusiastically by general or thoracic surgeons, who did most of the vascular surgery as well. The available technology consisted of needles placed directly into the target arteries. Carotid arteries were skewered, and rapier length aortogram needles were inserted into the abdominal aorta from the back in what now seems a spectacularly clumsy procedure, the translumbar aortogram. Always a low-prestige job among surgeons with full-sized egos, the angiogram was typically relegated to the junior member of the surgical group, and many young associates fresh out of residency made their livings doing angiography for the first few years of their careers. The procedure was nearly as crude as a battlefield amputation, with three or four members of the surgical team and radiology staff usually assigned to physically restrain the patient to prevent damage to the aorta during injection of the radiopaque dye. In 1951, the Swedish physician Sven Ivan Seldinger (1921–1998) introduced a technique using tubing and guide wires to improve the ease, safety, and qualitative results of the angiogram. Radiologists refined and perfected the equipment and techniques over the next 10 or 15 years until the procedure became unquestionably their own, and surgeons gladly surrendered it to them. Seldinger has since become lionized as the founding genius of the new subspecialty of invasive radiology.

As the fund of information and sophistication of surgical interventions in vascular disease broadened, the demanding technical skills needed for best results required full-time dedication to the knowledge and procedures of vascular work, and the general surgeons who performed the occasional vascular procedure started to get squeezed out. Concurrently, vascular surgery began to distinguish itself as a sub-specialty, developed its own fellowship programs, and defined conditions for the Certificate of Special Qualifications beyond general surgery boards. Vascular technology adapted intravascular access for therapy as well as anatomical diagnosis, and individual vascular surgeons gradually began to reclaim territory they'd once willingly ceded. Endovascular stent grafting dramatically changed vascular surgery's working relationships. The combination of the invasive radiologist's catheter expertise and the vascular surgeon's knowledge and ability in open arterial access and prosthetic grafts seemed ideally suited to endografting.[1] Vascular surgeons without much experience or skill in catheter techniques recognized that they had to improve their capabilities or be run out of business, and they sought fresh training in the art with the help of the medical device companies with whom they'd worked to develop endovascular grafts. Then they made catheter training a regular feature of their fellowship programs. Recent studies confirm that mixed-specialty endovascular teams can conduct endovascular procedures with the shortest operative time and the least blood loss.[2]

Among the three specialties in our scenario, the vascular surgeons have the most advanced clinical knowledge of peripheral vascular disease. Cardiologists see a good deal of it, because many of their patients have peripheral vascular disease associated with the conditions for which they've been referred, but their expertise in that area does not rival the vascular surgeons'. The cardiologists' vascular skills are largely acquired in treating the coronary arteries; their reapplication to peripheral vascular procedures is questionable, and many cardiologists seem to be burdened by a compulsion to treat every peripheral vascular lesion. The cardiologists' selective catheter placement skills are probably superior to those of both the other specialties, but the invasive radiologist has the least clinical exposure of the three disciplines. Radiologists have no advantage in endografting, but the most technical experience with peripheral vascular radiographic anatomy and techniques, performing peripheral vascular angiograms, placing vascular filters, and dilating and stenting peripheral stenoses. In 2004, an extraordinary cross-disciplinary study group representing the American College of Cardiology, the American College of Physicians, the Society for Cardiovascular Angiography and Interventions, the Society for Vascular Medicine and Biology, and the Society for Vascular Surgeons (ACC/ ACP/SCAI/SVMB/SVS) developed definitive guidelines, entitled "Clinical Competence Statement on Vascular Medicine and Catheter-Based Peripheral Vascular Interventions." Their report concluded that:

> ...it is important to emphasize that vascular surgery training provides in-depth exposure, not only to surgical and endovascular techniques, but also to the pathophysiology, diagnosis, and medical management of vascular disease. Indeed, for the past 50 years, vascular surgeons, in addition to performing operations, have functioned as principal care providers for patients with peripheral vascular disease.[3]

This training regimen includes natural history, the anatomy and physiology of vascular disease, the clinical diagnosis, understanding of imaging and laboratory tests, and, perhaps most important, the indications for intervention.

As hospital chief of staff, your ethical obligation to the institution's patients is always to ensure, through the clinical privileging process, that they are treated by the best-trained, most knowledgeable, and most widely experienced practitioners available. You are also ethically responsible for guaranteeing that each physician privileged within your hospital maintains the currency of his or her knowledge, skill, and experience so that the quality of care does not diminish with the passage of time out of formal training. Granting privileges to all the cardiologists will increase the number of invasive peripheral vascular faculty to 15, which, if the caseload remains stable, would provide an average of 10 procedures per practitioner per year. This would be far less than the minimum 25 cases per year recommended for continued competence by the Vascular Medicine Task Force,[3] and would threaten the credentialing eligibility of the surgeons and invasive radiologist as well as the newly added cardiologists. In some communities, physicians may hold clinical privileges at multiple institutions and be able to accumulate experience in several invasive radiology clinics, but our scenario describes only the one endovascular program in this city, and the requisite clinical caseload must be gathered here by all the privileged staff. Meeting privileging standards for the cardiologists, the surgeons, and the invasive radiologist would require a caseload increase of 250%, an unlikely event unless the clinic is padded with inappropriate patient referrals solely for the benefit of the newly-added staff. The Task Force does not agree that an otherwise well-qualified practicing cardiologist is qualified as an expert in the diagnosis and endovascular treatment of peripheral vascular disease. The Task Force recommends at least a 1-year training sabbatical under the supervision of a qualified vascular specialist for practicing internists, cardiologists, and vascular surgeons.[3] The American College of Cardiology, American Heart Association, and the Society for Vascular Surgery recommend that candidates participate in 50 therapeutic endovascular procedures and be the primary operator in 25 to qualify for clinical privileges in the field.[4] The workload of our hospital's clinic is inadequate to either train the cardiologists in peripheral endovascular procedures or to maintain the currency of their knowledge and skills were they to meet initial credentialing requirements by obtaining training elsewhere. The cardiologists' current expertise in peripheral endovascular procedures is not equivalent to that of the existing team, and the cardiologists' addition would not contribute any significant knowledge or skills that the program now lacks. This is not one of those specialty boundary incursions that heralds bold advances in the quality of the work at hand.

As chief of staff, you would therefore be correct in rejecting option (A), granting endovascular privileges to all the cardiologists, as a threat to your hospital's quality of care and a violation of your fiduciary relationship with the institution's patients. Option (C) would be no less incorrect for similar reasons; clinical privileges were never intended to be the currency with which to reward productive physicians who are not otherwise qualified to work in a specialty not their own.

Closing the invasive radiology suite would hammer this particular turf battle down, but it would assuredly cost the hospital its sole invasive radiologist and the community its only access to endovascular therapy. This would be neither an ethical nor an efficient way for the Chief of Staff to manage boundary disputes between physicians. Option (D) should be eliminated from consideration.

Option (E), appointing a committee to study the problem, is an ethically troublesome administrative ploy overused by indecisive leaders. It has been termed strategic procrastination.[5] Such hospital study panels have traditionally provided strongly polarized groups with an arena in which to exert political pressures toward their own interests, and perhaps succeed in gaining clinical privileges for unqualified physicians. When the decision is clear, alternatives to circumvent or delay it are unethical, ruling out option (E).

When it has something better to offer, one specialty's expansion into another's traditional area of practice can represent a significant advance in clinical medicine, as Dr. Seldinger's work did. More commonly, turf wars between physicians offer no improvements, usually only a manifestation of greed, sometimes involving money and sometimes just hubris and intellectual acquisitiveness. A little knowledge becomes literally dangerous when physicians believe they have skills and experience that they don't, or want what they should not have, with naive patients winding up at the wrong end of the bargain. As chief of staff, you would be correct in joining Dr. John Gregory in rejecting these turf wars as all about physicians and not at all about patients. Option (B), maintaining the existing alignment of clinical privileges, should be selected because it recognizes the integrity and value of a functioning program that provides patients with high quality care by physicians who meet rigorous professional standards for training, knowledge, technical skill, and experience. To do otherwise would be a violation of medicine's fiduciary relationship with the patients entrusted to its care.

References

1. Veith, FJ. Turf issues: How do we resolve them and optimize patient selection for intervention and ultimately patient care? *J Vasc Surg.* 1998; 28:370–372.
2. Mullenix PS, Starnes B W, Ronsivalle JA, Andersen CA. The impact of an interventional vascular specialty team on institutional endovascular aneurysm repair outcomes. *Am J Surg.* 2005; 189:577–580.
3. Creager MA, Goldstone J, Hirshfeld JW, Jr, Kazmers A, Kent KC, Lorell BH, Olin JW, Rainer, Pauly R, et al. ACC/ACP/SCAI/SVMB/SVS clinical competence statement on vascular medicine and catheter-based peripheral vascular interventions: A report of the American College of Cardiology/American Heart Association/American College of Physician Task Force on Clinical Competence (ACC/ACP/SCAI/SVMB/SVS Writing Committee to develop a clinical competence statement on peripheral vascular disease). *J Am Coll Cardiol.* 2004; 44: 941–957.
4. White RA, Hodgson KJ, Ahn SS, Hobson, RW, II, Veith FJ. Endovascular interventions training and credentialing for vascular surgeons. *J Vasc Surg.* 1999; 29: 177–186.
5. Chervenak FA, McCullough LB. Physicians and hospital managers as cofiduciaries of patients: rhetoric or reality? *J Healthc Manag.* 2003; 48:172–179.

· CASE 16 ·

Eyewitness to Incompetent Surgery

Let not mercy and truth forsake thee: bind them about thy neck;
write them upon the table of thine heart.
Proverbs 3:3

You are covering for a friend and colleague who has left town to attend a professional meeting. Two days prior he resected a rectal cancer and the patient has now developed an acute abdomen. In the OR you discover that the first surgeon clearly failed to properly construct the anastomosis during the original operation, thus precipitating the current life-threatening event. You have had other occasions to suspect gross errors in this surgeon's operative technique. After correcting the acute lesion and stabilizing the patient, you should:

(A) Enter your dictation of the operation in the medical record and take no further action.

(B) Report your findings to the chairman of the department of surgery.

(C) Report your findings privately to the first surgeon, including your observations concerning other technical problems.

(D) Report the surgeon to the State Board of Medical Examiners.

(E) Advise the patient and his family of your findings.

The techniques revealed to you when you revisited the operative site, the first operation's poor results, and the earlier technical errors you have witnessed appear to represent a pattern of incompetence that threatens the lives and health of patients. The problem must be urgently addressed as a matter of fiduciary responsibility to your colleague's present and future patients. While it is unlikely that this pattern is defensible, fairness and the need to be thorough mean that you should attempt to rule out incompetence by taking this matter up with your colleague without further delay. An overabundance of caution in this respect would lead you to option A, but this would abrogate the surgical profession's responsibility to exercise appropriate self-regulation.[1]

Option (D), reporting the case directly to the State Board of Medical Examiners, would constitute a premature assertion of malpractice and unfairly threaten the colleague's reputation. The first step therefore should be to advise your colleague of your legitimate and urgent concerns with his practice and ask him to explain the pattern you have observed to colleagues responsible for care at your institution.

Options (B) and (C), bringing the matter to the attention of the departmental chair and the Death and Complications Conference, and advising the patient and family that a surgical error requiring reoperation has occurred, are both necessary corollaries of the process that must be set in motion in such cases, but the primary responsibility for doing so resides with the surgeon who performed the first operation. Although you had an important role in the care of this patient, the original surgeon has the ethical obligation to reveal operative complications to the patient and to the professional peer group formally designated to evaluate the quality of surgical care. This peer group is also responsible for making informed recommendations for modifications in technique or judgment that will help avoid these kinds of errors in future similar cases.

Option (C) recognizes your ethical responsibility to acknowledge the integrity of your colleague and friend and initiates the essential process of professional self-regulation in surgical practice. This time-honored practice began with the Seal of Cause and Charter of Principles of the Royal College of Surgeons in Edinburgh in 1505, and was reaffirmed with the foundation of the American College of Surgeons in 1913.[2] Self-regulation within the surgical profession insures that high standards of practice will be established, monitored, and enforced by individuals who have the scientific training and clinical experience to do so fairly and knowledgeably, while protecting practitioners from the unwarranted criticism of those who do not. In addition to advising your colleague of your serious concerns with the operative management of this case, you should make clear that he must discuss the complications with the patient, and report them to the departmental D&C conference. Responsibility for evaluation and recommendation then properly devolves to the conference, which may or may not be guided by its findings to a pattern of earlier technical errors by this surgeon. Should your colleague fail to make these disclosures after your discussion with him, your fiduciary obligation to your colleagues' patients creates the inescapable obligation to make your concerns known immediately to the chief of surgery and to inform the patient about the reason for the second operation.

References

1. Jones RS, Fletcher JC. Self-regulation of surgical practice and research. In: McCullough LB, Jones JW, Brody BA, eds. *Surgical Ethics*. New York: Oxford University Press, 1998:255–279.
2. Brieger GH. Medicine as a profession. In: Reich WT, ed. *Encyclopedia of Medical Ethics*. 2nd ed. New York: Macmillan, 1995:1688–1695.

• CASE 17 •

Ethics of Operative Scheduling: Balancing Multiple Fiduciary Responsibilities

As members of a profession, physicians are expected to work collaboratively to maximize patient care, be respectful of one another, and participate in the processes of self-regulation, including remediation and discipline of members who have failed to meet professional standards.
—Physician Charter, 2002

You are a surgeon with an arduous operative schedule in a large private hospital. Your first two cases today took much longer than estimated, and your third case has been changed to "add-on" status. Your remaining patient is an indigent man with noninfected gangrene of the fifth toe and rest pain; he requires a femoral-popliteal bypass within 24 hours to avoid additional risk. All ORs except the trauma room are currently occupied. Staffing drops off with the shift change in 1 hour, and afterwards incoming trauma patients will probably delay the start of other cases. If your case is declared an emergency it will be started now, otherwise it must wait until a room opens. No cases are pending in the ER. Tomorrow is your clinic day and your operative schedule is full for the remainder of the week. What should you do?

(A) Do the case as an "add-on" after consulting the OR supervisor.
(B) Declare emergency status and operate in the trauma room.
(C) Cancel your morning clinic and operate tomorrow.
(D) Call your friend the chief of staff and apply pressure to operate now.
(E) Ask a colleague to do the case in the morning.

Large surgical services often experience periods when OR capacity is exceeded and the schedule becomes congested. Problems tend to cluster around first starts and the late afternoon, when everyone is pressing to complete the schedule. This patient urgently requires surgical management of serious vascular insufficiency to save his leg. If his gangrenous toe becomes infected, his condition could become life-threatening, with sepsis rapidly advancing through the ischemic tissue and compounding the risk of infection in the surgical graft. Declaring the case an emergency would heighten its priority and ensure rapid access to an operating room, starting before prime staffing time is over. Nevertheless, the definition of a surgical emergency in the Association of Operating Room Nurses (AORN) standards, uniformly accepted by American hospitals, is based on an absolute need for surgery within 2 hours to protect life and limb.[1] This patient's acuity level does not meet this standard: his need is urgent but not emergent.

The surgeon's primary fiduciary responsibility is to the patient, but that is not his or her only responsibility. There are secondary ethical obligations as well, and they must be honored. The surgeon has a clear obligation to observe and cooperate with the organizational and functional structures of the operating room, which are designed to insure that all patients will receive safe, timely, and complete operative care consistent with their clinical needs. Every hospital has established OR policies to efficiently utilize professional time, space, and equipment, while maintaining reserves in each category to handle the unforeseeable but inevitable emergency presentations. As a surgeon, you are expected to be an advocate for your patient, but not to the exclusion of all others, and particularly not at the peril of other patients with compelling needs. From an institutional viewpoint, surgery is a team enterprise, with mutually supportive roles intended to maximize every member's productivity and effectiveness[2].

It is well-understood that most surgeons would like to complete the day's operations as early as possible and clear the schedule for the next working day. With an established diagnosis of a potentially life-threatening condition, there is no question of this patient's legitimate demand upon the surgeon's attention. Nevertheless, option (B), declaring him a surgical emergency and commandeering the only unengaged operating room, is a deception primarily intended to satisfy the surgeon's impatience rather than improve the patient's prognosis, which will be substantially unchanged if he is operated on immediately, tonight, or tomorrow morning. Though the ER has no patients for emergency surgical referral, reclassifying your case as an emergency and taking him to the trauma room places any true emergency arriving while you are operating at potential mortal risk. Though no such cases may present, and though your primary fiduciary responsibility is to your current patient, professional integrity recognizes a concurrent obligation to support or change carefully crafted OR policies designed to anticipate the most extreme eventualities of patient care. Option (B) serves the surgeon's convenience without substantially improving the patient's prognosis, markedly imperils newly arriving true emergencies, and must be rejected.

Option (C), cancelling the next day's clinic and operating tomorrow to avoid a late case today, breaks faith with the patients who have arranged their own schedules, weeks or months in advance, to be seen by you. Many will likely be in significant need of your clinical attention, and could be placed at added risk by being asked to postpone their evaluation or postoperative care. Clinic cancellation on short notice is an imposition on the good will of patients and support staff alike, and is generally seen by referring physicians as a reflection upon one's professional reliability and integrity. Cancelling clinic should be reserved for those rare emergencies when a problem has no other solution. This one does, including proceeding with today's case later than anticipated, or asking another surgeon to operate for you. Option (C) should therefore be discarded.

Option (D), calling upon a personal friend in a position of higher authority to override the OR's contingency policies, imposes an unwelcome conflict of interest upon the chief of staff and generates all the other threats to emergency management just described, all to suit your own convenience without significantly improving your patient's situation. It should be rejected.[3]

Option (A) insures that surgery will be completed within necessary clinical parameters without misrepresenting the patient's acuity and creating a dangerous backlog should a true emergency present while you are operating in the trauma room. Though your day will be lengthened by waiting to add the legitimately "urgent" operation, your clinical and ethical responsibilities to your patient, the institution's other patients, and the OR team will all have been met.

Option (E), asking a colleague to operate on your patient in the morning, is a viable alternative if the prospect of a late operation after a long day causes you to be concerned about fatigue and the quality of your care. Surgeons determine the order of cases in the OR. Sometimes, the order is motivated by clinically irrelevant and therefore ethically unjustified considerations, such as the social standing of the patient, the source of payment, avoiding an inconvenient cancellation of a case, and others that are even more flagrantly self-serving. As the surgeon in this case, you are surely aware that you are scheduling an urgent case after two purely elective ones. This decision was entirely voluntary and unnecessarily created a potential ethical conflict that, if this patient's surgery is unduly delayed, will become an actual and serious ethical conflict. Through a failure of forethought or intentional disregard of appropriate scheduling priorities, you have now imposed a preventable hardship upon yourself, other surgeons, and the OR staff and management. The result is to put this patient, and perhaps other patients, at otherwise preventable risk of suboptimal care.

An organizational culture shaped by fiduciary responsibility and its professional virtues is an essential ingredient in a preventive approach to problems like this. Organizational culture includes the policies and practices of a working group, as well as its values and priorities, particularly as they become concrete in budgets and hiring and promotion decisions. Organizational culture is shaped by what leaders expect, inspect, reward, punish, and—perhaps most important—tolerate.

References

1. Association of Operating Room Nurses. Standards, Recommended Practices, and Guidelines. 2003.
2. Purtillo R, Shaw BW, Arnold R. Obligations of surgeons to non-physician team members. In: McCullough LB, Jones JW, Brody BA, eds. *Surgical Ethics*. New York: Oxford University Press, 1998:302–321.
3. Khushf G, Gifford R. Understanding, assessing, and managing conflicts of interest. In: McCullough LB, Jones JW, Brody BA, eds. *Surgical Ethics*. New York: Oxford University Press, 1998:342–366.

· CASE 18 ·

Do Unto Others: Justice in Surgical Education

You have scheduled a colleague who directs the surgical residency program at another local teaching hospital for an uncomplicated hernia repair tomorrow. She is now in your preoperative clinic and appears to be in otherwise excellent health. She asks that you personally perform the entire procedure without the assistance of your residents. When you explain that you will perform the procedure but would like a resident to be at the operating table with you to gain experience and provide you with help, she is firmly opposed. "If residents are in the OR, the temptation to allow them to actively participate is too great," she says. You should:

(A) Provide care as requested.
(B) Agree, but have your resident there as usual while you do the case yourself.
(C) Refuse to provide surgical care under the stated conditions.
(D) Refuse to provide care and say what you think of her attitude.
(E) Agree and follow your usual routine in the OR.

The adequate training of physicians requires that we provide students and residents with hands-on clinical experience. This has been regular practice since the 18th century, when medical students in Scotland and England became involved in the care of patients as part of their education.

In the English-speaking world of the 18th century, the first teaching hospitals were those that provided care for patients who were ill and impoverished. Chartered by the Crown, the Royal Infirmaries were founded by the owners of factories and mills that created the Industrial Revolution. These wealthy individuals wanted to insure that their ill or injured employees would receive sufficient medical care to insure their prompt return to work.[1] The Royal Infirmaries became the models for the first hospitals in the United States, founded in cities such as New York and Philadelphia near the end of the colonial period.

The medical school at the University of Edinburgh pioneered modern medical education in the second half of the 18th century, assembling many of the finest scientists and physicians in Europe and training students on the wards of the Royal Infirmary of Edinburgh.[1,2] In Colonial America, a similar practice developed at King's College (later Columbia University's College of Physician and Surgeons) and the New York Hospital. Dr. Samuel Bard, who went on to play a leading role in the American Revolution against English tyranny, argued that the sick poor should happily submit themselves as medical student training cases in exchange for their free care.[3]

Since the incorporation of the concept and practice of informed consent in medical law and ethics,[4] we can no longer assume that patients will implicitly accept an obligation to make themselves available as teaching material. The patients' informed consent for the involvement of trainees in their care must precede student or resident participation.

Medical ethics are not confined to the patient's entitlement to grant or withhold informed consent. It is arguable that patients are indeed obligated to participate in their medical care as teaching material, and there are at least two bases for such an argument. First, patients today benefit from the willingness of past patients to permit the participation of trainees in their care. To claim a right to the benefits of medical care without sharing the obligation to perpetuate medical knowledge and skills offends basic concepts of fairness and justice, which prohibit such an imbalance of benefits and burdens. Second, medical science and medical practice represent a culturally sanctioned accumulation and refinement of specialized knowledge, literally passed from hand to hand across the ages. The maintenance of that chain is a responsibility of all members of the society, each of whose lives has benefited, if not directly as a patient, then as a citizen of a world made safer by principles of public health and disease control. Unless patients are willing to play a role in training subsequent generations of medical professionals, each of us will be at risk for limited access to future medical care.

When the patient is a physician, the argument for reciprocity and fairness becomes even stronger. The colleague-patient in this case is a direct beneficiary of the willingness of patients to permit her participation in their care as a medical student, resident, and professional medical educator. To claim that she has not even a minimal reciprocal responsibility strains credulity. At a time when there is widespread concern about the potential exploitation of "clinic" or "public" patients, to grant colleagues the privileges of aristocracy further defiles the egalitarian standards of justice that define our culture.

Option (C) is the best response to your colleague, because her demand lacks any moral authority. Her condition is neither emergent nor life-threatening, and she may seek treatment elsewhere if she wishes. Honoring her refusal would ratify two disturbing precedents: First, the powerful and well-placed will surely receive the benefits of physicians' training but not contribute to perpetuation of the training system to gain access to that benefit. Second, this training director is rejecting the competence of surgical residents, the concept of surgical training, and the process of supervision, all of which she advocates for others in her professional capacity. Her authoritative voice constitutes a denial of surgery's well-structured training methods, and could threaten the willingness of others to participate in it. If your colleague's worry is confidentiality, you should remind her (and your team) that your obligation to her patient privacy will be fulfilled as with every patient.[5]

Option (A) is ruled out by this argument, but option (E) is even less ethically acceptable, because it involves frank deception, which is inconsistent with professional integrity and the requirements of informed consent. Option (B) is just slightly less deceptive, because the patient has refused consent for any trainee involvement. Exercising option (D) might soothe one's sense of righteous indignation at the patient's hypocrisy, but would personalize the issue and violate the sense of emotional removal necessary to one's professional demeanor and function.

References

1. Risse GB. *Hospital Life in Enlightenment Scotland: Care and Teaching at the Royal Infirmary of Edinburgh.* Cambridge: Cambridge University Press, 1986.
2 McCullough LB. *John Gregory and the Invention of Professional Medical Ethics and the Profession of Medicine.* Dordrecht, The Netherlands: Kluwer Academic Publishers, 1998.
3. Bard S. *A Discourse upon the Duties of a Physician.* New York: A. and J. Robertson, 1769.
4. Faden RR, Beauchamp TL. *A History and Theory of Informed Consent.* New York, Oxford University Press, 1986.
5. Marshall MF, Smith III, CD. Confidentiality in surgical practice. In: McCullough LB, Jones JW, Brody BA, eds. *Surgical Ethics.* New York: Oxford University Press, 1998:38–56.

• CASE 19 •

The Surgeon's Obligations to the Noncompliant Patient

Understanding is a well-spring of life unto him that hath it:
But the instruction of fools is folly.
Proverbs 16:22

A 61-year-old gentleman is referred with severe peripheral vascular disease marked by disabling ischemic rest pain. He is obese, diabetic, alcoholic, and smokes heavily. His target arteries are small, but can be bypassed. You have been following him for 6 months, and have attempted to reduce his operative risk by referring him to an endocrinologist for improved diabetic control, a dietician for weight reduction, a psychiatrist for treatment of alcoholism, and a smoking cessation program. All consultants have advised you that the patient has been noncompliant with their recommendations. This morning he is in your office, reporting severe pain unrelieved by oral analgesia and requesting either bypass surgery or an amputation. Your recommendation?

(A) Discharge him from your practice after referral to a competent colleague.
(B) Encourage him once again to participate actively in the recommended nonsurgical therapies.
(C) Admit him and amputate the affected limb.
(D) Admit him and do a femoral distal bypass operation.
(E) Consult your institutional ethics committee.

Noncompliance or poor compliance with recommended lifestyle changes are common among vascular disease patients; up to 75% of smokers were still smoking a year after a myocardial infarction.[1] In a survey of patients with symptomatic peripheral vascular disease (PVD), most attributed heart-lung disease to smoking, but fewer than half considered PVD to be smoking-related, and almost none thought that loss of limb was smoking-related.[2]

The rights of patients have been widely discussed in the last two decades, but the obligations of patients are less well understood by either patients or their doctors.[3] It would seem sensible to expect patients to follow their physicians' therapeutic instructions, but autonomous patients may be poorly compliant, particularly when the recommendations involve the effort associated with lifestyle changes. Patients who continue to pursue unhealthy lifestyles even as they seek treatment of self-inflicted disease can test the surgeon's beneficence and strain the doctor-patient relationship.

The authors of the American Medical Association's first Code of Ethics in 1847 conceived a compelling and still timely sense of patient obligations.[4] The Code's sixth article states: "The obedience of a patient to the prescriptions of his physician should be prompt and implicit. He should never permit his own crude opinions as to their fitness to influence his attention to them."[4]

This sternly paternalistic tone is mitigated by the authors' subsequent appeals to two essential concerns. First, a therapeutic regimen not closely observed nor fully completed by the poorly compliant patient may become ineffective or even dangerous. Second, as patients become asymptomatic, they may mistakenly think that they have fully recovered and prematurely terminate the treatment plan.[2] The first of these concerns applies directly to the case at hand: this patient's failure to discontinue tobacco use is highly likely to reduce the effectiveness of a bypass procedure. Long-term graft patency is an important endpoint in bypass surgery, and this goal is significantly imperiled by continued use of vaso-constricting tobacco products[5] and poorly controlled diabetes.

The AMA's first Code of Ethics also provides us with an account of the physician-patient relationship. The first of two major components in the relationship is the physician's commitment to a life of service by placing the patient's health-related interests ahead of the physician's self-interest. The second component is the concept of reciprocity, which proposes that the physician's acceptance of obligations toward the patient bestows reciprocal rights upon the physician: "As it is the duty of a physician to advise, so has he a right to be attentively and respectfully listened to."[4] In this case, the physician's right to be listened to entails a reasonable expectation that the patient will give due consideration to the added risk that his behavior poses to his health and to the effectiveness of the surgical intervention he seeks.

The authors of the original AMA Code of Ethics do not specify a physician's right to be obeyed, nor do they endorse terminating the physician-patient relationship when patients are noncompliant. Their argument for patient compliance is based in an appeal to prudence: the patient should calculate self-interest rationally and act accordingly by complying with a regimen of care that is reliably designed to protect and promote his health.

Patients are surely free to act imprudently. Assuming that this patient's tobacco and alcohol use are not refractory addictions, it is reasonable to conclude that he is indeed acting imprudently. Does this justify terminating the professional relationship with him? The answer to this question turns on the predicted effectiveness of the bypass procedure. The patient's global condition does not render surgery an intrinsically unacceptable risk. The bypass procedure can be successfully performed and therefore should not be understood to be anatomically or physiologically futile.[6]

The bypass procedure likely will provide him with some benefit, including pain control, in the short and intermediate term, though its long-term usefulness will be limited by his continued failure to follow medical advice. Thus, the short-term benefit is predictable, while the long-term risk of failure is conditional rather than certain, but long-term surgical benefits are always less predictable. If the requested operation is not assuredly futile, and does not otherwise violate surgical integrity, option (A) is not an appropriate response.

Option (B) appears to insufficiently appreciate the physiologically addicting properties of alcohol and tobacco, and the severe difficulty that even the best-intentioned individuals experience in terminating their use. Absent an absolute contraindication for surgery, insistence upon abstinence as a condition of care replaces clinical judgment with judgmental moralizing. Furthermore, this patient is experiencing profound chronic pain, which surgery can relieve well in advance of a lengthy substance abuse rehabilitation program. A better alternative would be to negotiate an agreement for the patient to begin an aggressive smoking cessation and alcoholism rehabilitation program in the immediate postoperative period, when the surgeon and team can help by controlling the patient's access to tobacco and alcohol.

Option (C) is based on an unfounded assumption that anything less than a scrupulously complete clinical regimen is of no value at all. The bypass procedure is not doomed to long-term failure, and will almost certainly have short-term advantages. Immediate amputation will obviously result in preventable, premature loss of major functional capacity, and is therefore ruled out.

Option (E) needlessly relieves you as the surgeon of responsibility for making a manageable decision. Referral to an ethics committee should occur when there is well-founded uncertainty about ethically acceptable alternatives, or when agreement between parties about the ethically appropriate course cannot be reached. Neither condition applies here. You should be able to organize your surgical thinking around principles of beneficence and patient autonomy to reach a clinically and ethically sound conclusion without consultation.

Option (D) is the preferable alternative. It acknowledges the limits of paternalism, honors the patient's autonomy, and seeks as much clinical benefit as the patient makes available, without insisting on the all-or-nothing approach. By making total compliance a condition of care, you would deprive the patient of the significant short- and mid-term benefits that the bypass procedure can provide. More than the surgeon, the patient is entitled to stipulate the conditions of care, provided those conditions do not completely neutralize the possibility of clinical benefit, render the risks of therapy greater than the possible benefits, or compromise your integrity as a surgeon. The surgeon must not interpret poor patient compliance as either a personal affront or as a challenge to the professional instinct to control a pathological process. Most importantly, you must not permit a sense of frustration to deprive the patient of those clinical benefits that can be achieved with or without the patient's full cooperation.

References

1. Rigotti NA, Singer DE, Mulley AG Jr, Thibault GE. Smoking cessation following admission to a coronary care unit. *J Gen Intern Med.* 1991; 6:305–311.
2. Bloom RJ, Stevick CA, and Lennon S, Patient perspectives on smoking and peripheral vascular disease. A veteran population Ethics of Operative Scheduling survey. *Am Surg.* 1990; 56:535–539.

3. Benjamin M., Lay obligations in professional relations. *J Med Philos*. 1985:10: 85–103.

4. American Medical Association. Code of Medical Ethics. Proceedings of the National Medical Convention 1846–1847: 83–106. Reprinted in: Baker RB, Emanuel L, Latham S, eds. *The American Medical Ethics Revolution: How the AMA's Code of Ethics Has Transformed Physicians' Relationships to Patients, Professionals, and Society*. Baltimore: Johns Hopkins University Press, 1999.

5. Giswold ME, Landry GT, Sexton GJ, Yeager RA, Edwards JM, Taylor LM, et al. Modifiable patient factors are associated with reverse vein graft occlusion in the era of duplex scan surveillance. *J Vasc Surg*. 2003; 37:47–53.

6. McCullough LB, Jones JW, Postoperative futility: A clinical algorithm for setting limits. *Br J Surg*. 2001; 88:1153–1154.

• CASE 20 •

The Ethics of Serving as a Plaintiff's Expert Medical Witness

The people's good is the highest law.
Cicero (106–43 BCE), De Legibus

Several years ago you developed and introduced a new surgical procedure, and are still considered the leading authority in its technical and theoretical application. At a recent national meeting, you were invited to discuss a paper on the procedure, and you criticized the authors' modifications as technical errors amounting to malpractice. Your unedited comments were published last month in the specialty's leading journal. Today you were called by an attorney representing a surgical patient who suffered chronic paralysis following the modified procedure which you predicted would increase the incidence of postoperative paraplegia. You have been sued twice in your career, with both claims dismissed without an award; you have otherwise assiduously avoided any involvement in litigation. The plaintiff's attorney asks you to serve as an expert witness against the surgeon in this case. What should you do?

(A) Refuse involvement.

(B) Explain that opinions expressed in your published critique represented intellectual jousting, not defensible scientific fact.

(C) Claim that you are too busy and decline to be involved.

(D) Agree to review the records objectively and be prepared to testify for the plaintiff.

(E) Testify and establish a Web page advertising your further availability as a plaintiff's witness.

With the advent of medical licensure in the 19th century, the medical profession has functioned within an explicit social contract which codified its ancient implicit one. In exchange for a monopoly over medical services, graduates of accredited schools of allopathic and osteopathic medicine, the only people eligible for independent medical licenses in the United States, have made assurance that the profession will regulate itself consistent with the public interest. This self-regulatory function is intended to maintain the quality of care by protecting patients from undertreatment, overtreatment, and mistreatment. Mistreatment caused by a physician's negligence, indifference, adventurism, or venal ambition, and resulting in harm to patients, is considered by the medical profession to constitute malpractice, and medical malpractice is considered by the legal profession to constitute a tort, or a wrongdoing for which compensatory damages may be sought.

No one in the medical profession likes medical malpractice actions. Physicians are properly troubled by what they see as a storm of frivolous claims, misplaced blame, disproportionate monetary awards, and vaulting insurance premiums. They believe that the medical tort system has ballooned costs, damaged the public's access to care, driven the medical profession nearer extinction, and impugned the good will and tormented the sleep of some of society's most talented, generous, and essential individuals. They are particularly aggrieved when insurers find settlement more expeditious than defense, leaving physicians with undeserved stains on their ability and integrity. Most blame trial lawyers for inflating awards, exaggerating patient pain and suffering, and ascribing malfeasance to every minor oversight or clinical misfortune. Nevertheless, in a profession overwhelmingly populated by highly intelligent, compulsively responsible, and vastly trained men and women, medical malpractice does occur, however rarely, and its results do palpable damage, not only to the immediately affected patients, but to every medical practitioner.

Some physicians believe that the damage done to the medical profession, and to individual professionals, by medical malpractice actions is so great that it vastly outweighs the consequences of the occasional instance of malpractice, and they disdain the entire tort process. Some highly prestigious professional medical societies covertly deny admission to any physician applicant who is reputed to have acted as a plaintiff's expert medical witness.

Should these hardened views prevail and medical experts withhold their knowledge and experience from the legal adversarial process as a display of professional solidarity, who then will fulfill medicine's obligation to self-regulate, and how will they do so? Internal hospital committees have an important role in reviewing and controlling poor practice, but their interests are inherently conflicted when findings of significant malfeasance reflect upon the institution as well as the guilty practitioner; nevertheless, this system represents a moderately well-functioning method of peer review. State medical boards, comprised of physicians, regulate qualifications for granting privileges well, but in actual practice withdraw many more licenses for infractions like substance abuse and sex with patients than for demonstrable malpractice. Most such boards are in fact too limited in their composition and activity levels to provide comprehensive oversight of the quality of care within their jurisdictions.

The wide remaining gaps are filled, likewise imperfectly, by the adversarial structure of the civil court system, which effectively encourages professional self-regulation by introducing opposite physician opinions of the same event. These obligations of the physician as citizen were recognized in the American Medical Association's Code of Ethics of 1847.[1]

Physicians commonly mistrust the legal system as an arbiter of medical disputes because attorneys and physicians use markedly different methods for resolving intellectual questions. The legal system utilizes an adversarial system, with advocates committing themselves in advance to opposing positions and presenting naive juries with selected evidence supporting their favored position. Physicians, conversely, engage scientific method to reach conclusions. They admit all possibilities, marshal all available evidence, challenge their own conclusions, and rule out individual explanations only when logical analysis so dictates. They specifically reject advocacy, and consider it a contaminant in the search for truth. The surgeon who rarely serves as an expert witness is more apt to maintain scientific objectivity and thereby influence the legal proceedings constructively. The Clinical Practice Subcommittee of the American College of Physicians warns against "small numbers of physicians spending disproportionate amounts of time testifying,"[2] as we often see today.

The surgical profession neglects an important element of its social responsibility if it utterly declines participation in this self-regulatory arena, or cedes to one or another opposing attorney, medical laymen, the opportunity to interpret medical information and judgment to a jury. Option (A) is therefore not ethically available; the quality of the medical tort system as an instrument of truth and justice can be only as good as the physicians who agree to participate in it. Protesting by declining participation will not stop the system from functioning, but it will make it more poorly informed and less just.

Option (B) reflects poorly upon your intellectual integrity and upon the system of professional meetings and journal publications we use to exchange information and expand our fund of scientific and clinical knowledge. If indeed your criticism of your procedure's modifications was merely a display of ego, and neither reliable nor useful to other surgeons, you are much to blame for having done so. If you have conjured this as an excuse to avoid testifying, you are now misrepresenting the important implications of your public and published statements, and are equally at fault.

Option (C), that you cannot spare time to defend a clinical improvement of your own devise against dangerous misuse, abandons your responsibility to the integrity of your important surgical advance, and to the patients whose suffering it may relieve. No one's interest is served by this posture, least of all your own.

Option (E), advertising your availability to plaintiffs' attorneys in future similar cases, creates the appearance of intentionally exploiting the misfortune associated with medical catastrophes to solicit fees for testimony. The ethical expert witness will provide the same testimony to either the plaintiff or the defendant. By limiting your availability to plaintiffs, you suggest a bias in your testimony that renders you unsuitable as an impartial expert professional.

Option (D), providing expert testimony on behalf of the patient consistent with your authoritative published opinions and after reviewing the case records, is the correct ethical course. It honors your responsibility to participate in the medical profession's self-regulation functions, insuring that medical judgments remain within the province of those competent to make them. You may help to protect future patients from similar injury, while articulating the medical profession's disapprobation of physicians who practice recklessly and despite the cautions of experts in their own specialty. As for the notion that expert testimony on behalf of a plaintiff betrays colleagues and weakens the medical profession, the process actually demonstrates how medicine places scientific truth and responsible treatment above the guild mentality of unquestioning self-protection. By confirming these ideals, we justify rather than diminish the public trust and the esteem in which our profession is widely held.

References

1. Baker RB, Emanuel L, Latham L. eds. *The American Medical Ethics Revolution: How the AMA's Code of Ethics Has Transformed Physicians' Relationships to Patients, Professionals, and Society.* Johns Hopkins University Press: Baltimore, 1999.
2. American College of Physicians. Guidelines for the physician expert witness. *Ann Intern Med.* 1990; 113:789.

• CASE 21 •

Standard of Care: What Does It Really Mean?

Injustice anywhere is a threat to justice everywhere.
Martin Luther King Jr.

As an expert witness testifying in a medical malpractice suit, you are asked if the defendant's performance fell below the standard of care. You are testifying on behalf of the defendant physician whom you supervised briefly during his residency. Your proper response requires reference to context, an understanding of complex physiologic relationships in the natural history of the disease, and an appreciation of the risks and benefits of therapy accessible to neither your attorney interrogator nor the laymen of the jury. A simple yes or no will not suffice. Under intensely pressured questioning by the plaintiff's attorney, you ask, "What exactly do you mean by the standard of care"? The judge interrupts. He makes it clear that the expert witnesses are expected to understand the meaning of their testimony and demands you "tell the court what you understand the standard of care to mean." Which of the following is your best response?

(A) Whatever the expert witnesses determine it to be. It can differ among different expert witnesses in the same trial or from the same witness in discussing different stages of care.

(B) Whichever expert's testimony the jury believes.

(C) In retrospect, whatever therapy would have resulted in the best clinical outcome.

(D) Whatever a majority of physicians would have done if faced with the same situation.

(E) It is complex, poorly understood by physicians, and has most value when unbiased expert witnesses define it by reference to evidence-based literature.

The legal and medical systems are superbly coherent intellectual constructs, theoretically. Problems with their application arise when physicians and attorneys whose thinking is less than perfectly coherent use the systems imperfectly. Oftentimes, the learned professionals, upon using them imperfectly, will claim the fault lies in the system. Despite some inevitable lapses, medicine and law provide society with the best available resources for resolving some of its most complex problems. The two disciplines directly confront one another in the medical tort arena.

The three legal criteria that must be satisfied for the plaintiff to be awarded damages are logical and direct but often manipulated. The patient must have (1) suffered compensable injuries or death as the (2) direct result of the defendant physician's treatment or failure to treat and, (3) in the provision of therapy, the physician's contractual professional responsibility was not met. The physician's contractual responsibility bears four implications: there must be a reasonable certainty that the patient will be clinically improved in some manner; the patient's best interests must be paramount; the surgeon must perform according to "the best in his power"; and the "best in his power" must have reached sufficiency[1]. Physicians gather, evaluate, introduce, and implement medical knowledge to clarify the patient's disease, injury, or disability and formulate therapeutic strategies. Because of biological variation, shortcomings in medical science, unanticipated correlates, and the huge volume of information needing to be considered, the practice of medicine is never fully mastered and there is always some risk that therapy can harm as well as heal. The conditions for malpractice come about when physician's decisions and actions depart significantly from those most other competent physicians would be likely to select and administer based on the amassed published experience of the profession. It follows that a practitioner who fails to maintain an adequate fund of current knowledge, practice conscientiously, or exceeds his or her abilities, then practices under conditions ripe for untoward patient consequences and redress within the tort system.

The critical legal benchmark in determining a failure to fulfill one's professional responsibility is the concept of the standard of care. The standard of care is breached whenever the physician fails to fulfill the minimal duty of care by failing to meet minimal levels of competence and to exercise minimal levels of judgment.[2] This concept, termed the "competence-based national standard of care," recognizes uniform requirements nationally for admissions to medical school, medical school curricula, residency training, and specialty boards. The quality of medical care proposed by this national standard should show minimal geographic variability with respect to such key components as the thoroughness of examinations, indicated laboratory tests ordered, consultations requested, therapy provided, and the promptness of administration of therapy. The resources-based caveat to the national standard slightly modifies its definition of the physician's duty to accommodate geographic variability in the availability of specialized medical facilities, services, and options as are "reasonably available".[2] A physician practicing without the availability of advanced radiological equipment cannot be expected to have promptly obtained a CT or MRI. However, there is no exemption for failing to refer to a more suitable facility or specialist when the patient's condition demands it. Thus, physician's practices are judged on the basis of his specialties' standards allowing for local variations in access to resources. The courts permit additional legal latitude in the respectable minority rule recognizing that science is not a democratic process nor is medicine unfailingly uniform. The appropriate therapy for a specific disease is not decided by majority vote, nor do majorities dictate the standard of care when equipoise exists; various standards of care can be reasonably established by several groups of competent physicians practicing independently of one another and not necessarily in a manner entirely consistent with the majority of practioners within a given specialty. Continual major scientific advances in clinical medicine historically have brought about many such situations.

That, however, is not the complete story. Several court cases have established that "should customary medical practice fail to keep pace with developments and advances in medical science, adherence to custom might constitute a failure to exercise ordinary care"[2]. Courts are beginning to hold physicians responsible for keeping up with the literature. The failure of the medical community and of individual physicians to adapt their practices in a timely fashion is no defense if substantial evidence supports the judgment that the prevailing practice should have changed. Particularly with the maturation of the digital age and its rapid dissemination of information, the standards of care are increasingly defined by the best available evidence rather than the local practice standard or the idiosyncratic opinions of expert witnesses. The world's medical literature is instantly available to anyone with a computer and a modicum of computer expertise.

The ethical expert medical witness understands that the standard of care should not be solely represented by the views of a particular well-compensated "expert" witness relative to their personal practice habits, although that is a common courtroom practice. Reading depositions of surgical "experts" taken under oath emphasizes the latitude in scientifically unsupported pronouncements currently flooding the courts. More to the point, standards of care are routinely interpreted oppositely by expert witnesses for the defense and plaintiff because counsel for both sides devotes considerable effort to screening and disqualifying consultant experts whose views do not represent the "standard" the attorney needs to make his case. The attorney is doing his job. The plethora of physician expert witnesses available to give programmed testimony is to the shame of the medical profession. The experts are expected to represent acceptable nationwide medical practice on the basis of their combined knowledge of their practice, the relevant evidence-based literature, from daily interactions with colleagues, and during participation at national professional meetings. The subjective elements of their testimony should be limited to an assessment of whether there was a significant variance from a well-known and established standard of care and whether clinical circumstances warranted the variance. Option (A) is therefore not an acceptable response, individually adjusting the standard of care for purposes of advocacy is grossly unethical with negative repercussions for patients and the profession alike.

Spencer noted these inherent system flaws when, "expert witnesses are actively pursued for their views, their presentation style, and their willingness to tailor their testimony according to the particular needs of the case".[3] Attorneys understand that the determination of malpractice is made neither by them nor by their experts; it is made by a lay jury weighing the credibility of medical experts for the plaintiffs and defendants who typically give contradictory testimonies. The most important characteristics of a medical expert for success in the courtroom, therefore, lies in his or her personal manner and believability. Sadly, option (B) is true in a practical sense but it exposes yet another theoretical fault of the legal system. It must be discarded as a choice for a definition of the standard of care. The medical expert who uses highly developed debating skills to convince jurors of a specious scientific opinion clearly is behaving unethically.

If option (C) were correct, more than half of the complications plaguing the practice of medicine would be classified legitimately as malpractice. Every surgeon who has attended a D&C conference has heard that "the retrospectoscope is always 100% accurate." Knowing the outcome and its effect on retrospective reasoning is termed hindsight bias; it enables the evaluator to connect the causal dots for a now-completed effect. Hindsight bias is likely to result in hypercritical reviews because clinical error is expected and searched for when the evaluator knows from the start that there has been a bad clinical outcome. Criticisms of physician reviewers of identical medical case histories varied significantly depending on what the clinician evaluators were told about the outcomes.[4] A subsequent study showed that the more experienced surgeons were the least influenced by hindsight bias, suggesting that this group would provide the most reliable and consistent expert testimony.[5] Surgeons need only remember the last spirited D&C conference they attended for a personal verification of the phenomenon. Hindsight bias influences case review with bad outcomes negatively. Accordingly, Hugh recommends that outcomes be omitted from expert's review material until after they declare their opinion of the care.[6]

Although conventional medical wisdom is usually correct, option (D) is not acceptable, as noted earlier scientific medial practice is not a democratic process; judgments grounded in evidence-based medicine are not made authoritative by majority opinion. Advances in medicine have often spent years in the obscurity of minority opinion.

Option (E) should guide the surgeon-witness in this case. The concept of the standard of care covers the range of clinical judgments, supported by the best available evidence at the time of the case. That evidence and the judgment derived from it, must strongly indicate that the procedure or other form of clinical management in question was reliably expected (1) to be life-saving or to prevent serious or irreversible disease, injury, or handicap to the patient, and (2) to involve manageable and acceptable risks that the surgeon took appropriate measures to minimize.[7]

The standard of care concept is currently embodied by physicians as a discredited legal term that has been long ignored by the medical profession. It is nevertheless at the center of medicine's opportunity to improve and formulate a sustained preventive ethics response to the professional liability crisis. Reliable judgments about what should be considered a standard of care are not adversarial; they are scientific and should be guided by the standards of high-quality

evidence-based medicine prevailing at the time the case occurred. Such judgments should be based on then-available high quality, evidence-based disease
management protocols and other clinical guidelines as well as rigorous review
of then-current peer-reviewed literature which categorically requires an unbiased expert witness. The American Association for the Advancement of Science offers independent experts to the courts to fix the meretricious testimony
of mercenary experts.[8] The federal courts have begun to accept this approach,
with the creation of "science panels" for expert testimony.[9] Physicians should
take the lead in advocating a similar approach in medical malpractice cases.
Thereby eliminating a great deal of the injustice to which both plaintiffs and
defendants are subjected by the existing system.

References

1. Cook, J., The delegation of surgical responsibility. *J Med Ethics*, 1980. 6:68–70.
2. Furrow, B., et al., *Health Law: Cases, Materials, and Problems*. 4th ed. 2001, St. Paul, MN: West Group.
3. Spencer, F.C. and K.S. Guice, The expert medical witness: concerns, limits, and remedies. *Bull Am Coll Surg*, 2000. 85:22–23.
4. Dawson, N, Arkos B, Sicilano C, Blinkdorn R, Laksman, C, Hindsight bias: an impediment to accurate probability estimation in clinicopathologic conferences. *Med Decis Making*, 1989. 8:259–264.
5. Herwig, R., C. Fangelow, and U. Hofferage, Hindsight bias: How Knowledge and Heuristics Affect Our Reconstruction of the Past. *Memory*, 2003. 11:357–377.
6. Hugh, T.B. and G.D. Tracy, Hindsight bias in medicolegal expert reports. *Med J Aust*, 2002. 176:277–278.
7. Chervenak, F.A. and L.B. McCullough, A comprehensive ethical framework for fetal research and its application to fetal surgery for spina bifida. *Am J Obstet Gynecol*, 2002. 187:10–14.
8. Brickley, P., Science v. law. A decade-old rule on scientific evidence comes under fire. *Sci Am*, 2003. 289:30–32.
9. Price, J.M. and E.S. Rosenberg, The war against junk science: the use of expert panels in complex medical-legal scientific litigation. *Biomaterials*, 1998. 19: 1425–1432.

INNOVATION AND RESEARCH

Surgery is perhaps the truest melding in any of the medical specialties of the objectivity of science and the subjectivity of art. Biological variability, and anatomical surprises, can make surgical art more important than surgical science in many cases. An individual "routine" for complex procedures is comprised of a complex series of individually developed algorithms. Surgical residents learn our craft by observing and repeating the techniques of the attending surgeons who teach them, but even before training is completed they will invariably begin to personalize the style of their procedures.

Operative skill subsets, known as maneuvers, are individually learned, sometimes through serendipitous intraoperative misadventure; when things don't go according to plan, surgeons must find a way to get them back on track. Failure is not considered an option in the OR. These urgent innovations, if successful and published, can become new operative standards. Surgeons perform only five basic tasks at the operating table—they excise, they connect or disconnect, they bypass, they remodel, or they replace—but to complete each of these objectives dozens if not hundreds of maneuvers must be done in proper sequence. The operative objective is the scientific plan, whereas the maneuvers to achieve it are individually determined. The oxymoron "controlled variation" describes the process well.

The objective of the Continuous Quality Improvement (CQI) methods introduced to industry by W. Edwards Deming (1900–1993) following World War II was quality control by eliminating unnecessary, especially uncontrolled, variation. Deming taught the postwar Japanese auto industry that the best-produced cars are made without variation. Once a product standard is established, variances from the standard constitute defects.

CQI techniques have since been adapted to the practice of medicine, forever changing the way medicine, especially surgery, is practiced. Total elimination of variance cannot be achieved in medicine. Moreover, excessive elimination of variance can become regimentation and eliminate the innovations that sometimes salvage operations and lead to important clinical advances. The goal in medicine is to progressively reduce those variations that do not improve outcomes. This CQI effort is being made through programs that have become institutionalized as clinical pathways, huge surgical databases that monitoring millions of operations, tracking and aligning hospital reimbursements, surgeons, and surgical outcomes with new standards of quality, termed pay-for-performance (P4P).[1,2] Although the prestigious Institute of Medicine has reservations about whether P4P will improve or worsen care,[1] methods of incentivizing physician behavior are currently popular and can be ethically supported if properly constructed.[2]

The moral conflict came to light when a perceived need for procedural uniformity, expansion of research oversight, and an increasing need for complete disclosure confronted traditional surgical autonomy.[3,4] The performance latitude at the heart of surgical autonomy is a continuum, accruing new standards and moral obligations as essential surgical innovation sometimes drifts into the realm of experimentation, then into research, and can eventually cross the line into reckless endangerment. The borders between these four conditions are recognizable, and the ethical duties once a border is crossed are clear. The practicing surgeon should be certain of the variable moral topography in daily practice, and the special responsibilities associated with each set of behaviors. As general rule, moral responsibility increases as the predictability of an action decreases.

The surgeon autonomously selects and discontinues preoperative medications, prophylactic antibiotics, and prep solutions, decides when to transfuse, where and how to make incisions and anastomoses, and which suture to use and how to tie it. Rational therapeutic decisions that don't alter the outcome and that don't violate established principles belong to the individual surgeon. The authors of descriptive text in every atlas of surgical procedures testify to the ubiquity of surgical individualism in regularly repeated captions reminding readers that the method described is "How I do this." These are judgments made on the basis of each patient's condition, operative indications, and the surgeon's personal experience and preferences for materials that are familiar and reliable.

When treatment proceeds entirely as anticipated, such idiosyncrasies are well within the range of normal variation seen in every practice. Neither individuality nor autonomy is a problem in and of itself while the surgeon is using materials and techniques that will afford his or her patient a highly predictable outcome. The decision-making authority to implement innovations, understood as adjustments in existing norms, is granted to the surgeon by society and by the patient. The authority is based substantially upon the understanding that the surgeon has completed a course of accredited training, accumulated experience in similar situations, and is well-prepared to make decisions likely to achieve a favorable outcome. The patient's written consent generally confers wide discretionary latitude with the common addendum, "and all other necessary procedures." The precise width of this latitude can be discerned by evaluating distinctions between innovation and experimentation.

Although surgical innovation is entirely discretionary, experimentation requires a more demanding set of ethical standards, because the outcome is not predictable. Experimentation requires prior informed consent, if possible, or subsequent transparent disclosure if prospective permission is not possible. Experimentation generally arises from the necessity of managing unanticipated events, early in the learning curve of new procedures or technologies, or when treating rare diseases that have no standardized therapy.

Radical intraoperative innovations should be limited to unforeseen circumstances when an unplanned or untested measure is considered necessary to resolution of an individual emergency or to correct a life-threatening misadventure. From time to time, a more seriously diseased aorta or more extensive spread of a neoplasm may be found unexpectedly during a procedure, altering the operative procedure and the preoperative estimates of mortality and morbidity. The preoperative informed consent no longer covers what needs to be done, but the surgeon's authority to proceed in the indicated but radically different direction is vital to the patient's recovery. Though revised consent of the anesthetized patient's surrogate may be properly sought before proceeding if time allows, the surgeon is mandated to make those adjustments that will most benefit the individual patient. If conditions have altered so the surgeon can no longer reliably predict the outcome of therapy, innovation becomes experimentation. The surgeon is obligated to inform the patient or surrogate at an appropriate subsequent time about what modifications have been added to the operation and whether the preoperative prognosis has changed.

Incremental changes in how a routine procedure is performed may be stimulated by reading the literature or conferring with colleagues. A small improvement in a conventional procedure as part of a rational evolutionary process is typically well within the bounds of acceptable clinical innovation. This may involve a variation in technique, but not a departure from the fundamental concepts of the procedure.[5] The skills developed versus skills required to perform an operation can demarcate the appropriate clinical boundaries between innovation and experimentation. New technologies require that even the most technically experienced surgeon submit to additional formal training. There is, inevitably, a learning curve in most cases, and with an identifiable learning curve, by definition, the surgeon learns new skills at the expense of early patients. As the surgeon seeks intellectual and technical familiarity with a new application that promises to improve care, existing standards must be maintained, and the patient must not be unknowingly placed at increased risk. Experimentation is taking place when an individual practitioner has insufficient data and/or experience to reliably predict the outcome of a procedure.[6,7] This means that the surgeon who fails to remain current with the available evidence-based scientific literature could be in a continual state of experimentation. This obviously places the quality of his care in jeopardy and increases the clinical risk to his or her patients. Hallmarks of the worst technical surgical surgeons are their *du jour* operative routines.

Intention and motivation denote the boundary between unshackled innovation and research, which requires significant limitations of surgical autonomy. Research alters the physician's basic therapeutic relationship with the patient. The outcome of the proposed care becomes unpredictable, raising the risk to the patient, and the fully informed patient must voluntarily embrace that unknown risk. Most important, because the randomization process and not the physician decides which of several therapies the patient will receive, the Institutional Review Board (IRB) assumes the role of patient fiduciary normally filled by the surgeon in clinical care.

The federal research regulations published by the National Institutes of Health, known as the "Common Rule," defines research as "a systematic investigation, including research development, testing and evaluation, designed to develop or contribute to generalizable knowledge."[8] Clinical innovation thus becomes research when an intervention is undertaken in conformity with development of a scientific protocol intended to widen the body of medical knowledge and put it into general application. As a clinical endeavor becomes research when conducted within a systematic effort to acquire knowledge, regulations require a detailed advance written plan, conformity with scientific method, approval by an IRB, and the patient's informed consent for research participation. The conduct of clinical research imposes behavioral obligations upon the surgeon. The surgeon engaging in research may not do so autonomously; he or she agrees to professional oversight, concurrence, critical outcome analysis, and restricted discretionary authority.

The conduct of research, therefore, entitles the patient to special protections not normally associated with individual variations in the judgment or procedural techniques of the autonomous surgeon. Tonelli concluded that the different nature of the informed consent can provide a test of whether a new treatment is experimental.[9] The consent process in conventional treatment includes a discussion of what is known, but in experimental treatment the discussion must concentrate upon what is not known. When uncertainty of outcome enters the informed consent process, the consent document and the surgeon's verbal explanation to patients must emphasize, above all else, this uncertainty and enthusiasm about the potential benefits to patient of study participation must be tightly controlled. The surgeon may legitimately recruit an appropriate patient for study enrollment, but he cannot aggressively sell enrollment to a reluctant patient.

Before beginning research, the surgeon must evaluate whether the question addressed is important enough, whether patient risks are minimized, whether prior data has been adequately studied, and whether the scientific methodology is sound. It is ethically and scientifically egregious to place patients at risk and to expend the extraordinary effort and expense research requires, only to acquire faulty data that will be of no use in advancing the practice of surgery. Information given the patient should be specific to the institution and surgeon. It is not sufficient in these circumstances to cite the number of such procedures other surgeons have done, or how they turned out. The patient should be informed of the number of these experimental research procedures done by the attending surgeon and his or her associated morbidity and mortality rates.

Innovation, experimentation, or research becomes reckless experimentation when therapeutic choice enters unknown territory without a well-established scientific foundation or without an adequate experiential basis. Taking unwarranted risks with the life and health of patients is always unethical.

By understanding and observing obligations in the variations required of surgical practice, the surgeon loses no legitimate autonomy and gains certainty about how to proceed with an ethical and more satisfying professionalism.

References

1. Institute of Medicine recommends new P4P system for Medicare. *Healthcare Benchmarks Qual Improv.* 2006; 13:133–137.
2. Jones JW, McCullough LB. Quality credentialing: Boon or boondoggle? *J Vasc Surg.* 2006; 43:1073–1075.
3. Michel LA. Evidence-based medicine, cost-containment, care effectiveness: Is it a new trilogy aimed at transforming the surgical mystique or the reality of double standards? *Acta Chir Belg.* 2001; 101:95–100.
4. Reitsma AM, Moreno JD. Ethical regulations for innovative surgery: the last frontier? *J Am Coll Surg.* 2002; 194:792–801.
5. Jones JW, McCullough LB. A surgeon's obligations when performing new procedures. *J Vasc Surg.* 2002; 35:409–410.
6. Jones JW. Ethics of rapid surgical technological advancement. *Ann Thorac Surg.* 2000; 69:676–677.
7. Jones JW. The surgeon's autonomy: Defining limits in therapeutic decision making. In: Reitsma M, Moreno J, eds. *Ethical Guidelines for Innovative Surgery.* Hagerstown, Md: University Publishing Group, 2006.
8. National Institutes of Health: Regulations and Ethical Guidelines. Title 45 Public Welfare, 2005.
9. Tonelli MR, Benditt JO, Albert RK. Clinical experimentation: Lessons from lung volume reduction surgery. *Chest.* 1996; 110:230–238.

• CASE 22 •

When Does Conventional Surgical Therapy Become Research?

Shun those studies in which the work that results dies with the worker.
Leonardo da Vinci (1452–1519)

A surgeon arranges with operating room nurses to alternate use of two FDA–approved and marketed implantable devices on odd and even operating days. This arrangement requires which of the following?

(A) No local review or patient consent, because both devices are FDA-approved and marketed.

(B) Institutional Review Board (IRB) approval and the informed consent of patients.

(C) Only the informed consent of participating patients.

(D) IRB approval, but not the informed consent of patients.

(E) IRB approval only if publication of results is intended.

Some ethical constructs, particularly those involving informed consent and the conduct of research, have been so uniformly accepted as essential to the rights of patients and the integrity of scientific method that they have been codified into federal regulatory law. Laws and medical ethics affecting research and patient consent are not limited to "investigational" compounds and devices. Although both devices proposed for use in our operating room scenario are approved for clinical care, the responsible clinician's selection of the best product with which to treat each patient would normally be based upon individual patient assessment, specific indications, and anticipated outcomes. The patients in our scenario will receive one or the other device based solely upon whether they come in on odd or even days, without regard to their unique characteristics and indications. The alternating assignment schedule is designed to serve the surgeon's research interests rather than the patient's clinical interests.

When the selection process for a medication, graft, or implant is randomized or preassigned, when the choice is not primarily governed by the patient's individual clinical characteristics, and when the clinical outcome cannot be predicted, the procedure must be considered clinical research rather than clinical care, and the laws and ethical considerations affecting research become applicable. The surgeon must modify his own behavior accordingly, and observe the legal and ethical conventions that ensure the integrity of scientific data and the safety of research subjects. The surgeon's plan to alternate use of the first and second devices is clearly intended to systematically collect data about the comparative performance of the two devices rather than to maximize the immediate benefit to each patient. The question of which device will provide the better clinical outcome is the subject of the research, to be answered by application of scientific method and statistical analysis of the resultant data. Option (A), proceeding with neither the patient's informed consent to participate in research nor approval of a scientific protocol by the IRB, is therefore neither ethically nor legally acceptable.

Option (C), proceeding with only the patient's informed consent, is appropriate to the conduct of routine clinical care, but not clinical research. Surgeons are permitted wide latitude in developing innovative operative techniques and typically function in a continuous quality improvement mode.[1] Structured investigative plans require the prior peer review and approval of IRBs to evaluate the scientific integrity of the study design and ensure satisfactory protection of human subjects. Similarly, option (D), IRB approval without the patient's specific understanding and consent that he is to participate in a scientific study, is not sufficient to meet the legal and ethical requirements for the conduct of research. In neither case is the requirement mitigated by the earlier FDA approval of the grafts to be studied. There are increasing concerns about the adequacy of the informed consent process in addressing whether patients understand that they are in a research rather than a therapeutic setting, that the physician's interest in adhering to the protocol could conflict with the patient's health-related interest, and that random group assignment is not influenced by the patient's specific clinical indications.[2] These potential misunderstandings must be specifically addressed during the informed consent process, particularly when such elements as FDA approval and market status may confuse the layman's understanding of whether the procedure is or is not investigative and subject to the special rules governing clinical research.

Option (E) erroneously associates the definition of research with publication or intent to publish. The results of much research remain unpublished for any number of reasons. Although patients have a legitimate concern that their privacy be maintained when research results are published, this is not the only risk to which they are subjected when they participate in clinical research. The requirement for prior IRB approval is in no way contingent upon whether or not study findings are ultimately published, as the potential risk to patients which IRBs attempt to minimize are not associated with the subsequent fate of study results.

Option (B), obtaining each patient's written informed consent for participation after the study plan is reviewed and approved by the local IRB for scientific integrity and effective patient protections, satisfies legal and ethical requirements for the conduct of clinical research.

References

1. Jones JW. Ethics of rapid surgical technological advancement. *Ann Thorac Surg.* 2000; 69:676–677.
2. Edward SJL, Lilford RJ, Braunholtz DA, Jackson JC, Hewison J, Thornton J. Ethical issues in the design and conduct of randomized controlled trials. *Health Technol Assess.* 1998; 15:1–132.

• CASE 23 •

A Surgeon's Obligations When Performing New Procedures

It is impossible for anyone to begin to learn what he already thinks he knows.
Epictetus (c. 55 AD–c. 135 AD)

A junior member of the surgery faculty has done two robotic total colectomies. Although he attended a standard 2-day training course conducted by the instrument manufacturer, performed several similar procedures in the animal laboratory, and read all the recent pertinent literature, technical errors resulted in significant morbidity in his first two patients. He proposes to use the technique once again on a hospitalized patient. His troubled chairman has called you for an opinion on whether an ethical question has now arisen. There are no specific credentialing standards for robotic surgery at this institution. Where might we most expect to see an ethical problem in the surgeon's management of the new case?

(A) In the level of training for robotic surgery.

(B) In the selection of patients.

(C) In the level of assistance sought from more experienced surgeons.

(D) In compliance with credentialing and Institutional Review Board (IRB) requirements.

(E) In disclosure to the prospective patient.

Since we embarked upon the new millennium and in the years just prior, the rapidity with which complex new technology has been introduced to surgery has surpassed the ability of the profession to validate it with evidence of safety and long-term effectiveness, before its widespread adoption. Trying to keep surgeons current with new advances in the profession, instruction courses in the operation of new technology are offered by most of our professional societies, many medical centers, and almost all medical device companies. A surgical profession without continuously evolving therapies would devolve to the age of Galen, and is unimaginable in the 21st century, but not every foray into unexplored ground represents an improvement in care.

Option (A) implies skepticism about the adequacy of the brief manufacturer-provided courses typically used to introduce surgeons to new technology. Surgeons and trainers alike usually find that these concentrated sessions provide sufficient hands-on experience with novel instrumentation. This training method has been generally successful and is widely accepted by the profession as effective and ethical. Group acceptance does not always mean adequacy, however, and this is a process that should receive more professional scrutiny than it does.

Option (C), concerning operative assistance, is related to option (A) in the sense that most manufacturers of surgical high technology will send a surgeon with extensive experience in using the new equipment to assist, and continue training, in the operating room during a surgeon's first few procedures with a new method. There is no evidence that our surgeon rejected available help. Nothing in the data we have here suggests that our surgeon, however young, has not selected patients with the proper indications for the colectomy procedures, eliminating option (B) from our areas of most concern.

Option (D), respecting credentialing and IRB authorizations, approaches a more difficult realm. With no specific criteria for the conduct of robotic surgery (or likely many other new procedures) included in the medical center's credentialing process, the usual "full privilege" designation permits the procedure. Centers using this blanket privileging terminology are skirting their oversight responsibility. There is a potential ethical breach here, but it resides with the institution, not the surgeon. Because this robotic procedure is not part of a structured research protocol, it will not normally be subject to IRB oversight, but a question arises about whether our case does in fact constitute experimentation. Innovation is sanctioned by the profession and society at large, which permits surgeons to make choices based upon clinical judgment. These choices include everyday decisions about prophylactic antibiotics and which incision to make. Innovation becomes experimentation when the outcome cannot be reliably predicted. This is the case when a surgeon uses a complex new technology requiring new surgical skills and knowledge or when a surgeon attempts a procedure he has never done before. The distinction changes the surgeon's obligations toward his patient regarding informed consent. Valid concerns that new surgical procedures are inadequately monitored have been articulated for many years.[2] Innovations may be required unexpectedly to meet intraoperative exigencies, but patients must be informed if they are to become participants in planned experimentation. Our surgeon has not done enough robotic-assisted colectomies to develop a statistical outcome profile. His results can therefore not be reliably predicted, the hallmark of experimentation. Difficult as such disclosure is likely to be for him in recruiting patients for the robotic surgery given his brief and not entirely successful experience with it, he should specifically disclose his previous results to each patient whom he proposes to operate upon with this method until he can be confident of expectations.

Option (E), the adequacy of patient disclosure, therefore presents itself as the area of greatest concern in this scenario. The ethical surgeon will not oversell the potential benefits of a new procedure while omitting what the patient most needs for informed consent—knowledge that the surgeon has very limited experience in the procedure and a high morbidity rate. The literature confirms that fully experienced surgeons have a learning curve when even slightly different skill sets are needed, increasing the likelihood that early patients will not realize the same quality of results as those treated after more experience has been gained. Until a favorable surgical outcome can be realistically anticipated, the learning period is effectively experimental. For it to be warranted, there must be the prospect of knowledge to be gained and adequate assurance that standards of care are maintained.

References

1. Jones JW. Ethics of rapid surgical technological advancement. *Ann Thorac Surg.* 2000; 69:676–677.
2. Spodick DH. Numerators without denominators: There is no FDA for the surgeon. *JAMA.* 1975; 232:35–36.
3. Lytle BW, Cosgrove DM, Loop FD, et al. Perioperative risk of bilateral internal mammary artery grafting: Analysis of 500 cases from 1971 to 1984. *Circulation.* 1986; 74: 11137–11141.

· CASE 24 ·

The Ethics of Innovative Surgical Approaches for Well-Established Procedures

To him who devotes his life to science ... his cup of joy is full when the results of his studies immediately find practical applications.
Louis Pasteur (1822–1895)

A surgeon with extensive experience in minimally invasive robotic procedures plans to use the robotic apparatus to treat a large splenic artery aneurysm. The patient is thin but otherwise in good health, and welcomes the prospect of less scarring, faster recovery time, and less pain and suffering than he might experience with the standard open procedure. He is furthermore eager to be among the first to receive this innovative operation. What special ethical obligations might the surgeon have when replacing a well-established operation with a new technological approach?

(A) He should provide an especially detailed description of the operation during the informed consent process, stressing that he has not used the robotic device to treat this condition before.

(B) He should observe the provisions of option (A), and send a note to the chief of surgery about his intentions.

(C) He should observe the provisions of option (A), and ask the chief of surgery to convene an ad hoc committee to consider a formal written plan of the proposed operation.

(D) He should provide the patient a generalized description of the operation he is planning. Technical details that could confuse or agitate the patient should be avoided.

(E) He should obtain prior approval from his institutional review board (IRB) and ethics committee.

A busier surgeon is a more efficient surgeon. Repetitive experiences are essential to the refinement of surgical skills; intellectual and technical mastery are accumulated during repeated performances. Even in the best hands, optimization of results awaits sufficient experience, or ascension of the surgeon's learning curve, while he refines new skills at the expense of early patients. In an analysis of 25,777 minimally invasive operations, surgeons further along in their laparoscopic experience had significantly shorter operating time, lower conversion and complication rates, and their patients had shorter postoperative hospital stays than surgeons who were early in their laparoscopic experience.[1] The learning curve is necessarily at its lowest point when any important element of the procedure is being performed for the first time. Although the learning curve is an unavoidable influence upon the surgical risk/benefit ratio, the profession and the individual surgeon are confronted with the potentially conflicting imperatives of ensuring that high standards of care be maintained early and late in the experiential process; that no patient is placed at increased risk, particularly unknowingly; and that the novel procedure is selected because it offers some special benefit to the patient, not just an opportunity for the surgeon to exercise his adventurous spirit or pad his case series.

The surgeon's autonomy should be regulated in direct proportion to the degree to which the outcome of elective surgery is uncertain.[2] When positive outcomes are effectively certain, the surgeon may select techniques, instruments, materials, and even procedural approaches from a standard armamentarium without prior peer review or other permission beyond the patient's standard procedural informed consent for operative care, and without explaining such details. These decisions are based on each patient's condition, indications, and the surgeon's preference for the familiar and routinely reliable medications and materials of prior experience. The patient provides informed consent for surgical treatment of a designated condition. If the procedural method is unusual, as with new applications of robotic minimally invasive surgery, then it, too, is likely to be specified in the written consent narrative, with special risks and benefits so designated.

When emergencies, additional pathology, or other unanticipated intraoperative findings or events require interventions not described during the informed consent process, the surgeon is compelled to autonomously proceed on the clinically indicated course. Of course, the surgeon is ethically obligated to subsequently explain his intraoperative case management to the patient or surrogate, including significant errors and complications, as well as the postoperative plan of care. Although untried methods may be employed to manage such exigencies, they are within the bounds of ethical clinical care.

Tailoring surgical therapy to a case involving a rare condition for which there is no standard treatment must be viewed as experimental, particularly because the outcome is unpredictable. Nevertheless, its intent is clinical rather than scientific, since it is unlikely that the condition will again be encountered and there is no intent to develop a systematic body of data from which to make scientific extrapolations.[3]

Treating a single unique patient may or may not entail greater risks than treating patients with common diseases, but the former will never constitute a learning curve. Surgical autonomy in clinical therapy of these very rare diseases is therefore limited only to the constraints inherent in the informed consent process. Clinical research clearly limits the surgeon's autonomy and imposes additional ethical and legal obligations. To ensure the scientific integrity of the research, as well as the safety of patients who become research subjects, the surgeon-investigator is ethically and legally obligated to seek and accept professional oversight, concurrence, critical outcome analysis, and restricted discretionary authority. The "Common Rule," the federal regulation that governs human subjects research, defines research as "a systematic investigation, including research development, testing and evaluation, designed to develop or contribute to generalizable knowledge."[4] Clinical innovation thus becomes research when an intervention is undertaken in conformity with a scientific protocol intended to widen the body of medical knowledge and put it into general application. As a clinical endeavor becomes research, conducted within a systematic effort to acquire knowledge, regulations require a detailed advance written plan, conformity with scientific method, approval by an IRB, and the patient's detailed informed consent for research participation. Our innovating surgeon is planning to transform a standard operation into an experimental one by radically revising its methodology. Because he has not performed this particular robotic operation before, the outcome is unpredictable and potentially bad. If successful, the operation may be reported in the literature, repeated by this or other surgeons, or become recognized as one of a small series of minimally invasive splenic artery resections.

The procedure, nevertheless, does not meet standard definitions of research for which advance approval by an IRB is required. This is not a controlled study with a standardized protocol, and an enrollment yielding statistically significant conclusions cannot reasonably be planned at this time; this case will have to be approached as individual clinical therapy.

Ineligibility for IRB review as a structured scientific study eliminates option (E) as an ethical guide, but the proposed procedure remains an elective experimental innovation. It may be argued that application of the minimally invasive technique to a standard procedure merely merges two established approaches and should therefore be considered neither experimental nor especially risk-laden. This view would make option (D) entirely satisfactory to fulfill the surgeon's ethical obligations, but it fails because it obscures the substantial distinctions that still exist between this robotic minimally invasive surgery and other more extensively used and refined laparoscopic techniques. The first proponents of laparoscopic cholecystectomy used similar arguments to minimize the difficulties of learning the distinctly different surgical skills required by the new method, and a clinical fiasco ensued. Surgeons who had long ago mastered open cholecystectomies were encouraged to embrace the new technology before they were adequately trained in it, and the increased rates of bile duct injuries inflicted on early patients were cruel reminders of the unforgiving principles of the learning curve. Robotic surgery shares some terminology and some techniques with the better-established laparoscopic operations, but its routine mastery within the profession is still years in the future, particularly for yet untried applications. The responsible use of the robotic equipment requires extensive training and repetitive practice under experienced guidance and well-controlled conditions.

As the most procedurally oriented of the medical specialties, surgery has been the most affected by a profession-wide laxity in defining the characteristics distinguishing new clinical therapies and structured scientific research. Major advances in surgical methodology have seldom been produced by the sort of carefully designed, large-sample, random assignment, double blind, placebo-controlled studies with which new drugs are routinely tested for safety and efficacy in advance of general availability. New operative techniques have historically had little or no regulation.[5] Many of the major advances in surgery have been the products of serendipity or desperate measures, and the slow deliberative scientific process which works well in drug trials is simply a poor fit in surgery.

McKneally and Daar have concluded that this mismatch suggests the need for a new paradigm to protect scientific integrity, the surgical professions, and surgical patients.[6] Experimental innovation in surgery that does not meet the other specialties' criteria for controlled research should nonetheless be answerable to the same ethical obligations and procedural safeguards accepted by our nonsurgical colleagues.

Option (A) is a good start and would suffice if the procedure were a single event never to be repeated. Option (B) adds the notification of a nominally controlling authority, but neither closely describes the proposed event nor invites critical evaluation of its many causes for concern. Option (D) describes what we fear is the current practice, giving patients little indication of their status as experimental subjects, which they most certainly are.

Option (C) proposes a method of thoughtful oversight that has not heretofore been widely applied in surgery. It meets the needs of the profession as an intermediary between complete absence of peer review and the IRB's traditional role as arbiter of studies with clearly delineated hypotheses, large samples of homogeneous subjects, and rigorously standardized procedures. It provides the patient with all the normal protections of the informed consent process, and supports them with a written plan to delimit the boundaries of the intervention. Furthermore, it adds the expert evaluative functions otherwise met by an IRB to ensure the proposal's medical and scientific plausibility, the adequacy of patient safeguards, and the legitimacy of its clinical rationale. The review by actual peers facilitates the surgeon's goal of providing good care, while fulfilling the surgical profession's ultimate ethical duty to protect the patients entrusted to its care. Requiring a formal review of peers before embarking on an experimental procedure necessitates a review of the literature. If our surgeon were to research the subject, he would find reports of splenic artery aneurysms being treated with minimally invasive techniques both by exclusion and resection.[7-9]

References

1. Dagash H, Chowdhury M, Pierro A. When can I be proficient in laparoscopic surgery? A systematic review of the evidence. *J Pediatr Surg*. 2003; 38:720–724.
2. Jones JW. Ethics of rapid surgical technological advancement. *Ann Thorac Surg*. 2000; 69:676–677.
3. Jones JW, McCullough LB, Richman BW. Ethics of surgical innovation to treat rare diseases. *J Vasc Surg*. 2004; 39:918–919.

4. Shelton J, Working Group of the Human Subjects Research Subcommittee of the National Science and Technology council. How to interpret the federal policy for the protection of human subjects or "Common Rule" (Part A). *IRB*. 1999; 21:6–9.
5. Reitsma AM, Moreno JD. Ethical regulations for innovative surgery: The last frontier? *J Am Coll Surg*. 2002; 194:792–801.
6. McKneally MF, Daar AS. Introducing new technologies: protecting subjects of surgical innovation and research. *World J Surg*. 2003; 27:930–934; discussion 934–5.
7. Watanabe Y, Sato M, Abe Y, Ueda S, Yamamoto T, Horiuchi A, et al. Three-dimensional arterial computed tomography and laparoscope-assisted splenectomy as a minimally invasive examination and treatment of splenic aneurysms. *J Laparoendosc Adv Surg Tech A*. 1997; 7:183–186.
8. Adham M, Blanc P, Douek P, Henri L, Ducerf C, Baulieux J. Laparoscopic resection of a proximal splenic artery aneurysm. *Surg Endosc*. 2000; 14:372.
9. Muscari F, Bossary JP, Chaufour X, Ghouti L, Barret A. Laparoscopic exclusion of a splenic artery aneurysm—a case report. *Vasc Endovasc Surg*. 2003; 37:297–300.

• CASE 25 •

Using Surgical Innovation to Treat Rare Diseases

Nothing is so conducive to greatness of mind as the ability to examine systematically and honestly everything that meets us in life.
Marcus Aurelius (121 AD–180 AD), *Meditations*

A gynecologist has referred you a 50-year-old woman with extensive intravenous leiomyomatosis. A tissue diagnosis of invasive low-grade malignancy is available, and the tumor extends into the renal and hepatic veins. You propose removing the tumor by hysterectomy, to be combined if necessary with an extensive venectomy. The patient has had multiple vascular procedures which have exhausted all her available autologous graft material. You will try to excise the tumor through a venotomy, but it is likely that reconstruction will require venous replacement with prosthetic material, for which you have chosen externally supported polytetrafluoroethylene. What is the ethical course of action?

(A) Initiate an especially detailed informed consent process, stressing the uncertainties and increased risks of such an operation.

(B) Advise the patient that the prognosis is not good, but there is no other choice.

(C) Provide a generalized description of what you propose. Technical details that may upset the patient are not necessary.

(D) Obtain informed consent and apply to the institutional review board (IRB) for approval of an experimental procedure.

(E) Obtain informed consent and IRB approval, and consult with the ethics committee.

Since ancient times, surgeons have individualized therapy to one degree or another without seeking supervision or prior approval by third parties. Past murmurings about excessive surgical autonomy, however, have culminated in recent calls for regulation of "significant" innovations.[1,2] Surgeons exercise autonomous judgment when they select, titrate, or discontinue medications, prophylactic antibiotics, and prep solutions; make transfusion decisions, incise, and anastomose; or choose a suture material and the way to tie it. These are judgments made in consideration of each patient's condition, clinical indications, and the surgeon's personal experience and preference for materials with which he has familiarity and confidence. When treatment proceeds without complication, such idiosyncrasies are well within the range of normal variation seen in every practice. Neither individual preferences nor autonomy are problematic in and of themselves when the surgeon is using materials and techniques that will afford his patient a highly predictable therapeutic result.

The decision-making authority to implement innovations, understood as adjustments to existing norms, is granted to the surgeon by the culture and by the patient. This authority is based substantially upon the understanding that the surgeon has completed a course of accredited training, has accumulated some experience, and is well prepared to make such judgments in order to achieve a favorable treatment outcome. The patient's provision of informed consent for the operation described is typically supplemented by the standard phrase "and all other necessary procedures," and confers upon the surgeon the wide discretionary latitude he needs to manage unforeseen complications or occult pathology revealed intraoperatively. To evaluate the boundaries of this latitude, we must distinguish between innovation and experimentation.

Defining our limits requires us to define our terms. What, then, do we mean by "surgical innovation"? The *Oxford English Dictionary*'s etymology of "innovation" offers the Latin root "innovatus," to renew or alter, implying revision or modification of something that is already established. If one accepts the limitations this definition places on the word "innovation," most innovation is not only acceptable but also desirable. Alternatively, innovation is recognized as the introduction of something entirely new. From this point of view, the phrase "surgical innovation" suggests necessary and desirable features as well as some that may be unnecessary and undesirable. Every surgeon has a clear idea of personal boundaries, but it is safe to say that the limits of acceptable innovation are neither widely accepted nor closely observed by the profession at large.[3]

Tonelli and associates[4] studied lung volume reduction surgery and concluded that the different nature of the informed consent can provide a test of whether a new treatment is experimental. The consent process in conventional treatment includes a discussion of what is known, but in experimental treatment the discussion must concentrate upon what is not known. When uncertainty of outcome enters the informed consent process, the concept of experimentation becomes a consideration. Because the present case involves a malignancy, experimental therapy is clearly indicated, but one should remember that, when not indicated, such therapy is "reckless experimentation." In rarely done procedures, the surgeon must evaluate whether data developed to resolve the uncertainty is sufficient and adequately studied to predict outcome of the proposed therapy. The patient always should be told how many such procedures the surgeon has done, as well as the associated morbidity and mortality rates. It is not enough to cite the statistics of other surgeons and institutions with similar procedures. When engaging in planned experimentation, the surgeon is obligated to obtain permission from the patient or his surrogate, after providing transparent disclosure of the uncertainty of outcome when appropriate to the operative conditions. If circumstances do not permit prior consent, then the patient or surrogate must be informed completely of the experimental nature of the surgery and the uncertainty of outcome at the first reasonable opportunity. This practice is common and well-observed among surgeons. Because of the unpredictability of the procedure and its outcome, the adequacy of the informed consent process is essential. It must make clear the limits of what is known and the relatively high degree of uncertainty. One must disclose that the types and rate of complications are uncertain as well.

Options (B) and (C) are inadequate for the purpose. Tailoring surgical therapy to rare diseases for which there is no standard treatment may be seen as experimentation, but its intent is clinical rather than scientific. The unusual nature of the proposed procedure imposes additional obligations upon the surgeon to ensure the patient's full prior understanding, but does not sufficiently resemble and organized research protocol, with multiple homogeneous subjects and systematic data collection, to require the prior review and approval of a scientific review panel or an ethics advisory board.

Options (D) and (E) are therefore eliminated as well. The now-venerable Belmont Report distinguishes between clinical practice and research on the basis of the clinician's intent.[5] "Practice" refers to interventions that are designed solely to enhance the well-being of an individual patient and that have a reasonable expectation of success. Innovation which "departs in a significant way from standard or accepted practice" is experimental, but becomes research only when its scope extends beyond the individual patient by producing generalizable knowledge.

There is no intent to include this patient in a series for purposes of systematically developing a new body of knowledge or surgical technique for future application to others with similar conditions; the intent is solely to provide clinical care. All associated clinical decisions are based entirely upon this patient's clinical indications; clinical options will not be limited by conformity to a standard research protocol and there will be no effort to establish scientific controls to produce replicable results. Since surgeon/patient autonomy is the cornerstone of legitimacy in experimentation, the completeness of consent is the single most important ethical consideration,[6] and option (A) is the most appropriate response. Some would propose that review of such therapies be mandatory, and we would agree if the procedure is used to treat diseases that are likely to be encountered repeatedly, but not for treatment of such rare conditions as we see in the present case. A surgeon, especially one newly minted, might be wise to informally consult with the surgeon-in-chief to insure supervisory support, but since all surgeons should be technically competent and none would be likely to have experience with the particular disease manifestation described, consultation couldn't be expected to add much practical guidance.

The Belmont Report suggests that radically new surgical procedures be made the objects of structured research soon after their introduction for purposes of scientific evaluation. The widespread occurrence of severe bile duct injuries following the unregulated combination of two established procedures, cholecystectomy and laparoscopy, to become laparoscopic cholecystectomy, is an oft-cited example.[1] Radically unorthodox surgical procedures applied without oversight when well-established effective methods are available are sharply criticized in the ethics literature.

References

1. Strasberg SM, Ludbrook PA. Who oversees innovative practice? Is there a structure that meets the monitoring needs of new techniques? *J Am Coll Surg*. 2003; 196: 938–948.
2. Frader J, Caniano D. Research and innovation in surgery. In: McCullough LB, Jones JW, Brody BA, eds. *Surgical Ethics*. New York: Oxford University Press, 1998: 216–241.
3. Reitsma AM, Moreno JD. Ethical regulations for innovative surgery: The last frontier? *J Am Coll Surg*. 2002; 194:792–801.
4. Tonelli MR, Benditt JO, Albert RK. Clinical experimentation: Lessons from lung volume reduction surgery. *Chest*. 1996; 110:230–238.
5. U.S. National Commission for the Protection of Human Subjects of Biomedical and Behavioral Research. The Belmont Report: ethical principles for the protection of human subjects of research. Washington, DC: Dept. of Health, Education and Welfare (US); 1979 Apr. Report No. (05) 78–0012.
6. Gillett G. Ethics of surgical innovation. *Br J Surg*. 2001; 88:897–898.

• CASE 26 •

Ethics of Introducing New Operating Room Technology

Leadership and learning are indispensable to each other.
John F. Kennedy (1917–1963), 35th President of the United States

Before beginning the procedure this morning, Dr. B. Reddy had been given to understand that the circulating nurse was familiar with a new fiber optic probe with guided imagery. She had attended a 2-hour training session provided to all operating room (OR) nursing staff by the equipment manufacturer. Dr. Reddy had himself attended the weekend expense-paid hands-on training course offered by the company at its Arizona headquarters, a seminar available only to surgeons. The procedure was nevertheless delayed by more than an hour this morning because neither the surgeon nor the circulating nurse knew how to recalibrate the machine properly when a malfunction occurred after anesthesia induction. The manufacturer was contacted by phone to trouble-shoot the problem while the patient remained anesthetized. Dr. Reddy com-plained to the nursing supervisor that the circulating nurse had failed to manage the new equipment. The nursing supervisor responded that the nurse had taken the brief course and passed the in-service exam, neither of which referred to the kinds of problems encountered that day. During the training course in Arizona, Dr. Reddy had felt that it was more important for him to focus on the operative techniques demonstrated than on the instrument's cali-bration. Who bears ethical responsibility for this problem?

(A) The surgeon-in-chief ultimately has the responsibility.
(B) OR nurses are responsible for OR equipment.
(C) It is an equally shared responsibility between the surgeon and the cir-culating nurse.
(D) The OR supervisor is responsible and must make certain that the cir-culating nurse is adequately trained to operate new equipment.
(E) As the attending surgeon, the physician must be the most proficient of the OR team in understanding new equipment, and is most responsible.

The surgeon's first and most fundamental ethical obligation as patient fidu-ciary is to be competent in the services offered. In simpler times, this meant only that the surgeon should possess the fund of knowledge and clinical skills required to diagnose patients' conditions and perform procedures within a specified area of expertise. Although these functions remain the surgeon's core competencies, they no longer constitute an adequate inventory of what is needed to provide patient care in the context of technological surgery. Surgery is a team per-formance with ever-increasing complexity and demanding roles for everyone involved. The surgeon is nevertheless the captain of the team.[1] Effective team leaders represent ideals of intellect, ability, and fairness. The surgeon's responsibility for promoting team morale and high performance is a direct extension of his patient care responsibilities. Surgery has come often to require advance planning with others who will be in the OR, including other surgeons, anesthesiologists, trainees, nurses, and technicians. As team captain, the surgeon properly oversees the integration of the supporting professionals' knowledge and abilities toward the conduct of a safe, efficient, and effective operation. Legitimate oversight requires close familiarity with each team member's duties. Self-assuredness is a necessary component of the surgical persona and enhances the effectiveness of the OR team. This effectiveness diminishes when the surgeon, because of poor planning or insufficient knowledge, cannot resolve a basic glitch in the operative procedure, like trouble-shooting new equipment.

Surgeons have always needed lots of help, to hold down terrified patients in the days before anesthesia, or to pass instruments, hold retractors, and run pumps and operate equipment in a modern OR.[1] The surgical team has become essential, because no single person can be expected to perform simultaneously all of the differentiated tasks and skills involved in today's surgery. In this context, there might be a tendency to assume that all of the trained and certified people in the OR will know and perform all elements of their individual assignments equally well. A sense can develop that fiduciary responsibility has become diffused throughout the team. It hasn't. It is always the surgeon's operation: no other team member directly enters the ethical professional/patient relationship.

Surgery is not unique among the medical specialties in having to address the ethical challenges of team care, especially the diversity of skills sets and consequent diffusion of responsibility and potential lack of accountability. We find direct parallels in obstetric ultrasound, where sonographers operate sophisticated imaging equipment and interpret resulting images. It has been argued that the physician ultrasonologist should have at least the fund of knowledge and skills of the sonographer in order to adequately supervise and evaluate the sonographer's work and promote continuous quality improvement.[2,3] Self-sufficiency is an essential constituent of the surgeon's character, along with dexterity, decisiveness, diligence, veracity, and intellect, and should be developed rather than relinquished.

As supervisor of the operating team, the surgeon loses self-sufficiency when another member performs an essential task and the surgeon is without knowledge or appreciation of it. By concentrating on those elements of the technical training that interest them and leaving those that do not to team members less lavishly courted by equipment manufacturers, surgeons abandon their leadership role. Our surgeon surrendered his moral authority by blaming the nurse for the same lapse of which he was guilty. His responsibility for knowing how to calibrate and operate the essential equipment may in fact be greater than the nurse's, because he had the more extensive training course and took it under conspicuously more favorable learning conditions.

Option (B) therefore represents an abrogation of not only the doctor's supervisory responsibility as the attending surgeon and team captain, but the responsibility for personal competence he assumed when he scheduled a case requiring this technology and then failed to prepare himself for any intraoperative eventuality. Option (C), shared responsibility, is consistent with the team concept, but the division of shares is not necessarily equal. Given that the greater share of the training resources in this case was provided to the surgeon, and that the surgeon will be the most highly rewarded member of the team for his contributions to its success, it must be realistically concluded that the greater responsibility for the machinery's operation, including its calibration, is expected of the surgeon as well, with a lesser portion of responsibility assigned to the less fully-trained nurse. Every member of every team knows the pattern in which rewards are distributed among the group, and the morale and effectiveness of every team correlates highly with the demonstrable competence of those in its lucrative leadership roles. It should not be left to medical device and equipment manufacturers to define those roles for medical professionals. Surgeons who want to maintain leadership of their OR teams must do so by demonstrating every day that their authority derives from mastery of everything that occurs in direct relationship to the operation.

Option (D) represents another abandonment of the surgeon's supervisory responsibility. The nursing supervisor has used the available objective measures—course attendance, course content, and in-service exam results—to develop a reasonable assurance that the circulating nurse is adequately prepared to operate the new equipment in the OR. The nursing supervisor's oversight responsibilities are qualitatively different from the surgeon's because she does not have the latitude to cross disciplines to ensure full coordination of efforts within the OR. She has likely not been authorized, for example, to insist that surgeons pay better attention during the equipment training courses to avoid the sort of problem that occurred in this case.

Option (A) is pertinent, but cannot replace option (E) as the correct ethical response. The surgeon-in-chief is responsible for ensuring that the operating staff is adequately trained and credentialed to do their jobs. Too many surgical programs credential their physicians in general terms like "block privileges" or "all other privileges within this specialty," surrendering appropriate oversight and patient safeguards to administrative expediency. Though advances happen quickly in high-tech surgery, privileging documents can be amended or supplemented just as fast to keep up. Surgeons can and should be specifically credentialed by their institutions in the use of each of the advanced technological instruments with which they operate. Lasers, laparoscopic equipment, robotics, and the rest of the innovative machinery introduced after most of us completed our formal training require new skill sets and should be individually privileged. The elements of their use should properly and specifically include adjustments, calibrations, settings, and trouble-shooting as well as their direct operative applications. These considerations should be met not only to ensure the integrity of supervision within the OR, but to guarantee, as with existing privilege formats, that patients get a good operation. This responsibility encompasses the equipment and technology used directly by the surgeon in the performance of the operation. The anesthesia machine, the extracorporeal pump, and portable x-ray equipment, on the other hand, are supportive technology, and responsibility for their operation properly remains with the specialists extensively trained to use them as the primary tools of their professions.

References

1. Purtillo R, Shaw BW, Arnold R. Obligations of surgeons to non-physician team members and trainees. In: McCullough LB, Jones JW, Brody BA, eds. *Surgical Ethics*. New York: Oxford University Press; 1998:302–321.
2. Chervenak FA, McCullough LB. Ethics in obstetric ultrasound. *J Ultrasound Med*. 1989; 8:493–497.
3. McCullough LB, Chervenak FA. *Ethics in Obstetrics and Gynecology*. New York: Oxford University Press; 1994.

• CASE 27 •

Patenting Surgical Procedures

"Reputation is what other people know about you. Honor is what you know about yourself."
L. M. Bujold, "A Civil Campaign," 1999

Dr. A. Droit developed an operative technique that can permanently repair aneurysms with no significant risk to patients. The technique does not involve a new medical device, only a readily available tissue adhesive already approved and marketed. The technique is easily mastered. The inventor-surgeon has devoted years of effort to the project, sometimes to the neglect of his practice and income. He is now considering patenting the procedure and realizing a return on his invested effort. He confides the details of his project and plans to you as a respected colleague and friend. You should advise him that:

(A) He could ethically patent the idea if he donated a portion of the royalties to charity.

(B) He has every right to patent and receive compensation for a valuable idea.

(C) His discovery should be published and freely shared among fellow surgeons.

(D) He should patent the glue used by disguising it and sell it for a premium.

(E) He should form a company that he owns and have the company patent the operation.

Prior to the early 19th century, the ancient tensions between medicine's entrepreneurial and professional aspects were usually resolved in favor of the former, as characterized by the widespread practice of preparing and promoting the sale of secret remedies and nostrums. Snake oil salesmen traveled the country offering panaceas to the unsuspecting. The concoctions were usually little more than alcohol or opium-based placebos. In the late 18th century, physician-ethicists John Gregory in Scotland and Thomas Percival in England argued that the physician should be the patients' fiduciary, dedicated first to the protection of patients' health, and only secondarily to his own self-interest.[1] Consistent with these professional ideals, The Council on Ethical and Judicial Affairs (CEJA) of the American Medical Association has advanced a detailed argument against patenting surgical procedures.[2] CEJA first appeals to the "open exchange of information without the expectation of financial reward for advancing medical science," a spirit, the Council claims, which has existed among physicians "since the time of Hippocrates." The claim stands when corrected to the late-18th century. CEJA rightly notes that the patenting of surgical procedures is likely to diminish professionalism by promoting self interest, limiting patient access to care, inhibiting the development of new medical procedures by placing physicians at risk for unknowingly violating a patent, shielding "trade secrets" from peer review and evading quality improvement processes, and increasing the cost of medical care.

Surgical therapy is an intellectual and technical craft made possible by a centuries-old tradition of information completely and freely taught to all in the profession, regardless of the financial impact on the teacher. Entrepreneurial craftsmen have historically trained their successors and eventual competitors in apprenticeships paid for with years of hard servitude. Surgical training differs significantly from other technical crafts because its ultimate goal is perpetuation of the profession and its ability to altruistically extend human life and health, upon which no one can fix a price. The better cabinet constructed by a superior cabinet maker brings a higher price when it goes to market. The artisan who made it is not obligated to teach his colleagues how to improve their cabinet-making skills, nor does he function under a moral imperative to advance the art and function of cabinetry. Most importantly, the life and health of the community do not depend upon the quality of its cabinets.

The surgeon, on the other hand, whose ability represents a distillation of many generations of hard-won but generously shared knowledge and technique, has a solemn responsibility not only to practice well, but to teach and broaden the principles of surgery, anatomy, physiology, instrumentation, asepsis, hemostasis, anesthesia, pharmacology, and transfusion medicine.

This ever-accumulating archive of information is gathered, tested, and distributed by a medical profession that has functioned in a continuous quality improvement mode throughout human history. Ideally, the surgical specialties attempt to disseminate knowledge so well that a collective professional consciousness is developed, within which information and wisdom are shared, expanded, and advanced by our own and subsequent generations of surgeons. This system appears to have worked well thus far, as suggested by the enormous expansion of surgical capability witnessed in the last half century. The cost of this dissemination is distributed among the entire culture, in almost every part of the world, with only the smallest fraction borne by the trainee himself. The surgical profession has established structures like residency training, morbidity and mortality conferences, scientific journals and textbooks, medical libraries, professional websites, CME programs, and scientific meetings for the sole purpose of perpetuating and advancing this body of knowledge and ensuring its availability to future generations of physicians, who are expected in turn to identify and communicate additional refinements in the care of the sick and injured. The inclusionary nature of surgical education is intended to make therapeutic methodology rapidly accessible to physicians and the patients who need them. Patents are by their nature exclusionary, intended to limit access to essential knowledge to paying customers and enrich the patent holder. A surgical patent holder violates the sacred traditions of surgery by using its accumulated body of knowledge not to advance the profession, but to advance his own prospects, much like the cabinet maker. Unlike the developer of novel medications or equipment, the surgeon who discovers and patents an innovative procedure is unlikely to have invested millions in capital; he very likely refined his concept on routine patients in hospital operating rooms. His fund of basic information, his subjects, and his laboratory have all been provided to him by the existing medical establishment, and he has probably received his regular fee for the surgery.

In Europe and the United Kingdom, "methods of treatment of the human or animal body by surgery" are excluded from patent protection.[3] The United States is one of the few highly developed countries that allows patenting of surgical procedures.

By hoarding for sale the information the patent holder gains, rather than sharing it to advance the profession that prepared him to make the discovery, he violates his ethical obligation to broaden the scope and ability of surgery to serve its patients. Although your colleague may have developed a useful idea, the ethical traditions of the surgical profession call for him to share it through publication or presentation rather than sell it.

This conclusion eliminates option (B) and favors option (C) as the correct response. Donating some of the royalties to charity does not mitigate any of CEJA's objections, eliminating option (A) from consideration. Option (D) involves an attempt to patent an already patented product and a frank deception, both of which are illegal as well as unethical.

A newly formed company wholly owned by your colleague is intended to disguise him and limit his liability; it does not eliminate the inherent conflict of interest and adds to it an unacceptable element of deception which renders option (E) ethically unsupportable.

References

1. McCullough LB. *John Gregory and the Invention of Professional Medical Ethics and the Profession of Medicine*. Dordrecht, The Netherlands: Kluwer Academic Publishers, 1998.
2. Council on Ethical and Judicial Affairs, American Medical Association. Ethical issues in the patenting of medical procedures. *Food Drug Law J.* 1998; 53:341–357.
3. Meltzer D. Patent protection for medical technologies: Why some and not others? *Lancet.* 1998; 351:518–519.

• CASE 28 •

Sham Surgery in Research

We give a placebo with one meaning; the patient receives it with quite another. We mean him to suppose that the drug acts directly on his body, not through his mind....Placebo giving is quackery.
Richard Clark Cabot (1868–1939), *JAMA* 47:982,1906

As the only surgeon appointed to the Institutional Review Board of a large private teaching hospital, you are asked to review a research protocol submitted by an orthopedic colleague. The study proposes to compare a patient group receiving a well-established arthroscopic procedure to a control group with the same pathology randomized to receive a sham surgical procedure. You determine that the question to be answered is important, the scientific design is solid, the informed consent appropriate, and risks to patients in both groups are minimized. Patients in the control group will be sedated rather than anesthetized in the OR. Your recommendation to the committee is:

(A) Sham surgery has no role in the ethical conduct of surgical research, and the proposal should not be approved.

(B) Sham surgery is an ethical research instrument if the likely benefit to future patients substantially exceeds limited risks to the control group.

(C) Sham surgery is essential to the evaluation of surgical therapy, and the proposal should be approved.

(D) Your institution should not be among the first to explore this controversy.

(E) All randomized studies are unethical because they do not individualize care based upon patient evaluation.

"Sham" derives from a Middle English variant of "shame," and, as the word suggests, sham surgery has always been ethically controversial. Most everyone's first impression is that it is not ethically defensible to subject a patient to the risks of anesthesia and a painful invasive surgical procedure with no apparent counterbalancing clinical benefits.[1] Research involving sham or placebo surgery would therefore appear to violate the ethical principle of nonmaleficence, the obligation not to harm patients.[2] On closer examination, however, this objection to sham surgery as a legitimate tool in clinical research rests on an assumption that current surgical techniques have been reliably shown to be clinically beneficial. In fact, surgical procedures are most often developed and accepted as the standard of care without benefit of the rigorous controlled clinical trials required for the introduction of new medications.

The ethics of innovation in surgery without conformity to the discipline of scientific method has received recent critical attention in the literature.[3,4]

Some writers have based their ethical objections to research using sham surgery controls on assumptions that the controls will be at greater risk than the designated treatment group, that they will be left with both their ailments and the pain of surgery, and that they will receive no benefit from study participation. By utilizing a sham surgery controlled study model, investigators in a recent investigation were able to conclude that a widely-used orthopedic operation was ineffective, thereby eliminating the surgical risk and expense to which 50,000 patients a year had been needlessly subjected.[5]

The "placebo effect" is widely acknowledged in medicine but generally disregarded in surgery. The placebo is usually thought of as an inactive compound administered to a naive patient as if it were medication. The deception underlying a placebo effect is generally considered unethical in the clinical practice of surgery. Nonsurgical specialties diligently compare new medications to placebos in similar groups of subjects to factor out the placebo response, producing the often beneficial effect of the patient's desire to become well and optimism about the treatment provided. Surgeons, too, must properly recognize and study these powerful psychophysiologic effects. Well-designed sham-controlled clinical trials of innovative surgical interventions could improve the quality of surgical science in the same way that pharmaceutical placebos improve the evaluation of new medications. Because research using sham surgery is not inherently more harmful or less beneficial than unproven active surgery, it cannot be considered intrinsically unethical, and option (A) can therefore be firmly set aside. There is an essential ethical requirement that the sham surgery must pose less risk to subjects than the procedure being tested, which eliminates from eligibility in sham-controlled surgical studies the critically ill, the acutely traumatized, and patients whose conditions can be successfully resolved with a proven safe and effective procedure. Our profession's defining ethical principles require that no surgeon perform a procedure of no possible benefit to patients. When conditions for limiting risk are met, when the effectiveness of the active procedure is uncertain, and projections of future benefit seem realistic, sham surgery can be an ethically and scientifically acceptable research instrument.[1]

Present risks to study subjects must be balanced by potential benefits to future recipients from the knowledge to be gained. Participation in the sham surgery study group must not prevent the patient from subsequently receiving an effective surgical procedure. With assessed risk to sham surgery subjects lower than that of patients in the study's active surgery arm, control group patients benefit when outcome measures find the active procedure ineffective.

Observing these conditions, option (B) is the best recommendation. Option (C) errs in its absolutism. Sham surgery can be, but is not always, critical to a well-designed and well-conducted surgical clinical trial. Horng and Miller restrict the use of sham surgery to trials in which the subjectivity of measured outcomes cannot be eliminated by alternative study design.[1] Furthermore, the research question to be answered should be estimated to be of sufficient benefit to future patients that it exceeds the level of risk to the current subjects, which in all events must be thoroughly minimized. It was for this reason that the control group in our scenario received sedation rather than anesthesia. The sham-controlled study is but one of many effective research models available to surgical scientists. As with other methods, it should be selected only when it is the instrument best-suited to test a particular scientific hypothesis.

Option (D) avoids well-reasoned ethical analysis and ensures that the scientific work will not be accomplished, failing the medical profession on both counts. Clinical research in every medical specialty is by its nature intellectually challenging, and is unlikely to be well-conducted by those without an aptitude for confronting imperfections in the status quo.

Option (E) confuses clinical research and clinical care. The purpose of clinical research is to develop improved treatment methods for future patients. A properly administered informed consent process makes clear to prospective study subjects that they may derive no clinical benefit from study participation, and that study procedures are uniformly determined by the protocol and not by the individual patient characteristics that normally guide clinical care. Likewise, sham surgery in clinical research should not be confused with sham surgery in clinical care, where it has no legitimate or ethically supportable role, even when no effective therapeutic modality is available. We know how to design and conduct clinical trials that are ethically consistent with the additional patient risks inherent to them. As an argument against controlled surgical research, option (E) therefore misses the mark.

You and the other IRB members have a heightened responsibility to ensure that sham-controlled surgical studies are methodologically sound, address important questions, and are scrupulous about limiting patient risk. Properly designed and carefully conducted placebo surgery should present no greater or lesser ethical dilemma than other methods of scientific control.

References

1. Horng S, Miller FG. Is placebo surgery unethical? *N Engl J Med*. 2002; 347: 137–139.
2. Beauchamp TL, Childress JF. *Principles of Biomedical Ethics*. 5th ed. New York: Oxford University Press, 2002.
3. Frader JE, Caniano DA. Research and innovation in surgery. In: McCullough LB, Jones JW, Brody BA, eds. *Surgical Ethics*. New York: Oxford University Press, 1998:216–241.
4. Jones JW. Ethics of rapid surgical technological advancement. *Ann Thor Surg*. 2000; 69:676–677.
5. Moseley JB, O'Malley K, Petersen NJ, Menke TJ, Brody BA, Kuykendall DH, et al. A controlled trial of arthroscopic surgery for osteoarthritis of the knee. *N Engl J Med*. 2002; 347:81–88.

• CASE 29 •

Stem Cell Research: Obligations When Religious Values Conflict with Professional Values

Science without religion is lame, religion without science is blind.
Albert Einstein (1879–1955), 1941

You are a recognized expert in surgical therapy for ongoing acute strokes secondary to carotid artery arteriosclerosis. Such cases are referred to you emergently. A cell biologist with a laboratory in the hospital has approached you with a proposal for a collaborative study involving injection of neuroblastic stem cells developed in her laboratory into patients who are stroking. The randomized model appears scientifically sound, with the potential for improving treatment of a serious disorder. Embryonic material was obtained from aborted embryos, and the procedure has been shown to improve the neurologic status in a murine model. Your religious denomination considers abortion immoral, however. What is your most ethical reaction to the request for collaboration?

(A) Participate after institutional review board (IRB) approval.
(B) Insist that the matter be reviewed by the ethics committee as well as the IRB if you are to participate.
(C) Decline participation outright.
(D) Consult your clergyman.
(E) Consider whether matters of individual conscience permit ethical participation in the project.

As the surgeon recruited for the scientific investigation, you must consider two separate ethical issues: first, whether or not the project is ready and appropriate for clinical trials (a question of professional conscience), and second, how to resolve the conflict the proposal poses between your religious beliefs and your dedication to advancing the therapeutic abilities of the surgical profession (a question of individual conscience). Understanding the historical basis of clinical research is critical to evaluating whether the study is appropriate. Early in the 17th century, the British philosopher of science and medicine, Francis Bacon (1561–1626), lamented what he believed to be the inadequate, if not decrepit, state of medicine. Rather than being based on "experience" (Bacon's nascent concept of what has come to be known as the scientific method), medicine was based on appeals to authority and custom. Bacon called on physicians to incorporate careful, disciplined investigation into their regimens and remedies to determine which ones actually worked, and then to refine them to improve their therapeutic capability.[1] Physicians led by John Gregory, at the University of Edinburgh, took up Bacon's challenge.

Gregory called for physicians to study, distill, and expand medicine's clinical capacities through research while remaining mindful of the iatrogenic risks. Gregory's point was that carefully designed and rigorously conducted clinical investigation of medications could produce incremental advances with acceptable levels of deleterious side effects, with risks offset by therapeutic advances. In taking this position about the modest but steady progress that medical science should be expected to make, Gregory cautioned against "enthusiasm"— excessive expectations for how rapidly and well medicine could expand its capacity. He railed that thousands of patients had been sacrificed needlessly on the altars of enthusiastic physicians and surgeons.[2] Such headlong enthusiasms for rapid and dramatic advances in medicine remain with us today.

The role of professional conscience in clinical research has developed considerably over the last three centuries, becoming formalized with IRB review and governmental regulations.[3] However, the individual physician's moral stance remains the cornerstone of the professional conscience. As a counterweight to excessive enthusiasm about when clinical studies of stem cell injections should begin and how they should be designed, the rigor used in examining the research from the perspective of professional conscience should be in direct proportion to the investigator's eagerness to undertake the study.

Physicians naturally have individual as well as professional consciences. They bring to their medical and surgical practices ethical principles and convictions not solely influenced by their lives in medicine, including the sum of their education, acculturation, and experience in the world at large, as well as their personal religious orientation. For physicians and surgeons of serious religious conviction and practice, the protection of individual conscience from ethically unjustified violation is categorically a matter of legitimate self-interest.[4] Conflicts between the requirements of professional and individual conscience are oftentimes very real and must be responsibly managed.

Medicine is a secular profession in the sense that its intellectual and moral warrants do not appeal to any transcendent reality nor, therefore, to any revealed tradition or sacred texts. There is a sharp distinction between modern evidence-based, scientifically oriented medical practice and the spells, dances, and potions of our professional ancestors, the shamans, who dealt in placebos and occasional good luck. Your patients come to you for your secular persona; otherwise, they would have sought clergy. The intellectual warrant for medicine is biomedical science with its evidence-based standards, which has been understood to be secular since Bacon successfully argued that it should be, if medicine were to become effective in "relieving man's estate." The moral warrant for medicine is the physicians' commitment to fiduciary responsibility— to becoming competent and using clinical knowledge and skills primarily for the benefit of patients.[1] Boards and societies license and certify physicians to practice in accordance with established standards and actions of the medical profession, not as individuals enacting idiosyncratic beliefs and personal ideologies. Responsible management of conflicts between professional and individual conscience compels the physician to act primarily on the basis of professional, not individual, conscience.

Secular science and medicine are not necessarily hostile to religious belief, but as technological advances occur, there is considerable potential for tension between the two. Science and religion come into conflict when each professes to be the sole means of discerning truth. Since they are the two most powerful influences over thoughts and ideas in the world, their struggle is to shape the world's future ideologies. Total dominance of either has historically resulted in a constricted and lesser world. The American psychologist and philosopher William James (1842–1910) understood the tension to result from differences in the way "isolated systems of ideas (conceptual systems)...framed the world to verify experiences."[5] He concluded, "But why in the name of common sense need we assume that only one system of ideas can be true?"

That tension emerges in this case because the use of stem cells from aborted embryos raises matters of profound moral significance for a physician who subscribes in individual conscience to the religious teaching that abortion is immoral and that anything deriving from it, such as fetal tissue, is equally tainted and must be rejected outright.[6] A physician who personally accepts religious authority prohibiting a particular medical procedure on doctrinal grounds may feel ethically justified in withholding participation, even if that participation might advance the medical profession's capacity to care for heretofore untreatable conditions. If you believe the use of tissues obtained through moral violations to be wrong, then you must refuse to participate.

The solutions to morally difficult situations require an intellectually disciplined search for truth by examining tradition, but tradition is an imperfect ethical standard. Had tradition continued unimpeded, many sordid practices, such as cannibalism, would persist today as morally correct actions.

Option (C) offends professional conscience by failure to examine tradition. Although you subscribe to the doctrine that abortion is intrinsically evil, you have not been a party to what you view as a moral wrong and the stem cells proposed for the study lack the potential to differentiate into a person. "Some stem-cell enthusiasts think that even antiabortion absolutists can support stem-cell research, since it uses surplus embryos that are doomed anyhow," Michael Kinsley notes, "But that logic would justify Nazi experiments on doomed Jews in the concentration camps."[7] However, being doomed to die, which we all are, is not the exact equivalent of having no potential for meaningful existence. Stem cells, unlike Jews in prison camps, have never been and will never be conscious or feel pain. The stem cells described lack even potential without which they are no more human than a bacterium. The principle question becomes whether it is wrong to use stem cells obtained by a wrongful act. The argument could arise that successfully reducing neurologic deficits would encourage others to obtain more aborted tissue. But are prohibitions against doing good because it might encourage others to do evil justified? Most great scientific advances have the potential to be used by others for good or for evil purposes; their discovery, being ethically neutral, is thought blameless.

Religious principles have been used wrongly as well to encourage evil, and religious sages are absolved when their teachings are misused. Compare the ethics of stem cell therapy to the ethics involved when transplanting organs from a murder victim. Murder is intrinsically evil but provides the means for good through transplantation. Even those deeply against abortion would consider discarding transplantable organs from a murdered donor to be an unethical act. If after careful analysis of whether participation in this stem cell research, permissible in professional conscience, would be consistent with the requirements of individual conscience, you are ethically justified in refusing to accept your colleague's offer of collaboration on the basis of individual conscience. Both consciences require fulfillment.

If you refuse, you should make it clear to your colleague that your moral inability to participate in her clinical trial stems from individual conscience. Option (E) is therefore the correct response. By refusing to participate, you are not prohibiting the study as being done by others, so refusal does not violate professional conscience. Option (D), consulting with your clergy, is always an acceptable option in cases such as this, so that you have the opportunity to clarify what your individual conscience should include and require of you. In doing so, be aware that the clergy may be bound by tradition with both its advantages of comfort and clarity and its inherent resistance to change.

Options (A) and (B) concern whether your colleague's research meets current, accepted scientific and ethical standards. Rigorous IRB review and approval should be sufficient for you to have confidence that participating is consistent with your professional conscience. While IRB approval is crucial for judgments based on professional conscience, such approval, with or without additional layers of review, is irrelevant to judgments based on individual conscience. If you believe the study should be done and are troubled by refusal on the basis of personal morals, referral of eligible subjects to others doing the study would be required as a matter of professional conscience. Science through technology is beginning to delve into and lay bare the encryptions of life itself. As the potential of molecular medicine increasingly becomes reality, we can expect many more such ethical conflicts between professional conscience in surgical research and practice and individual conscience.

References

1. Bacon F. *Novum Organum*. C. Montague, ed. Philadelphia, PA: Carey and Hunt, 1844.
2. McCullough LB. *John Gregory and the Invention of Professional Medical Ethics and the Profession of Medicine*. Dordrecht, the Netherlands: Klwuer Academic Publishers, 1998.
3. Brody BA. *The Ethics of Biomedical Research: An International Perspective*. New York: Oxford University Press, 1998.

4. McCullough LB, Chervenak FA. *Ethics in Obstetrics and Gynecology*. New York: Oxford University Press, 1994.

5. James W. *Varieties of Religious Experience: A Study in Human Nature*. New York: Collier Books, Macmillian Publishing Co., 1961.

6. Cahill LS. Abortion: Religious traditions: Roman Catholic perspectives. In: Reich, W, ed. *Encyclopedia of Bioethics*. 2nd ed. New York: Macmillan, 1998:30–34.

7. Kinsley M. Stem cells: Uninformed clowns in the limelight again...the false controversy of stem cells. *Time* May 31, 2004. Available at: http://www.time.com/time/archive/preview/0,10987,1101040531–641157,00.html

• CASE 30 •

Ethics of Odd Ideas, Good Science, and Academic Freedom

They called me mad at the university.
Dr. Victor Frankenstein

A religiously devout junior faculty member, recently recruited out of residency, seeks approval and departmental funding from the chair of surgery in a major academic medical center for a proposed study of relationships between religiosity and good surgical outcomes. Her hypothesis, patient selection criteria, assessment scales, and data management plans are not fully polished but appear basically sound. The chair nevertheless believes this to be very soft science. He quietly suspects that the young surgeon may be pursuing an intensely held personal bias. He thinks that patients' religious activity, like visits from the hospital chaplain, may stimulate transient positive mental states, but that scientific evidence of actual clinical improvement can only be illusory and nonreplicable. He also fears that work of this sort could reflect badly on the department's well-earned reputation as an outstanding clinical research center. He tells the assistant professor that he'll think her ideas over and let her know. The chair is your long-time friend, and he seeks your advice before deciding whether or not to approve the study. What should you suggest?

(A) Disapprove the research.
(B) Approve and fund the research.
(C) Tell her to write and submit a National Institutes of Health merit review grant application.
(D) Recommend a pilot study.
(E) Advise her to conduct the project at a religiously affiliated medical institution.

Research is often highly controlled in academic surgical departments, where the chair or division head can kill or stimulate a faculty study proposal well before an Investigational Review Board ever gets the chance to consider it. Most senior surgeons selected for leadership positions in academic surgical programs are established scientists as well as outstanding clinicians. Effective chairs and division heads regularly call upon their own experience as investigators to make wise mentoring decisions in developing the careers of young faculty. In doing so, they typically influence the entire department's research agenda, guiding faculty toward studies they believe are ripe for intellectual exploitation and valued by granting organizations, recruiting and nurturing highly motivated surgical scientists, fostering cross-stimulation, and otherwise nourishing a favorable academic research reputation for the department and the faculty. In most departments and in most cases, this top-down system works well to encourage and foster ideas, people, and research productivity. By the same token, it can also discourage and inhibit research, especially innovative and unorthodox research, and thereby smother academic freedom. By restricting research projects to areas of personal expertise or conventional interest, well-meaning department executives can stifle some of the most creative and forward-thinking hypotheses.

Academic freedom is the privilege "to teach and do research in any scholarly discipline without constraint," and "to discover and promulgate new ideas no matter how controversial."[1] The intellectual principle has been developed and defended against many assaults in the full understanding that it yields a great deal of dust and a much smaller cache of diamonds, but that the diamonds would not otherwise be found.

Academic leaders are ethically obligated to protect their faculty members from threats to academic freedom that arise from within and outside the university, and to be alert to the possibility that they can themselves become those threats. Academic freedom supports our culture's long-term interest in protecting ideas that may at first seem unpopular, unrealistic, or even outlandish, but may later prove valuable, either in and of themselves, or by opening connecting doors to unexpected and ultimately important new concepts.[1]

Academic freedom becomes an especially compelling consideration in surgical ethics when teaching and research that are undertaken to standards of intellectual excellence also happen to be controversial or against the grain of a department's traditional orientation. Surgery is still a craft in which individual innovation plays a vital role in the improvement of methods and techniques, and, perhaps more than most of our fellow medical specialists, we must continue to prize the academic freedom to explore everywhere and question everything. Your friend the chairman may believe that the proposed research is not scientific and therefore not subject to the protections of academic freedom in a medical school. Nontheists often suggest that the various forms of deism (belief in a creator-god, but not in the god of any particular denomination), or theism (the belief in a particular denomination's god) are illusions, and the benefits to health claimed for religious belief and practices are equivalent to a placebo effect, if they occur at all. It logically follows from such a view that a nonexistent god could not occultly influence the clinical outcomes of surgical patients, and that even if a controlling god did exist, there is no available scientific way to study or confirm supernatural causation. The very mention of theistic beliefs in recent times causes many nontheists, especially those in science and the media, to cringe.

Perhaps a skeptical response to the nontheist is in order. It appears that although science is indeed incapable of confirming the existence of the God-concept or supernatural causation, it can rigorously assess relationships between religious practices and clinical outcomes. In large longitudinal studies of religious denominations, Mormons, Seventh-Day Adventists, and Jews have been found to experience reduced mortality rates during the study period, compared with the general population in the United States.[2] Environmental factors such as disciplined lifestyles, dietary restrictions, and discrete gene pools may provide conventional explanations for these findings.

Some intriguing data have nevertheless been derived from using the frequency of attendance at religious services as a presumptive indicator of religiosity. These studies have examined correlations between religiosity and health status and controlled for confounding variables. Religious attendance is independently associated with decreased mortality when other factors known to influence survival are accounted for.[2–13] In one large study conducted across three decades, infrequent attendees at religious services with similar health habits and prior health status had higher rates of mortality from circulatory, digestive, and respiratory conditions during the period of the study.[10] In another study with a 28-year follow-up, frequent attendees at religious services had 36% lower mortality rates than occasional or nonattendees, but they also smoked less, exercised more, and socialized more frequently.[12] When their healthier lifestyles' effects on mortality were mathematically excluded, the frequent attendees retained a 23% reduction in mortality. Koenig et al.[5] followed almost 4,000 adults over 63 years of age for 6 years and compared those attending services weekly to those who did not attend weekly. They found an overall 46% survival benefit that decreased to 28% when the benefits of healthier lifestyles were factored out.[5]

In 1992, Bryant and Rakowski[14] reported that mortality among African-Americans who did not attend religious services was twice that of weekly attendees. In a smaller study that estimated religiosity using variables other than service attendance, little improvement in overall lifestyle was found,[15] but elsewhere the same investigators noted that Protestant males smoke less but have a higher body mass index.[16]

It appears that religiosity, as measured by frequency of attending formal religious services, may or may not promote healthier behaviors, but has an added health advantage not explained by conventional associated factors. Patients who are ill have been found to suffer significantly higher mortality if, by their report, they are psychologically engaged in a "religious struggle" involving uncertainties about their relationship with God.[11]

Although 80% of patients believe God acts through doctors to cure them, and 69% want to discuss their psychological condition when they are seriously ill, only 3% wish to do so with a physician; most of the rest seek the guidance of a clergyman.[17]

It appears that it is possible to scientifically study hypothesized correlations between religiosity and health outcomes, using well-selected objective behavioral indicators, as our assistant professor is proposing. As a legitimate evaluation using measurable parameters and scientific method, not subjective advocacy of magical, miraculous, or otherwise supernatural events to confirm personal beliefs, her proposal should indeed be protected by the concepts of academic freedom. Moreover, if she conducts the research rigorously and objectively, the results cannot be predicted. Hypotheses about correlations between religiosity and improved clinical outcomes of surgery may or may not be validated. Discouraging faculty members from pursuing innovative and even unconventional hypotheses, despite an objective study design and a careful methodology, is contrary to the ideals of science. Option (A) is therefore a poor choice.

The chairman has been offered only the rough outlines of a proposal and is not yet fully persuaded that the study is feasible. From the information he now has available to him, his caution is neither imprudent nor contrary to his responsibility to uphold academic freedom. Furthermore, despite his own extensive research experience, he cannot at this time realistically predict either the study's total cost or the novice investigator's competence in managing a large patient sample and complex body of data through the acute and lengthy follow-up phases. Option (B) is therefore premature.

Large unfunded studies are no longer economically possible. With little research history or published work in the area of her new idea, there is little likelihood that a novice investigator can successfully compete for an approved and funded national merit review grant. Suggesting that she make the attempt at this stage of her career is a sort of buck-passing, relieving the chairman of the unpleasant responsibility for turning her down but guiding her into certain eventual disappointment after she invests the extraordinary effort required to prepare a merit review application. Although this in itself may be part of a young professional's learning process, it might negatively affect the rest of her career. The ploy is furthermore an act of dishonesty and therefore an ethical breach by the chairman. Option (C) is to be avoided.

For the same reasons that the chair should overcome his own preconceptions toward the value and validity of this kind of study, the work must be protected from bias at the other end of the belief spectrum. Conducting the study at an institution with a strongly religious orientation could introduce a poorly controlled variable into the process, or at the very least cause results endorsing a clinical benefit for religiosity to be viewed skeptically by the medical community. Option (E) is not a good choice.

Recommending a modest pilot study fosters the budding investigator's creativity and gives her an opportunity to refine her hypothesis and research skills while improving her study design, data collection and analysis methods, patient management techniques, and budgetary expertise. A pilot study will also permit her to sharpen the overall goals, specific aims, and feasibility of her study to ensure that results will be scientifically meaningful and replicable should she go on to conduct a full-scale investigation. Option (D) best fulfills the chair's ethical responsibility to stimulate innovative thinking within his academic department, support academic freedom, and ensure the soundness of the faculty's scientific productivity. Academic freedom has served us well in the search for truth and improved quality in clinical care. Academic freedom is not a luxury to be reserved to those who pursue safe or approved ideas or those endorsed by the established seats of power and authority. Careful review of research proposals by experienced department leaders, institutional review boards, and peer review committees remains essential to scientific integrity and the quality of the work scientists produce, but these processes need not work at cross purposes with the bold, groundbreaking, or otherwise peculiar ideas that sometimes lead us to our most important advances.

References

1. Robinson G, Moulton J. Academic freedom. In: Becker L, Becker C, eds. *Encyclopedia of Ethics*. New York: Garland Publishing, Inc., 1992.

2. Hummer RA, Ellison CG, Rogers RG, Moulton BE, Romero RR. Religious involvement and adult mortality in the United States: Review and perspective. *South Med J.* 2004; 97:1223–1230.

3. Comstock GW, Partridge KB. Church attendance and health. *J Chronic Dis.* 1972; 25:665–672.

4. Hummer RA, Rogers RG, Nam CB, Ellison CG. Religious involvement and U.S. adult mortality. *Demography.* 1999; 36:273–285.

5. Koenig HG, Hays JC Larson DB, George LK, Cohen HJ, McCullough ME, et al. Does religious attendance prolong survival? A six-year follow-up study of 3,968 older adults. *J Gerontol A Biol Sci Med Sci.* 1999; 54:M370–M376.

6. Levin JS, Vanderpool HY. Is frequent religious attendance really conducive to better health? Toward an epidemiology of religion. *Soc Sci Med.* 1987; 24:589–600.

7. Matthews DA McCullough ME, Larson DB, Koenig HG, Swyers JP, Milano MG. Religious commitment and health status: a review of the research and implications for family medicine. *Arch Fam Med.* 1998; 7:118–124.

8. Musick MA, House JS, Williams DR. Attendance at religious services and mortality in a national sample. *J Health Soc Behav.* 2004; 45:198–213.

9. Oman D, Reed D. Religion and mortality among the community dwelling elderly. *Am J Public Health.* 1998; 88: 1469–1475.

10. Oman D, Kurata JH, Strawbridge WJ, Cohen RD. Religious attendance and cause of death over 31 years. *Int J Psychiatry Med.* 2002; 32:69–89.

11. Pargament KI, Koenig HG, Tarakeshwar N, Hahn J. Religious struggle as a predictor of mortality among medically ill elderly patients: A 2-year longitudinal study. *Arch Intern Med.* 2001; 161:881–885.

12. Strawbridge WJ, Cohen RD, Shema SJ, Kaplan GA. Frequent attendance at religious services and mortality over 28 years. *Am J Public Health.* 1997; 87:957–961.

13. Strawbridge WJ, Cohen RD, Shema SJ. Comparative strength of association between religious attendance and survival. *Int J Psychiatry Med.* 2000; 30:299–308.

14. Bryant S, Rakowski W. Predictors of mortality among elderly African-Americans. *Res Aging.* 1992; 14:50–67.

15. Kim KH, Sobal J. Religion, social support, fat intake and physical activity. *Public Health Nutr.* 2004;7:773–781.

16. Kim KH, Sobal J, Wethington E. Religion and body weight. *Int J Obes Relat Metab Disord.* 2003; 27:469–477.

17. Mansfield CJ, Mitchell J, King DE. The doctor as God's mechanic? Beliefs in the Southeastern United States. *Soc Sci Med.* 2002; 54:399–409.

• CASE 31 •

The Ethics of By-Lines: Would the Real Authors Please Stand Up?

What rage for fame attends both great and small!
Better be damn'd, than not be named at all.
John Wolcot (1738–1819), 1793
Lyric Odes to the Royal Academicians, Number IX

A young faculty member in an academic surgical department has completed a manuscript for submission to a professional journal with a high impact score. The concept, involving outcome comparison of two techniques for intestinal anastomoses, was entirely his own. He prepared the IRB submission, collected the data, and wrote the first draft of the resultant paper. A senior faculty member made periodic helpful suggestions throughout the design and data-gathering phases, and offered sensible editorial advice after reading the manuscript. A departmental statistician ran the data. The mentor and the statistician suggested that the principal investigator add some faculty colleagues to the by-line of the journal submission, pointing out that this time-honored practice would likely result in his own inclusion as an author on their subsequent publications, with the thickening of his curriculum vitae and the hastening of his eligibility for faculty promotion and tenure. One of the faculty members suggested for honorary authorship publishes widely, and it's pointed out to the young investigator that this man's prominence may very well improve the paper's chances of acceptance by the journal. The other man recommended for inclusion as an author has not had a single article appear in the literature for years, but performed the surgery on about half the patients the investigator used for one of his comparison groups. Neither the statistician nor either of the people recommended as "honorary" coauthors have read the manuscript. What should the young investigator do?

(A) Cite as authors only himself and the senior faculty member who advised him.
(B) Include as authors the senior adviser and the statistician.
(C) Include the adviser, the surgeon who operated on the study patients, and the widely-published faculty member.
(D) List only himself as the paper's author.
(E) Include as authors the adviser, the statistician, and both recommended faculty.

There's very little confusion about who wrote such complex works of individual imagination as *Paradise Lost or The Canterbury Tales*, but even the most mundane of medical research projects require a division of responsibilities within a group, and that's where trouble begins. Someone in every group inevitably does a lot, someone else does less, and in the confusion there has arisen in medical research a tradition of those who do nothing. The inclusion on publication by-lines of colleagues who have done little or no work in the conceptualization or development of a scientific project has been called "gift authorship," "guest authorship," "honorary authorship," "gratuitous authorship," sometimes "ghost authorship," and more. The fact that the practice has drawn so many appellations, and that all of us know just what each of them means, is evidence enough of how wide-spread and deeply institutionalized it is within the medical profession. The additional fact that none of these terms is inherently pejorative is further evidence of the practice's tacit acceptance among almost all of us.

Objective and accurate publications, carefully written by knowledgeable and responsible investigators and thinkers, are how the medical profession expands and distributes its most important information. The process relies entirely for its authority upon the personal integrity of the participants, a confidence that physicians and scientists will practice medicine and conduct research consistent with standards of intellectual and moral excellence.[1] The falsification of research results in exchange for fame, promotion, or money is a considerable affront to the profession and its processes, because it sends colleagues down dead-end paths and ultimately imperils the health and lives of patients and research subjects whom the medical profession exists to protect.

But does a little fudging on a paper's by-line, some generosity in the distribution of credit for authorship, really sink to the level of data falsification? Or is it ultimately a victimless crime, and one that greases the wheels of the academic medicine business, builds working alliances, lends prestige, settles small debts, and stimulates future cooperation?

The prevalence of gratuitous authorship in medical publications has been closely studied, and it is breathtakingly high, ranging on individual papers from 48%[2] to 60%,[3] dependent upon the type of article and the particular journal. The gift of a coauthorship on a paper published in one of the most prestigious of the refereed journals is, expectably, more dearly prized than one in an obscure throwaway, and there's been a historic tendency for extraordinary lists of authors to pile up on papers appearing in the profession's leading periodicals; all have issued stern admonitions to prospective contributors. Department Chairs and Division Chiefs have shown a marked proclivity for attaching their names to papers they had no role in producing, usually in the last, or senior author, position. There appears to be a saturation phenomenon at work here, as Chairs with more than 10 years' tenure appear in the senior author position significantly less often than those still getting themselves accustomed to the thin air of medicine's aristocracy.[4] At the lower elevations of academic departments, faculty may pass honorary authorships around among themselves to help one another with organizational pressures to publish, with expectations of appreciation or future considerations, or to insure that referral sources remain obligated. Coauthorship is often the currency offered in exchange for essential functional help like provision of tissue samples or a special lab test.

These may seem like pretty good reasons, given the realities of academic medicine, to give or receive a gratuitous addition to an authorship list, but it actually violates standards to which we hold others who function all around us. If we piously issue failing grades, or even expel from the institution, those of our students found plagiarizing the course work they submit, how can we wink gleefully when we mirror the practice by representing someone else's work as our own? Our deception is in fact quite a bit more consequential than that of a plagiarizing student, because it is not done in the context of a training exercise, a trial run, but as an actual contribution to the professional literature, intended to guide other professionals in their clinical work or direct their future scientific studies.

But still, who's hurt by this? It's been going on practically everywhere in medicine for years, and no one seems to have really been injured, right? The primary reason for gift authorship is just the cultivation of pride. The principal author offers inclusion in an article's by-line to a colleague as an appeal to pride, and it is accepted accordingly. Surgery is filled with hard-charging personalities with a well-developed sense of self-esteem who like to see their names in print, the more the better. But after we gaze lovingly at our names neatly printed on gleaming heavy stock paper, we add that article to our curriculum vitae (CV), where it serves forever after as evidence of our merit. If we send the CV to another medical school in search of a more favorable faculty position, a higher rank or a better salary or a bigger lab, we're using that unearned citation to misrepresent ourselves to others in the interest of material gain. If we submit it to a national institute to prove our worthiness for a competitive grant that will advance our careers, we've done much the same. When our credentials are reviewed by our own tenure and promotions committees, or when we bask in an introduction from the podium at a national meeting as the author of 200 publications when we really worked on only about 75, we have in fact stolen something, and diminished the general integrity of our profession. The professional deception always erodes professional integrity. In the case of gift authorship, it does so by asserting authority for people who do not deserve it, and by courting a misplacement of trust, the most valuable single commodity that we have to sell in the medical profession. The crime is not victimless.

The donor of the "gift" is no less at fault than the recipient. If a primary author adds a well-known colleague to the by-line in hopes of positively influencing the journal's reviewers, he is misrepresenting the work, and offering it on something other than its scientific merits. If he adds the names of other faculty members with influence in his department to curry their favor and perhaps cut a few corners on the path to promotion and tenure, he is equally to blame. He may be overwhelmed by the tyranny of a department executive elbowing himself into an unearned slot on the by-line, but he should not be forthcoming with an offer for purposes of ingratiating himself. The principal author who rewards a clinical referral source with gift author-ship on a scientific paper might just reveal that maybe he isn't the kind of person who should be trusted with another doctor's patients after all.

NIH guidelines suggest that, "Those persons designated as authors should make a significant contribution to the conceptualization, design, execution, and/or interpretation of the study, and be willing to accept responsibility for the study."[5] Coauthors should work as a team from inception of the project until completion of the manuscript for submission. The International Committee of Medical Journal Editors is only slightly less demanding in its standards for authorship of professional publications. They propose that "Authorship credit should be based on (1) substantial contributions to conception and design, or acquisition of data, or analysis and interpretation of data; (2) drafting the article or revising it critically for important intellectual content; and (3) final approval of the version to be published. Authors should meet all three conditions."[6] At a minimum, each coauthor of a published article should be able to explain the article in detail and defend it against critics.[7]

Option (C) is the wrong choice for several reasons. It assigns two coauthors who don't meet the minimum criteria for that designation. Its use suggests that the young principal author is courting favor and a subsequent *quid pro quo* from an uninvolved senior colleague, misleading the journal about this respected investigator's role in the research, and mischaracterizing the routine clinical work of a colleague who had no intellectual involvement in the study. The functional contributions of the operating surgeon might be properly mentioned in an acknowledgments section at the conclusion of the published article.

Option (E) should be similarly eliminated, and it and option (B) both become further disqualified by the presence of the statistician, who was absent until the end of the study and has neither read nor can explain the manuscript. Had the statistician been closely involved in designing the study method-ology and substantially influencing how the data should be conceptualized, organized, and evaluated to best determine whether the study hypothesis had been substantiated, coauthorship would have been a legitimate consideration. As described in this case, that has not happened, and the statistician's duties have been effectively limited to loading a computer program and mechanically running data through it. Recognition of her contribution should also properly appear in the article's acknowledgments section.

Our young faculty member conceived of, effectively implemented, and substantially described the research project, clearly meeting all the criteria for authorship, and specifically primary authorship, of the resultant publication. Option (D), sole authorship, is not, however, his correct choice. Option (A) is. The young investigator did not, and likely could not, have completed the project as well as he had alone and without the guidance, from beginning to end, of his experienced mentor. Having significantly contributed to the study design, data-gathering methods, and preparation of the manuscript for journal submission, the senior faculty member has met all the legitimate criteria for coauthorship, despite having offered some bad advice about adding some "honorary" authors. His contribution should be so-noted with an author's citation in the second position. Principal investigators can sometimes lose sight of how valuable the listening, encouragement, and editorializing of a colleague can be in patting a scientific project into shape and bringing it to fruition. Recognizing the mentor as the paper's second author is ethically sound, not only because his contributions have been genuine, but because none of the principal investigator's motivations for doing so are deceptive, irrelevant to the scientific project, or intending toward secondary gain, the fallibilities that commonly distort the process of assigning multiple authorship in medical publication.

If the most exacting of the NIH guidelines were to be honored, the by-lines of our professional publications would almost certainly become substantially shorter and more accurate. That seems to us to be a pretty good idea.

References

1. McCullough LB, Jones JW, Brody BA. Principles and practice of surgical ethics. In: McCullough LB, Jones JW, Brody BA, eds. *Surgical Ethics*. New York: Oxford University Press, 1998:3–14.
2. Mowatt G, Shirran L, Grimshaw JM, Rennie D, Flanagin A, Yank V, et al. Prevalence of honorary and ghost authorship in Cochrane reviews. *JAMA*. 2002; 287: 2769–2771.
3. Bates T, Anic A, Marusic M, Marusic A. Authorship criteria and disclosure of contributions: comparison of 3 general medical journals with different author contribution forms. *JAMA*. 2004; 292:86–88.
4. Shulkin DJ, Goin JE, and Rennie D. Patterns of authorship among chairmen of departments of medicine. *Acad Med*. 1993; 68:688–692.
5. Benos DJ, Fabres J, Farmer J, Gutierrez JP, Hennessy K, Kosek D, et al. Ethics and scientific publication. *Adv Physiol Educ*. 2005; 29:59–74.
6. International Committee of Medical Journal Editors. Uniform requirements for manuscripts submitted to biomedical journals: Writing and editing for biomedical publication, updated 2004. Available at: http://www.icmje.org/ (accessed July 11, 2007).
7. Johnson C. Questioning the importance of authorship. *J Manipulative Physiol Ther*. 2005; 28:149–150.

· CASE 32 ·

When the Data Won't Get You There: The Ethics of Scientific Error, and Worse

I was crazy with work. I could see nothing in front of me. I saw only one thing, and that was how my country could stand straight in the center of the world.

Dr. Hwang Woo Suk, 2006

A surgical scientist, Dr. B. Slack, is informed by his research assistant and statistician after they've reviewed data for a new publication that the conclusions of a previously published paper may be incorrect. The prospectively collected data were assembled from experiences at several hospitals. The criteria for inclusion were not precisely observed, and a number of experimental-arm patients at one institution were mistakenly excluded from the analysis after enrollment. A computer glitch has corrupted much of the original data and the backups are not to be found. Huge study samples and data sets, and the long interval since the data were collected, make chart retrieval effectively impossible. The study's conclusion did not alter conventional surgical practice; it supported current assumptions and techniques. The statistician now cannot confirm whether the data did or did not support the conclusions. The people who worked on the project all feel that even if the contaminated data were excluded, the recalculated data would support the published paper. But a recalculation is not possible. What should the surgeon do?

(A) Send a retraction to the journal that published the original paper.

(B) The paper does not change the practice of surgery. He should forget it.

(C) The paper's problems were discovered by a fluke. He should forget it.

(D) Friends at his institution advise against a retraction. They say it will unnecessarily damage both his and the institution's reputations. He should forget it.

(E) Confer with friends on the journal's editorial board about what should be done. If they agree to let the paper stand as published, he should forget it.

Since the turn of the new century, editorial staffs of the leading scientific journals have worked harder than ever to forestall publication of tainted material. The most prominent peer-reviewed journals have made substantial progress in ridding their pages of data manipulated for private advantage by industry, gift authorship, and multiply-published data. Editorials, policy statements, authorship verification forms, certifications of authorial independence in industry-sponsored studies, confirmation of IRB approval, and disavowals of conflicts of interest have lately become commonplace. These are indeed important measures to ensure that the distribution of scientific information is governed by honesty, integrity, and care.

As important as valid authorship and disclosure of conflicts of interest are, the veracity of scientific publication is entirely dependent on the authors' data management procedures. Peer reviewers have to assume that the study was conducted as described. They assess whether the methodology seems scientifically sound, whether the data accurately support the conclusions, and whether those conclusions seem sufficiently important to warrant their journal's imprimatur. There is almost no feature of the peer review system designed for the detection of intentional fraud or scientific incompetence if the investigators have somehow managed to make their methods, data, and conclusions look internally consistent. Objective and accurate publication, carefully written by knowledgeable and responsible investigators and thinkers, is the primary medium through which the medical profession distributes its most important information. The process relies entirely for its authority upon the personal integrity and effectiveness of the participants, a basic trust that physicians and scientists have practiced medicine and conducted their research consistent with standards of intellectual and moral excellence.[1]

The scientific community joined the public at large in amazement when Dr. Hwang Woo Suk's claims to have successfully cloned a human embryo in his South Korean lab were exposed as false in January of 2006. As unpleasant news so often seems to cluster, other prominent international scientific frauds have lately come to light.

- The *New England Journal* found that the authors of a Vioxx study it had published had intentionally failed to report an unusual incidence of heart attacks among study patients.[2]
- A Norwegian, Jon Sudbo, published an article in *The Lancet* featuring fabricated data that he gathered from "thin air" on the lifestyles of 900 nonexistent subjects.[3]
- A Japanese biochemist's work was declared science fiction when it could not be reproduced.[4]

The current champion of serial scientific fraud appears to be Eric Poehlman, who has admitted to 54 counts of falsifying data and has retracted 10 published papers.[5] In each of these cases, discovery and discredit followed skeptical inquiry by others, usually offended associates, not spontaneous remorse and recantation by the charlatans.

The immediate damage done to the authenticity of the scientific literature is only the most obvious consequence of these wicked shenanigans. Sox examined the fallout of Poehlman's publications and found his papers cited 3,700 times. Incredibly, this serial fraudster's papers continued to be quoted even after retractions had been published![6] Hwang Woo Suk has done more to cause public mistrust of scientists than Dr. Frankenstein, and his malfeasance has given aid and comfort to the factions promoting complete bans on stem cell and cloning research and favoring other manifestations of antiscientific, anti-intellectual neo-know-nothingism. Fraudulent reports send subsequent researchers down blind alleys, waste the precious time and resources of reputable scientists who work to replicate work that isn't replicable, and shoulder the pretenders to the head of the line in competing for scarce grant support to which they haven't earned entitlement, while denying it to legitimate investigators. Scientific fraud is a very serious crime, with the potential to threaten the health and lives of every one of us.

Falsifying data is surely the most egregious offense to scientific integrity, but it is only one of many ways in which distortion can be introduced to the scientific system.[7] Generated errors can be located in the design, conduct, analysis, or reporting of a study. Overinterpretation of the significance of findings in small trials, selective reporting of results in the abstract, cavalier methodology, failure to report negative outcomes that don't support the hypothesis, and use of multiple statistical methods until positive results are obtained all assault the integrity of the scientific process.

There is a dangerous blind spot in the surgical literature, the honest mistakes that can happen when reporting a large operative experience. The mainstay of the surgical literature is retrospective analysis of large clinical experiences. The subject cases are usually accumulated over a long period of time, perhaps an entire career, and at different institutions. Busy practicing surgeons usually have data collected, maintained, and analyzed wholly or in part by surrogates, fellows, residents on research rotations, lab assistants, and statisticians. The clinical "experience" can be packaged into categories of treatment that may be only loosely scientific, but are still susceptible to quantification and statistical analysis if the methodology is clearly published. These potential sources of creeping error absolutely require the senior surgeon to be more closely involved in the data gathering and preparation process than many currently are. Specific data sets that have been used for other publications cannot automatically be pooled for another article before reassessment of the individual data confirms alignment with the study protocol and definitions. This certainly accounts for data derived from different centers.[8]

"Integrity" is derived etymologically from the same root as integer, indicating wholeness or completeness, with nothing hidden or missing. It can be used to mean the comprehension and fidelity necessary to the enactment of sound moral principles. Scientific and clinical integrity, the basic professional virtue of surgeons, requires rigorous adherence to time-tested standards of research methodology, especially when no one is watching. The integrity of the scientific process depends vitally on such self-monitoring and self-mastery. Most of us have a tendency to want to see our hypotheses supported at the conclusion of a research study, but that taint of pride in our own cleverness and insightfulness can be a terrible blind spot, and ultimately a contaminant to good science. Surgeon-investigators must therefore closely monitor themselves for bias and, worse, a tipping of the data to confirm a prior supposition. The publication of negative data will seldom be as exciting as a startling new finding, and in fact even the best journals are less apt to accept such articles, but other investigators and ultimately our patients depend upon the accuracy of our reports, and upon our comprehensive integrity. The surgeon with whom we began this discussion needs to get it right. An explanation of the errors and a retraction of the paper should be prepared and sent to the journal forthwith. Option (A) is the ethically correct course of action.

The argument that the accuracy of the publication in our opening scenario is inconsequential, and can be safely ignored because the article does not influence current clinical practice, forgets that science is a continual hunt for truth, not a destination. Science denies the existence of ultimate truth, and none of us can conceive of a condition at which the state of knowledge will be considered complete and further inquiry redundant. If the paper was important enough to publish in the first place, it is important enough to correct. A bad paper can stifle subsequent advances by misdirecting investigators who use it to prepare for some next inquiry, or by leading them to believe that a problem has been solved when it has not.

Does it not seem odd to repeatedly find large published clinical studies totally contradicting each other's conclusions more often than in literature of other nonclinical disciplines? Reproducibility is a scientific necessity to determine truth, the violation of which should lead to questions, as in the case of the just-mentioned Japanese biochemist who was found guilty of fraud. In clinical medicine, we perfunctorily dismiss clinical contradictions as "different" experiences from different institutions. How much equipoise in surgical literature is related to data problems? If an inaccurate report does not affect patient care now, it likely will later. Option (B) must be rejected.

How the inaccuracies were discovered clearly makes no difference at all to how our surgeon should react to them. Many of medicine's greatest discoveries were serendipitous. Surely no one would suggest that penicillin should not have been used in patient care because its effectiveness was discovered by accident. Reject option (C).

A prevalence of faculty colleagues who recommend unethical behavior may indicate a serious institutional defect. Avoiding potential damage to one's reputation is a legitimate concern; most of us work very hard to establish good reputations within our profession, and none of us would lightly dispense with them. But good reputations are properly earned and kept by striving to advance the profession's ideals and body of knowledge, not by striving to advance personal egos. Admission of a mistake will always be a lot less damaging than discovery of a fraud. Certainly a scientist's reputation and future credibility would be elevated within the profession by admission of imperfections in a publication so long as they were inadvertent, not intentional, or repeated. Dr. Hwang, who kept his dark secrets, is unlikely to ever again be believed or respected within the scientific community. Option (D) is the wrong choice.

Once the investigator has found that a paper is of questionable reliability, the temptation to manipulate professional friendships to gain absolution has to be resisted. The investigator who has published a significant error is properly embarrassed, but he must recognize that he has placed the journal and its editors in an embarrassing situation as well. Our most trusted journals have gained their exalted status within the profession by printing work of consistently high quality, rigorously conducted and absolutely trustworthy. Journals that publish articles that don't meet these standards are called throwaways. Our surgeon must not add insult to injury by asking the editors whom he's embarrassed to somehow mitigate his error and soften his embarrassment. Option (E) should be rejected. The errant author must request retraction of the flawed paper without presuming to further compromise the journal's institutional integrity.

Retractions of publications are very rare in the surgical literature. Searching the literature for withdrawals of articles published in peer-reviewed journals yielded a dozen cases, most of which involved medical devices, not surgical techniques. Could so few surgeons have discovered errors in their published data, or just so very few who honestly corrected what they found after publication?

References

1. McCullough LB, Jones JW, Brody BA. Principles and practice of surgical ethics. In McCullough LB, Jones JW, Brody BA, eds. *Surgical Ethics*. New York: Oxford University Press, 1998:3–14.
2. Curfman GD, Morrissey S, Drazen JM. Expression of concern: Bombardier et al., Comparison of upper gastrointestinal toxicity of rofecoxib and naproxen in patients with rheumatoid arthritis. *N Engl J Med*. 2000; 343:1520–1528. *N Engl J Med*. 2005; 353:2813–2814.
3. Marris E. Doctor admits Lancet study is fiction. *Nature*. 2006; 439:248–249.
4. Fuyuno I, Cyranoski D. Doubts over biochemist's data expose holes in Japanese fraud laws. *Nature*. 2006; 439:514.
5. Dahlberg JE, Mahler CC. The Poehlman case: Running away from the truth. *Sci Eng Ethics*. 2006; 12:157–173.
6. Sox HC, Rennie D. Research Misconduct, Retraction, and Cleansing the Medical Literature: Lessons from the Poehlman Case. *Ann Intern Med*. 2006; 144:609–613.
7. Al-Marzouki S, Roberts I, Marshall T, Evans S. The effect of scientific misconduct on the results of clinical trials: A Delphi survey. *Contemp Clin Trials*. 2005; 26: 331–337.
8. Jacobs MJ, van Eps RG, de Jong DS, Schurink GW, Mochtar B. Regarding "Prevention of renal failure in patients undergoing thoracoabdominal aortic aneurysm repair." *J Vasc Surg*. 2006; 43:428–429; discussion 429.
9. Jacobs MJ, van Eps RG, de Jong DS, Schurink GW, Mochtar B. Prevention of renal failure in patients undergoing thoracoabdominal aortic aneurysm repair. *J Vasc Surg*. 2004; 40:1067–1073; discussion 1073.

· 5 ·

Conflicts of Interest
and Conflicts of Commitment

Medical practice abounds with conflicts of interest and conflicts of commitment. Conflicts of interest occur when there are conflicts between the physician's obligations to the patient and the physician's self-interest. Conflicts of interest arise because surgeons have multiple self-interests that they cannot or will not abandon in their role as physicians. Conflicts of commitment exist when the surgeon's obligations to the patient collide with responsibilities to people other than the patient or himself. Conflicts of commitment often arise when the physician simply cannot excuse himself or herself from these obligations, many of which are not related to his professional persona.

The inviolability of the professional relationship must be the primary ethical consideration when the medical care of a patient is involved, but it is not the only consideration. As a general rule, conflicts of interest can be readily resolved because the physician is free to independently relinquish elements of self-interest that conflict with professional responsibility toward the patient. This is not always the case for conflicts of commitment, because there are typically more relationships involved than just those between the surgeon and the patient. This feature frequently makes their ethical resolution more difficult to manage than ordinary conflicts of interest.

The best management of conflicts of interest and conflicts of commitment, as with so many other ethical challenges, is preventive. Before making a decision to obligate oneself, a brief consideration should be given to whether or not previous obligations will prove to be conflictual. Even surgeons with the most highly developed anticipatory skills will invariably experience these conflicts in their practices at one time or another. The responsible management of these conflicts hinges on the ability to prioritize the importance of one's self-interest and the importance of one's obligations to the patient and others before making decisions. Although the surgeon's fiduciary responsibilities toward his or her patient are paramount, there are complexities, limitations, and even exceptions in any relationship. We will explore some of them here.

We start this chapter with the physician's most insidious manifestation of conflict of interest: intentional overtreatment to increase billings. We label this "unmentionable" because it is clearly wrong, and because so many of us are plagued by gnawing suspicions that our competitors across town, about whose practices we probably know very little, do it all the time. Conflicts of commitment can be occur when family members demand information or decision-making authority about other family members in your care, and the surgeon must balance courtesy and empathy against issues of patient confidentiality and autonomy. Conflicts of commitment can also arise when important events within the surgeon's own family, or within his network of nonprofessional personal friends, come up when patient care responsibilities seem inescapable.

The Medical/Industrial Complex, with which we are all inextricably entangled, has developed a nearly infinite variety of slick marketing tactics to mask the conflicts of interest they impose upon us to challenge our patient care responsibilities. Some pharmaceutical and equipment manufacturers dangle honoraria for very little work, "training sessions" in luxurious vacation resorts, research grants without associated study protocols, and high-salaried "consultation" positions before the successful surgeon as bald elements of their marketing programs. Most have devised fascinating and innovative ways to disguise conflicts of interest, financial and otherwise, that we know test the boundaries of ethical behavior.

Some have permitted the allure of romance with patients or members of patient's families to complicate their clinical responsibilities. The prohibition dates as far back as the Hippocratic Oath, and in modern times discovery may result in the loss of medical licensure when the matter is brought to the attention of state medical boards.

Despite the sometimes unrealistic esteem in which our patients hold us, physicians have lives outside medicine, and the elements of those lives are seldom fully consonant with the selflessness and total devotion which many fantasize for our profession. This inescapable fact of professional life creates sometimes very challenging conflicts of commitment. We will explore some of the most ethical ways to manage collisions between surgical practice and the enticements and demands that our other roles, as family members, friends, and ordinary people needing personal time to pursue healthy recreational interests, present to us.

• CASE 33 •

Intentional Overtreatment: The Unmentionable Conflict of Interest*

It is asking more than human perfection to assume that a surgeon's judgment may not be influenced unconsciously by a pressing financial need.
Edwin P. Lehman, M.D., *Surgery* 1950 28:595

Dr. I. R. Tepid, highly regarded in residency, joined the group practice 9 months ago. His practice lacks the volume anticipated by the practice partners. He has not covered his expenses thus far and has 15 months remaining to receive a lucrative contractual salary, benefits, office help, and a nurse assistant. Everyone except Dr. Tepid gets their salary from professional fees after expenses. The three other senior vascular surgeons are overloaded with work while the new associate goes to meetings and studies for his boards. Dr. C. Ponzi, a founding partner who championed the hiring, wants Tepid released. What should be done?

(A) Give him time to get known in the area.
(B) Start encouraging him in a jocular manner to operate more.
(C) Hire a leg-biter attorney to connect his salary and trip taking to productivity.
(D) Send more of the group's patients needing vascular consults to him.
(E) Separate him from the group.

No other secular profession exceeds medicine in having so many potential conflicts of interest and in which the stakes of remaining clearly focused on the interests of those served are so high, except perhaps military officers in combat situations. The medical profession is as close as secular gets to sacred but, as with all whom society idealizes, medicine is at risk of rapidly becoming profane if exploited. Professionalism is medicine's morality codified. Medical professionalism has standards set by values that protect the patient's interests by subordinating the physician's to those of the patient.

Professional conflicts of interest (COI) are temptations that blur objectivity crucial to evidence-based medical practice. COI can involve nonmonetary interests such as convenient hours, time for activities other than medical practice, and one's religion or beliefs, but most often, and most identifiable, are conflicts involving money in some form or another. Professional conflicts of interest threaten the fiduciary obligation of the physician to protect and promote the patient's health-related interests by practicing medicine in

---

* This case scenario was suggested by a similar one from Charles G. Wells, a medical student at the University of Alabama.

an unbiased fashion and keeping one's own self-interest systematically secondary.[1] The present case emphasizes a conflict at the palpable marrow of medical practice. Arising astride waning clinical volume, particularly when beginning anew, personal financial pressures may directly influence recommendations of care. Overtreatment is rarely overt; it slips in beneath watereddown indications.

What wisdom do our guiding professional documents offer? The Hippocratic Oath emphasizes beneficence (doing good) and nonmaleficence (avoiding intentional harm) indicating the "correctness" of therapy as, "I will apply dietetic measures for the benefit of the sick according to my ability and judgment; I will keep them from harm and injustice."[2] Not openly prohibiting overtreatment, those Oath takers in ancient Greece did not possess the expensive therapies available today. The Declaration of Geneva is more general implying that COI must be responsibly managed: "the health of my patient shall be my first [but not only] consideration." Another popular reworked version of the Oath by Louis Lasagna pins down the message as, "I will apply, for the benefit of the sick, all measures [that] are required, avoiding those twin traps of over-treatment and therapeutic nihilism."

Intentional overtreatment is such an obvious ethics breach that it is the medical equivalent of a four-letter-word. Overtreatment is considered extensively by politicians, insurance executives, and economists, rarely by physicians. Overtreatment occurs when the patient is subjected to diagnostic or therapeutic interventions that, in evidence-based clinical judgment, should not be expected to benefit the patient clinically. They result in net iatrogenic harm. We consider auto mechanics as potential black-hearted scoundrels every time our cars require repair, and some are, but even the worst only cheat us of money. Medical overtreatment can cost and then injure, maim, or even kill; it is fraudulent antiprofessionalism.

In a follow-up to "Code of Professional Conduct," the American College of Surgeons Task Force on Professionalism suggested that considerations of the effect of expensive on communities be considered[3] by stating, "We, as surgeons, frequently perform expensive therapy. The interests of our individual patient may conflict with the resources available to other patients and to the community at large. We, as advocates for our patients, must remain sensitive to the limited resources available in our hospitals and our communities." This is an important consideration but only nudges the stoop of overtreatment.

The Charter on Medical Professionalism, from nonsurgeons, recognizes that medical treatment can be overdone and, forcefully urges that it be avoided. "The physician's professional responsibility for appropriate allocation of resources requires scrupulous avoidance of superfluous tests and procedures. The provision of unnecessary services not only exposes one's patients to avoidable harm and expense but also diminishes the resources available for others."[4]

End-of-life provides a fertile area to examine overtreatment, those patients are desperate.[5] When questioned about what they witnessed, medical students perceived, "that the medical system is over-treating patients and sometimes causing harm to dying patients."[6] Earle examined Medicare claims of 28,777 patients 65 years and older dying of cancer and found 15.7% received chemotherapy within the last 2 weeks of their life.[7] In a study typical of current literature on patients having advanced pancreatic cancer, after 45 cycles of chemotherapy, the median survival was a paltry 6.8 months![8] The authors' Panglossian conclusions were, "Treatment with NFL chemotherapy is well-tolerated in patients with advanced pancreatic cancer...survival in these patients with poor prognosis compares favorably with other treatment options." There are aggressive oncologists who administer therapy costing 100% more than those less aggressive and despite the increased cost and morbidity, survival is the same.[9]

In a more general sense, economists developed and studied the target-income model of Supplier-(Physician)-Induced-Demand early in Medicare's fee regulation era. As fees were decreased by Medicare managers, physicians did in fact compensate by increasing their services to Medicare patients, enough to replace from 40%[10] to 70%[11] of lost income. Medical care consumption in the more lucrative private insurance sector was also increased during this period, perhaps to an even greater degree, as doctors scrambled to catch up.[10] When physicians weren't making additional interventions to compensate for the lowered profitability of some Medicare-targeted procedures, they made up the difference by applying their time to something else. A 10% decrease in Medicare's physician payments for cataract removal caused a 5% increase in the incidence of noncataract procedures.[12] In a community that fluoridated its water, dentists compensated for the reduction in corrective dental services by increasing their restorative work.[13] This is disturbing evidence of irresponsibly managed economic COI.

Few data are available concerning surgical procedures and nonsurgical data implies rather than impeaches. And it generally appears that increases in procedural utilization are in the gray areas rather than being unindicated. When increased utilization of angiography was examined according to guidelines proposed by the College of Cardiology, the increase was in the group that angiography was marginally useful and effective not in the unindicated group.[14]

Our scenario is oft-repeated as practices grow and new associates are recruited. We have all heard of newly added surgeons "not working out" after a few years. "Not working out" has multiple causality; personality clashes, moral issues, newly minted surgeons passing through professional adolescence, and the new surgeon becoming too successful, to name a few. However, the majority of surgeon's group practice spats involve money. Most surgical groups do a good job with their new additions but other groups have great difficulty in finding someone "good enough."

This case contains the pressure of personal financial need and moral trespass of the senior surgeons who are behaving at best insensitively and at worst unethically. If the new surgeon has sufficient foundational knowledge and any moral worth, he is operating on referrals that have proper indications for surgery and following those patients who do not. Nudging Dr. Tepid to do more operations, without providing him more referrals, pressures him to lower his threshold for recommending surgery putting his patients at systematic risk of unethical overtreatment. If Dr. Tepid is lazy, or lacks standards of talent desired by the group, correct those deficiencies or let him go but do not ask him to marginalize his fiduciary duty. Option (B) attempts to cover a serious moral breach; it overtly pressures while deceptively seeming not to do so, it obviates dialogue as how to correct a serious group practice rift by honest communication. Afterward, neither side will have learned how to avoid repetition of one of the most unpleasant series of events that can be encountered in group practice.

Terminating a contract or changing the terms when the contract lacks stipulations about productivity levels as mentioned in options (C) and (E) are inappropriate moral and legal responses because they would violate the fledgling surgeon's rights. Groups seeking to recruit new members should study their practice dynamic and be prepared to commit to helping new members to become successful. Taking on new members only to lessen on-call pressures or other reasons unrelated to patient care quality violates fiduciary responsibilities.

In all except the largest medical staffs, a new surgeon should be known by a normal gestation period, especially in a high-profile specialty. The other partners in the group have not properly introduced him to the community. Waiting an additional time without helping him get known will only make things worse. Option (A) does not explicitly include provision of the needed help, is therefore not acceptable.

A group practice should be just that; members of like abilities and mindsets who share equally in the work loads and ultimately in the rewards of the practice. New members of a group practice should share in a referral system they did not create with every expectation that they will create opportunities for a next generation. Option (D) implements these ethical considerations and should be adopted in this case.

The first rule of professionalism should read, "honest medical fiduciaries will never intentionally under- or overtreat nor encourage others to do so." It overrides all others and conflicts with none.

References

1. Speece R, Shimm D, Buchanan A. *Conflicts of Interest in Clinical Practice and Research.* New York: Oxford University Press, 1996.
2. Jones W. *Hippocrates.* Loeb Classical Library. Cambridge, Mass: Harvard University Press, 1923.
3. Barry L, Blair PG, Cosgrove EM, Cruess RL, Cruess SR, Eastman AB, et al. One year, and counting, after publication of our ACS "Code of Professional Conduct". *J Am Coll Surg.* 2004; 199:736–740.

4. Medical professionalism in the new millennium: A physician charter. *Ann Intern Med.* 2002; 136:243–246.

5. Jones JW, McCullough LB, Richman BW. Truth-telling about terminal diseases. *Surgery.* 2005; 137:380–382.

6. Karlsson M, Milberg A, Strang P. Dying with dignity according to Swedish medical students. *Support Care Cancer.* 2006; 14:334–339.

7. Earle CC, Neville BA, Landrum MB, Ayanian JZ, Block SD, Weeks JC. Trends in the aggressiveness of cancer care near the end of life. *J Clin Oncol.* 2004; 22: 315–321.

8. Garcia AA, Leichman L, Baranda J, Pandit L, Lenz HJ, Leichman CG. Phase II clinical trial of 5-fluorouracil, trimetrexate, and leucovorin (NFL) in patients with advanced pancreatic cancer. *Int J Gastrointest Cancer.* 2003; 34:79–86.

9. Hoverman JR, Robertson SM. Lung cancer: A cost and outcome study based on physician practice patterns. *Dis Manag.* 2004; 7:112–123.

10. Rice T, Stearns SC, Pathman DE, DesHarnais S, Brasure M, Tai-Seale M. A tale of two bounties: The impact of competing fees on physician behavior. *J Health Polit Polic.* 1999; 24:1307–1330.

11. Yip W. Physician response to Medicare fee reductions: Changes in the volume of coronary artery bypass graft (CABG) surgeries in the Medicare and private sectors. *J Health Econ.* 1998; 17:675–699.

12. Mitchell JM, Hadley J, Gaskin DJ. Spillover effects of Medicare fee reductions: evidence from ophthalmology. *Int J Health Care Finance Econ.* 2002; 2:171–188.

13. Grembowski D, Fiset L, Milgrom P, Conrad D, Spadafora A. Does fluoridation reduce the use of dental services among adults? *Med Care.* 1997; 35:454–471.

14. Guadagnoli E, Landrum MB, Peterson EA, Gahart MT, Ryan TJ, McNeil BJ. Appropriateness of coronary angiography after myocardial infarction among Medicare beneficiaries: Managed care versus fee for service. *N Engl J Med.* 2000; 343:1460–1466.

• CASE 34 •

Patient Responsibilities, Family Responsibilities

Live in such a way that you would not be ashamed
to sell your parrot to the town gossip.
Will Rogers (1979–1935)

As a senior partner in your area's leading vascular surgical group, this morn-ing you repaired an otherwise healthy 75-year-old woman's thoraco-abdomi-nal aneurysm using left-heart bypass. The operation went well, the patient regained consciousness, moved her lower extremities, and was extubated before you left the hospital for the day. Clotting studies were normal and there was less than 200 ml of chest tube drainage. This evening you are preparing to accompany your wife to a banquet at which she'll receive an award from her professional association. You receive a call from the ICU reporting that the patient's chest tube drainage was 600 ml over the last hour. The equally experi-enced vascular surgeon who assisted you in surgery is taking call for the group this evening. What should you do?

(A) Return to the hospital and take care of the problem.
(B) Tell the ICU staff to look more closely at the on-call schedule and to page the proper surgeon.
(C) Page your on-call partner, explain the situation, and ask him to accept a transfer of responsibility for the case during the on-call period.
(D) Go to dinner with your wife and plan to look in on the patient later.
(E) Tell the ICU nurse to repeat the clotting studies, monitor the output carefully, and call you in 2 hours.

The physician has fiduciary obligations to his or her patient, and must therefore accept protection and promotion of the patient's health as primary concerns and commitments. In this life of service, protection and promotion of the surgeon's self-interest become necessarily and systematically secondary. The fiduciary role is largely defined by such professional virtues as integrity (practicing medicine to standards of intellectual and moral excellence), com-passion (empathic therapeutic response to pain and suffering), self-effacement, and self-sacrifice (of time, effort, convenience, and even health to meet patient needs).[1]

The first virtue, integrity, does not admit of compromise. Compassion must be modulated by dispassion sufficient to permit effective action in emotion-ally-laden situations, but is ultimately the motivating principle of the medical profession. Self-effacement and self-sacrifice, by contrast, have limits, and their limits are as ethically necessary as their obligations. The totally self-abnegating surgeon would soon become an exhausted, overwhelmed, and ineffective surgeon, capable of serving neither the interest of others nor of himself. Making reliable judgments about when obligations to others in one's life should be protected and fiduciary responsibility limited can be one of the physician's most difficult ethical challenges. Because the surgeon's role can so often affect a patient's actual survival, the weight of decisions about the responsible management of conflicts of commitment can be particularly heavy upon our specialty.

Given its relatively greater time requirements, the frequency of unanticipated emergencies, and its demands upon the physician's physical as well as intellectual stamina, the practice of surgery will place extraordinary stress upon conflicting obligations. All of us have lives outside of medicine, and in our capacities as spouses, parents, children, siblings, and friends we incur moral responsibilities, just as we do in our roles as surgeons. The ethical obligations attendant to those relationships are part of what define us, and everyone expects us to honor them. It is unlikely that many of our patients could be comfortable in their trust of us if we were known to behave irresponsibly in all our other interpersonal transactions. Fulfilling significant obligations in our family and social lives contributes to the sense of self respect and self confidence that every surgeon knows is essential to the practice of our craft; if it happens that we derive personal satisfaction and enjoyment from doing so, and from otherwise finding respite from our uniquely demanding work, we strengthen ourselves.

Returning to the hospital immediately in response to the call, option (A), would disappoint your wife upon an important occasion and ultimately violate your ethical obligation to provide her with emotional support, particularly at significant junctures in your life together. Although a surgeon's spouse has likely suffered many such disappointments and knows there will be more, our families are entitled to have their own realistic expectations met when other options are available for managing patient emergencies.

Option (B), petulance and impatience with the ICU staff, will neither resolve the problem nor earn you their unblemished future cooperation. The staff is correct in first calling you as the attending surgeon to determine how you want the patient care problem handled.

Option (D), honoring your obligation to your wife but thoroughly abrogating your responsibility to a patient with an impending emergency, clearly violates the legitimate boundaries of professional responsibility in surgical practice. The surgeon may ethically fulfill his or her spousal commitment only after the interest of his patient has been assured.

Temporizing by ordering redundant tests and observation (option (E)) to briefly extend the time you can spend with your wife is clearly poor medical practice and probably poor home practice, because neither patient nor spouse will receive the full measure of attention to which they are entitled. Transferring care to a competent surgeon who knows this case and with whom you have recently reviewed it (option (C)) is likely to achieve as satisfactory a result as if you went in and handled it yourself. Insuring a good outcome for the patient is the crux of this ethical and clinical dilemma, not who must be most self-abnegating. The on-call system as it is designed throughout the medical profession is intended to substitute one physician's abilities for another's and provide all with opportunities for scheduled rest and recreation. The steps you would take to gain control of this complication (repeat clotting studies, drainage monitoring, CXR, medical management, or return to the OR as indicated) are those that would be taken by virtually any surgeon in attendance. If there were an idiosyncrasy of this patient, or a feature of your operative technique, which you are uniquely equipped to address in the face of this complication, then you are ethically obligated to go to the hospital and take personal charge of the case management. If you can otherwise insure a satisfactory outcome and maintain your obligation to a family member, your decision to do so is ethically correct.

References

1. McCullough LB, Jones JW, Brody BA. Principles and practice of surgical ethics. In McCullough LB, Jones JW, Brody BA, eds. *Surgical Ethics*. New York: Oxford University Press, 1998:3–14.
2. Khushf G, Gifford R. Understanding, assessing, and managing conflicts of interest. In McCullough LB, Jones JW, Brody BA, eds. *Surgical Ethics*. New York: Oxford University Press, 1998:342–366.
3. Jones JW, McCullough LB. Surgeon-industry relationships: ethically responsible management of conflicts of interest. *J Vasc Surg*. 2002; 35:825–826.

• CASE 35 •

Nonfinancial Conflicts of Interest

Oh! that I were a dog, that I might not call man a brother.
Henry "Light-Horse Harry" Lee (1756–1818)

You are contacted by an internist who reports that his patient has specifically requested referral to you for placement of a Hickman catheter for home intravenous antibiotic administration. The internist explains that Mr. I.N. Solent is an attorney who represented a former patient in a malpractice action against you 2 years earlier. The case went to court and a jury found no malpractice, denying the plaintiff an award. The patient has told the internist that despite losing the case, he was particularly impressed by your professionalism and command of information during the trial, and would like you to perform his procedure. You recall that in his role as plaintiff's attorney the man now seeking your care intentionally mischaracterized your actions and motivations in his remarks to the jury during the trial, and attempted to confuse and intimidate you on the witness stand. You concede to yourself that you have bitter feelings toward him. The proper response to the referring internist is which of the following?

(A) Thank him for the referral and immediately schedule the patient for the procedure.
(B) Explain that you have a potential conflict of interest and suggest another local surgeon who can take the case.
(C) Tell the internist that your schedule is filled for the next several weeks.
(D) Refuse without explanation.
(E) Refuse the referral on the grounds that you would never provide surgery to lawyers who sue doctors.

The physician–patient relationship is both fiduciary and contractual.[1] As fiduciaries, physicians are obligated to be competent, to possess expert knowledge and clinical skills, and to use their competence primarily to protect and promote the health-related interests of the patient, making the pursuit of self interest in patient care a systematically secondary consideration.[1] The physician–patient relationship is also a contractual relationship that, except in emergencies, the physician is free to enter at his or her discretion.[2] In emergencies, the physician's fiduciary obligation to aid patients in need overrides the normal contractual options.

It is with respect to their fiduciary role that physicians can confront and must responsibly manage conflicts of interest between their fiduciary obligations to their patients and their personal self interest.[3] In general, physicians are expected and ethically obligated to manage conflicts of interest in a manner favorable to patients and the provision of care, even when some degree of self sacrifice is involved. The medical ethics literature has been heavy with discussions of economic conflicts of interest.[4,5] As a rule, unless the economic sacrifice is intolerable, physicians are expected to absorb it in the care of patients.

Less attention has been directed to conflicts of interest that do not involve money, and to whether such nonfinancial conflicts of interest justify refusing the referral of a patient with an established need for the kind of care you provide. Several forms of self interest are in play for the surgeon in this case. First, although the possibility of surgical complications in a minor procedure like this is minimal, the need for a Hickman catheter may suggest the presence of serious illness that could result in subsequent complications. You may also have a proper concern that your lingering resentment could consciously or unconsciously influence the quality of care you provide. You might even be at risk for serious clinical error by overcompensating and being too meticulous, practicing defensive medicine by overtreating. In either event, it will be essentially impossible to treat this as a routine case, and this factor almost always increases patient risk. The proposed patient has an established history of interpreting medical complications as medical malpractice, and you are justified in not wanting to place yourself in his path.

The attorney's request for your services may be a conciliatory gesture or an expression of his feelings about the boundaries between personal and professional behaviors. He likely views your last encounter as thoroughly professional and dispassionate, but in the exercise of his professionalism he has impugned yours, electing to distort and otherwise misrepresent your ability and your character without consideration of the pain this has caused you. A desire to avoid further relationship with the source of such bitterness is a legitimate manifestation of rational self-interest.

Is there any reasonable prohibition against acting on these quite understandable and therefore legitimate forms of self-interest? The patient's condition is not emergent, so the emergency exception does not apply. Other surgeons are immediately available in your community to perform the procedure. Because you have never provided care to this person, there is no extant fiduciary relationship that obligates you to him. If there were, you would have to dispense with considerations of self interest and self protection—or any element of antipathy or compromised standards—that could influence your conduct of the procedure. It is justifiable to refuse to perform any medical procedure when it is not indicated, that is, when it cannot be reliably expected to benefit the patient clinically,[2,6] but this procedure is clearly indicated. Refusing to accept a patient because of irrelevant and invidiously discriminatory factors such as race, gender, religious beliefs, or sexual orientation is not acceptable,[2] but this attorney is not a member of an oppressed minority, nor are you prejudging him in some invidiously discriminatory way. The forms of self interest just described are rational and legitimate. They are neither harmful to the man in need of care nor do they deprive him of any right.

Option (E) would indeed represent an act of unfair discrimination against a class of persons, because the grounds invoked are clinically irrelevant. Free-floating and irrational antagonism toward the plaintiff's bar is inconsistent with standards for rational self-interest. Option (A), accepting the patient on referral without carefully evaluating the potential personal conflicts of interest or revealing them to the referring physician, would be a fatuous denial of their reality. The argument made thus far justifies refusal of the referral but does not ethically proscribe its acceptance if you are so minded, provided you assess your conflicts of interest and conclude that you have the self mastery to manage all elements of them and provide the patient with your accustomed high quality of care. Option (C) is an unnecessary fabrication, and it demeans all involved, including yourself. Option (D), refusing without explanation, is rude and could both embarrass and insult the referring physician. Like option (C), it suggests that you have given your decision insufficient thought and are uneasy with it. Your colleague, his patient, and ultimately you, should know exactly why you have reached your most appropriate conclusion, option (B).

References

1. McCullough LB, Jones JW, Brody BA. Principles and practice of surgical ethics. In: McCullough LB, Jones JW, Brody BA, eds. *Surgical Ethics*. New York: Oxford University Press; 1998:3–14.
2. Sugarman J, Harland R. Acute yet non-emergent patients. In: McCullough LB, Jones JW, Brody BA, eds. *Surgical Ethics*. New York: Oxford University Press, 1998: 116–132.
3. Khushf G, Gifford R. Understanding, assessing, and managing conflicts of interest. In: McCullough LB, Jones JW, Brody BA, eds. *Surgical Ethics*. New York: Oxford University Press, 1998:342–366.
4. Rodwin MA. Medicine, money, and morals: Physicians' conflicts of interest. New York: Oxford University Press, 1993.
5. Speece RG Jr, Shimm DS, Buchanan AE, editors. *Conflicts of Interest in Clinical Practice and Research*. New York: Oxford University Press, 1996.
6. McCullough LB, Jones JW. Postoperative futility: A clinical algorithm for setting limits. *Brit J Surg*. 2001; 88:1153–1154.

• CASE 36 •

Ethics of Overscheduling: When Enough Becomes Too Much

A man's got to know his limitations.
Harry Callahan, Magnum Force, 1973

You are a busy surgeon who takes emergency room call in a large private hospital with resident staff. As usual, your first two cases took longer than expected, and you are getting ready to start a third case before the elective schedule closes and operating room staffing drops off. Between cases, you were consulted to perform a percutaneous tracheotomy on a patient in the ICU, and now can either join a chief surgery resident who is waiting to perform the procedure or start your third elective case. The resident is highly skilled, and has done many such procedures successfully. You have plans to attend your daughter's gymnastics meet. You have a busy clinic scheduled tomorrow. How should you handle this?

(A) Go to the ICU, and if the OR won't allow you to start the remaining case promptly, declare emergency status.
(B) Go to the ICU and do the OR case later as an "add-on"
(C) Cancel your morning clinic and do the tracheotomy tomorrow.
(D) Do the OR case and tell the resident to go ahead with the tracheotomy.
(E) Ask a colleague to supervise the resident and promptly start the third OR case.

Busy surgeons occasionally experience periods where they allow their capacity to be exceeded, especially on Friday afternoons and just before holidays. As the workload increases, most surgeons simply work longer and harder. Although the need to add on cases during a workday can feel flattering to a surgeon who delights in having his skills acknowledged with abundant referrals, it complicates the work schedule, often more for others than for the surgeon.

Surgeons are typically self-centered in their work habits, perhaps because they have not usually been adequately trained in making surgical work-processes efficient. After the first case of the day, over 50% of operating room cases start late, which is why first-case starts are so highly valued. The most important cause of poor punctuality in the OR is the surgeon's inaccurate estimations of the time they'll need to perform specific procedures.[1] "Compressing" their estimates of anticipated operating times so that what needs doing gets scheduled is a widely accepted ruse. At one prestigious hospital, surgeons were very accurate in their estimations of procedural durations, except when booking, when 50% of cases exceeded booked times. As a result, there was considerable waste, with one-third of scheduled cases cancelled.[2]

Agreeing to do additional cases when one is already too overloaded to fulfill standing supervisory and personal obligations is not an act of laudable self-sacrifice. Overscheduling should, instead, be understood as a lapse of judgment., of which surgeons are usually exceptionally competent. Surgeons should understand that overscheduling is generally preventable, but does the obligation to avoid it actually have an ethical component?

The surgeon's primary fiduciary responsibility is to his or her patient, but that is not the surgeon's only responsibility. There are institutional and personal ethical obligations as well, and they must be honored. Surgeons have a clear obligation to observe and cooperate with the organizational and functional structures of the operating room, which are designed to ensure that all patients will receive safe, timely, and complete operative care consistent with their clinical needs. Every hospital has established OR policies to efficiently utilize professional time, space, and equipment, while maintaining reserves in each category to handle the unforeseeable but inevitable emergency presentations. Attempts to game this responsible management of the scarce resource of OR time inevitably creates delays in other patients' access to the OR when they need it. These delays mean unnecessary additional costs and inconvenience for other surgeons' patients, and for one's own patients, thereby violating the profession's fiduciary responsibility toward all patients. Advocacy for an individual patient justifiably is limited when patients with more compelling needs are put in clinical peril by an overscheduled OR.[3]

"From an organizational perspective, surgery is a team sport, with mutually supportive roles intended to maximize every member's productivity and effectiveness."[4] Declaring the case an emergency would heighten its priority and ensure rapid access to an operating room, starting promptly after prime-time staffing. Nevertheless, the definition of a surgical emergency in the AORN standards, which are uniformly accepted by American hospitals, is based on an absolute need for surgery within two hours to protect life and limb.[5] This patient's acuity level in our scenario does not meet this standard; his need is elective, not emergent. Option (A) would be ruled out if only it involved deliberate deception. But matters are made worse by its self-centered dishonesty, misuse of physician autonomy and authority, waste of resources, and resulting potential harm of other patients not receiving timely care for which they've been prepped. This option is unethical and should not be adopted.

It is well understood that most surgeons would like to complete the day's operations as early as possible and clear the schedule, especially for important family obligations. Obligations to family members often come into conflict with fiduciary responsibility for one's patients, as we discussed at some length earlier in this chapter. This is known in professional medical ethics as a conflict of commitment. As a rule, such conflicts should be resolved in favor of fiduciary responsibility to one's patients when meeting their clinical needs cannot be postponed or otherwise satisfied with safe and effective management of their condition or problem. That is not the case here, and so the conflict of commitment can be justifiably resolved in favor of one's family obligations. One must avoid inappropriate use of our "professional obligations" to sidestep nonprofessional responsibilities, like attending a child's important function. Option (B) would fail to meet family obligations without sufficient ethical justification, assuming that the additional case can be safely completed by another surgeon.

Option (C) would delay suitably meeting the ICU patient's care and would inconvenience a number of others to accommodate your bad judgment. The attending physician in ICU has every right to expect prompt treatment for his patient, and has a fiduciary obligation to ensure that the needed intervention is performed in a timely fashion. You should have had the foresight to ask if a delay would create a problem. It is unlikely that forgoing a case for a good reason would imperil future referrals, and more likely that frank disclosure of previous professional and personal obligations would be considered praiseworthy. Rational self-interest is poorly served by option (C).

It is unlikely that the resident has full hospital privileges. Moreover, there is a fiduciary obligation to the ICU patient to properly supervise residents when indicated. You are also obligated to comply with hospital staff bylaws that are in place to assure patients that their physicians are qualified to do the procedures they accept. Knowingly circumventing this protection is morally wrong, eliminating option (D).

Option (E), arranging timely and judicious supervision by another competent attending surgeon of the resident fulfills your obligation to the ICU patient and to the hospital bylaws. Completing the third case will not prevent you from fulfilling your family obligation, so the conflict of commitment is effectively managed. You can justifiably proceed with the last OR case within the elective schedule as you first intended. These considerations make option (E) the ethically preferable resolution of your scheduling problem.

We underscore the fact that surgeons' cynical gaming of OR schedules to suit their own predilections unfairly imposes upon patients, colleagues, and other support professionals working in the area, and is therefore inherently unethical. We readily acknowledge that a busy schedule rewards both the surgeon and the patients treated. A busy surgeon's dexterity is whetted to its sharpest and there is no incentive to extend indications for therapies. There exists, however, a flashpoint at which stress and fatigue limit one's effectiveness, when fiduciary obligations are forgotten, and when conflicts of commitment are unnecessarily created and poorly managed. To insure that patients receive the surgeon's best care, surgeons should keep themselves reminded that scheduling workload is not merely a bureaucratic issue of no real importance. It is an unappreciated arena for properly fulfilling fiduciary obligations to patients, family, and co-workers.

References

1. Lebowitz P. Why can't my procedures start on time? *Aorn J.* 2003; 77:594–7.
2. Pandit JJ, Carey A. Estimating the duration of common elective operations: implications for operating list management. *Anaesthesia.* 2006; 61:768–776.
3. Jones JW, McCullough LB, Richman BW. Ethics of operative scheduling: Fiduciary patient responsibilities and more. *J Vasc Surg.* 2003; 38:204–205.
4. Purtilo R, Shaw B, Arnold R. Obligations of Surgeons to Non-physician Team Members and Trainees. In: McCullough LB, Jones JW, Brody BA, eds. *Surgical Ethics.* New York: Oxford University Press, 1998:302–321.
5. Association of Operating Room Nurses. AOOR: Standards, recommended practices, and guidelines. 2003.
6. Jones JW, McCullough LB, Richman BW. Patient responsibilities, family responsibilities. *J Vasc Surg.* 2003; 37:698–699.

• CASE 37 •

An Impaired Surgeon and Supervisory Responsibilities

The shifts of fortune test the reliability of friends.
—Cicero (106–43 BCE), De Amicitia

You are the chief of surgery at a major urban medical center. A 67-year-old general surgeon on staff, Dr. A.B. Norm, has been your close friend since you were residents together, and has had excellent clinical results throughout his long career. During the last year, however, you have been hearing anecdotal reports from several sources that his behavior has become somewhat erratic. Cases reviewed in the departmental D&C conference suggest that his complication rate may have risen slightly during this period. This Monday morning, a surgeon with a well-known long-standing dislike of Dr. Norm has come to your office to report indignantly that he detected the odor of alcohol when your friend and colleague came in for an emergency case the previous afternoon. What should you do?

(A) Refer the matter to the hospital chief-of-staff.
(B) Meet with Dr. Norm about the report, interview the other parties, document your findings, and refer him for counseling if indicated.
(C) Appoint an investigative committee, which you will chair.
(D) Meet with Dr. Norm and document your findings carefully.
(E) Make extensive notes and wait to see if it happens again.

Drug and alcohol abuse, with their associated functional impairments, are the leading cause of physician sanction by professional oversight bodies in the United States. More than one in every seven physicians is affected by substance abuse at some time in their careers.[1] Within all the medical specialties, the surgical patient is potentially at the greatest risk in the care of a cognitively or physiologically impaired physician, because the surgeon's role requires simultaneous application of fine neuro-muscular, cognitive, and intellectual skills, as well as the emotional composure and critical judgment to make urgent decisions, and the physical endurance to stand for long hours at the operating table. When overlaid upon the standard risks associated with invasive care of an acutely ill patient, the personal limitations of a physician affected by acute or chronic substance abuse are clearly ethically and medically intolerable.

The history of medicine has been characterized by constant attention to and reexamination of the physician's obligations to become and remain intellectually, technically, and morally competent in the performance of his or her patient care duties. This tradition has been central to the practice of medicine for so long that it predates the influence of scientific method. A physician's competence is assessed by his or her ability to maintain an extensive fund of information, retrieve and evaluate it, and apply it judiciously to the ailment of the individual patient lying before him. The competent physician's clinical judgment is grounded in evidence or rigorous evaluation of the processes and outcomes of care. The technically competent physician has mastered the physical and cognitive skills and requisite experience to successfully conduct the diagnostic and therapeutic procedures common within his specialty. Surgeons are generally understood to be the leading exemplars of procedural medicine. Dr. John Gregory wrote that the essential qualities of, "a resolute and Collected mind, a good Eye, and Steady hand, are the Qualifications... to make a good operator in Surgery."[2] Dr. Thomas Percival addressed the delicate ethical question, over three centuries ago, of when a physician should consider withdrawing himself from operative practice. Specifically, Percival suggested that when a physician loses, through aging, illness, or other impairment, the ability to retain the baseline intellectual and manual skills required to fulfill his ethical obligation, he should cease clinical practice to protect and promote the health-related interests of his patients. This "rule of conduct," Percival wrote further, "is still more necessary" in the case of surgeons, "for the energy of the understanding often subsists much longer than the quickness of eye-sight, delicacy of touch, and steadiness of hand, which are essential to the skilful performance of operations."[2]

Percival first appeals to a sense of professional responsibility to justify his conclusion. The medical profession is a "public trust" that should be relinquished when the physician or surgeon no longer possesses the skills essential to clinical care. He next appeals to the court of individual conscience, requiring the insight to know when to retire.[3] The first appeal remains relevant, but the second has become increasingly inadequate. Discussing impaired physicians, Verghese observed, "the doctors had one common feature—namely, exquisite denial that allowed them to believe they could still care for patients perfectly well."[4] With the development of modern health care organizations, which apportion the responsibilities of clinical care among teams, and quality is focused upon economic interests as well as clinical outcomes, the concept of accountability for the quality of patient care has become ever more indistinct. Furthermore, Percival may have been overly optimistic about our personal abilities to banish self-deception and embark upon a program of disciplined self-scrutiny that would lead to our voluntary withdrawal from a lucrative practice, an admired social role, and a personal identity one has spent a life-time constructing. The bitter truth is that we are often the last to know when time, fading health, and bad habits start coming around to collect their back taxes.

Having accepted accountability for the quality of patient care as one of the defining obligations of medical professionalism, what is to be done about our apparently weakening friend? Though the source of today's allegation may be malicious and even untrue, the anecdote is consistent with a pattern of reports and clinical evidence that has been unfolding for some time. If the aging surgeon is indeed impaired secondary to alcohol abuse, his prognosis with treatment is excellent; physicians undergoing substance abuse rehabilitation programs record far better recovery rates than the general population, typically as high as 80–90%.[1]

Without therapy, your friend and colleague can seriously injure patients entrusted to his care, be professionally destroyed and emotionally devastated by malpractice suits, defame his institution and colleagues, and eventually lose his license to practice medicine, even before succumbing to the personal medical ravages of his disease. Enough suggestive evidence has been accumulated to demand that a rapid intervention be made to protect the interests of everyone in this surgeon's orbit, including especially himself. Options(D) and (E), efforts to further temporize and exercise caution, are therefore not the proper ethical courses in this case.

It is now well understood that those in senior positions of accountability should undertake their investigation of all such reports and allegations of professional impairment in a fashion that is scrupulously fair to all concerned. There is, furthermore, a strict common law duty to do so. Central to that duty is judgment unimpeded by personal conflicts. Although your position as surgeon-in-chief would normally bear this responsibility, your career-long personal friendship with the subject of any inquiry constitutes a clear and undeniable conflict of interest, without which option (B) would be an entirely suitable choice. Option (C) holds inherent risks to confidentiality, and could be precipitous without reliable evidence of past or imminent harm to a patient. Dependent upon the outcome, some may believe that you have overcompensated for your personal affection with undue harshness, or some may believe that you have been improperly protective of a friend. Option (C) is not a good response to the problem.

The values of professionalism, justice, and accountability validate option (A) as the best ethical response. Option (A) recognizes, implements, and supports all three values. Reporting the matter to the chief of staff and asking him to resolve it impartially should not be seen as an evasion of one's own responsibility as the surgeon-in-chief, any more than is a judge's decision to recuse himself from a case in which he sees a potential conflict of interest. Ethical leadership and responsibility for the welfare of others may sometimes be best acknowledged in the recognition that others are sometimes better situated for the performance of a particular role. The important issues here are protection of the hospital's patients, a fair regard for the rights of an honored surgeon whose career and reputation are in the balance, and the community's ongoing confidence in the integrity of the institution to provide safe and effective care. It is much less important who has the final word in such matters than that the final word be accurate, fair, and definitive.

References

1. Boisaubin, EV and RE Levine, Identifying and assisting the impaired physician. *Am J Med Sci.* 2001; 322:31–36.
2. McCullough LB, ed. *John Gregory's Writings on Medical Ethics and the Philosophy of Medicine.* Dordrecht, The Netherlands: Kluwer Academic Publishers, 1998.
3. Percival T. *Medical Ethics, or a Code of Institutes and Precepts, Adapted to the Professional Conduct of Physicians and Surgeons.* London: Johnson and Bickerstaff, 1803.
4. Verghese, A. Physicians and addiction. *N Engl J Med.* 2002; 346:1510–1511.

• CASE 38 •

Surgeon–Industry Relationships: Ethically Responsible Management of Conflicts of Interest

There is gold for you. Sell me your good report.
Shakespeare (1564–1616), *Cymbeline*, Act 2, Sc. 3

A representative of Medflow Corporation brings breakfast to all of the morning surgical conferences and talks regularly with residents and faculty. She also provides educational travel funds to you as Chair for departmental use. Some of Medflow's medical products are used at your institution. Which of the following most accurately characterizes the ethical implications of this relationship?

(A) Accepting gifts from commercial sources is always wrong within the medical profession.

(B) Since you would already be using Medflow products, there is no conflict.

(C) You do not have a serious conflict of interest if you have minimal purchasing authority and accept only minor gifts from vendors.

(D) Physicians with any influence on medical purchases are nearly always violating their fiduciary obligations to patients and their institutions by accepting gifts from product manufacturers.

(E) More of our educational funding must be provided by sources other than faculty clinical practice, and industry support is welcome.

The surgeon is understood to have a fiduciary relationship with patients which underpins the professionalism of medical ethics. This means that the surgeon makes reliable judgments about the patient's health, promotes and protects the patient's health as a primary goal, and sublimates his or her own self interest to his patient's in that regard. A conflict of interest can occur even when the surgeon's legitimate and necessary self interest, including concern for personal time and an adequate income, conflicts with his or her fiduciary obligation to give primacy to his patient's interests.[1] The surgeon's professional integrity compels him or her to maintain standards of intellectual and moral excellence in his practice. Intellectual excellence means that one's clinical judgment is based upon the best scientific and clinical information available. The commitment to intellectual excellence is central to the first of the three components of fiduciary responsibility, the reliability of the surgeon's medical decisions. A commitment to moral excellence provides the basis for the second and third components of fiduciary responsibility, dedication to the patient's health and to the primacy of his needs. Accepting money or other gifts from medical equipment and pharmaceutical manufacturers creates the potential for conflicts of interest. In a classic discourse, Waud[2] recognized gifts from the medical industry to be "bribes to physicians" because physicians order the products; they do not pay for them.

Options (B) and (E) represent two common rationalizations for accepting these gifts and denying the element of bribery. Option (B) is unacceptable because a potential conflict of interest resides in the possibility that the company's gift could influence future decisions to continue purchase of its products, even if another manufacturer makes available a model with improved patient-care features. Subtly affected by the donation, the surgeon may even unconsciously respond to a sense of future obligation toward the company. Option (E) fails to recognize that economic conflicts of interest can be created even in the process of meeting real and important institutional needs for revenue in support of medical education. The utilitarian argument of an important unmet need does not justify an inappropriate response. The unspoken obligations created by such seemingly altruistic educational support can gain a competitive advantage for the donor company unrelated to the patient-care qualities of its products. At the very least the gift buys product name recognition, a commodity highly valued by manufacturers and campaigning politicians in influencing future choices. Option (D) best addresses this multifaceted problem, because it alerts the surgeon to the core issue of economic conflicts of interest.

Option (C) fails to consider that even though the financial value of the contribution is insubstantial, the company's intent is always to create some sense of good will, indebtedness, or obligation that will ultimately manifest itself in increased or continued product sales. Physician administrators and members of pharmacy and equipment committees are not the only ones who influence purchases. Every physician who writes a prescription or suggests a new device to his clinical service chief is affecting some company's profitability.

Option (A), which implies severance of all financial ties with industry, is one emphatic approach to protecting the fiduciary integrity of an academic program or private practice. Accepting grants for scientifically sound, independent research, and arms-length sponsorship of scientific meetings can remain acceptable, however, if their provision can be shown to be solely dedicated to the advancement of medical knowledge, and entirely without encumbrance or hope of future gain. These altruistic impulses can best be demonstrated by anonymous donations to institutions working to further these goals. Travel funds, honoraria for nominal "consultancies," lunch for our students and residents, elegant dinners accompanied by product demonstrations, and guest lecturers with favorable views of donors' products are all suspect, and all threaten our integrity as well as our ability to think first of our patients in our medical decisions. Graduate and professional schools in other intellectual disciplines less lavishly courted by marketers seem somehow to fulfill their functions, after all. No one should assume that economic conflicts of interest are benign; they are volatile and potentially predatory on fiduciary integrity.

References

1. Khushf G, Gifford R. Understanding, assessing, and managing conflicts of interest. In: McCullough LB, Jones JW, Brody BA, eds. *Surgical Ethics*. New York: Oxford University Press, 1998:342–366.
2. Waud DR. Pharmaceutical promotions—a free lunch? *N Eng J Med*. 1992; 327: 351–353.

• CASE 39 •

Relationship Funding of Professional Foundations: Just a New Black Sheep?

Sir Winston: "Madam, Would you sleep with me for 1 million pounds?"
Unknown woman: "Yes sir, I think I would"
Sir Winston: "Well, how about 1 pound?"
Unknown woman: "Winston! What sort of woman do you think I am?"
Sir Winston: "Madam, that matter has already been solved.
Now we're just haggling over your price."
Apocryphal anecdote about Winston Churchill (1874–1965)

As a member of the pharmacy and medical device committee at a leading hospital, you are part of a discussion considering whether or not varieties of coronary artery stents should be limited, and if so which ones should be chosen. The hospital representative has endorsed a particular stent from a contractual cost basis. The cardiologist member strongly recommends a particular company's product. His stated reasoning is that the recommended manufacturer contributes heavily to the Penumbral Heart and Vascular Foundation which funds various local research projects. A number of local leading physician members are on the company's suggested speaker panels and clinical advisory board as well. The cost of the stent recommended by the cardiologist member would be higher than using another product, but it is argued that the prestige of the medical staff and the institution would decline with a possible reduction in referrals. What should be done?

(A) Everyone has biases. Approve the recommendations of your cardiology colleague.
(B) Let the deciding factor be a poll of all the cardiologists practicing at your hospital.
(C) Demand that the cardiologist recuse himself and make the decision on the recommendations of cardiologist advisors who have no conflicts.
(D) Conflicts aside, the product must be the best or your nationally-known colleague would not be using it. Approve his recommendations.
(E) Report the matter to the ethics committee of your county medical society.

We have lately been subjected to what seems like a constant bombardment of dark social ills served up by the daily news, including family violence, hate crimes, public malfeasance, and corporate thievery. Whether this societal degeneracy is newly hatched or was conveniently ignored in the past, one can only hope the increased level of media awareness can lessen these immoralities. Physicians are hardly immune from the press finding sewage in their mainstreams, usually involving professional conflicts of interest.[1-4] These professional conflicts of interest usually involve some medium of exchange and the innovative ways some physicians appear willing to compromise professional integrity to supplement their already comfortable incomes constantly astonishes.

Reed Abelson, one of the *New York Times'* most talented medical sensationalists, published a recent article entitled, "Charities Tied to Doctors Get Industry Gifts."[2] The article opens not with a deflectable jab but with a solid right cross to the ethical snout of medicine, beginning with the story of a cardiologist reporting at a conference in March this year that a $14,000 ultrafiltration device removed fluid better in heart failure patients than diuretics. Hardly surprising, and a Ferrari goes faster than a Ford, but to what avail? Although prominent researchers questioned the study's conclusions, the presenting doctor remained adamant. "We believe these results challenge current medical practice and recommendations," said the presenting physician, who predicted many patients might benefit."[2] The doctor somehow neglected to disclose that the company making the device had donated $180,000 to a foundation she and 50 associates staffed, funded the study, and paid her a salary as a consultant, three potential conflicts of interest against her and her credibility as an unbiased scientist.

We don't know at this point if this therapy could eventually become the standard of care, but look at the implications if adopted. According to the National Center for Health Statistics, 1.09 million patients were discharged (not just admitted) from hospitals in the United States with a diagnosis of heart failure in 2003.[5] Because the population is aging, the number is higher today. If universally adopted then, the therapy would have added a 15.3 billion dollar bloat to health care. The late Senator Everett Dirksen's mockery of those who waste big comes to mind: "A billion here, a billion there, and pretty soon you're talking real money."

The science and practice of the group, the foundation, and the data may well be legitimate, but there are quite a few possible improprieties. Let us count the ways: the influence of industry money upon the individual physician's research and practice; the influence of industry money upon the general group practice; the influence of personal relationships between industry representatives and the investigators, affronts to the legitimate charitable foundations of major medical societies and colleges; suspect business practices of the medical company sponsors; a possible tax dodge for a capital enterprise masquerading as a charitable foundation, and, not least at all, a prestigious platform for distributing conflicted information about the safety and efficacy of expensive new medical technology.

Elsewhere we have decried intrusions by industry on medicine's professionalism.[6-9] Consider the least objectionable financial relationship, receiving seemingly insignificant gifts from medical companies.[7] What difference can a free medical book, a nice pen or pencil, or dinner to discuss the latest drugs or devices make? It can create a sense of obligation that clouds the physician's medical judgment, that's the difference it can make. It can make one choose a more expensive therapy without patient benefit, expand unsupported indications for therapies, or lead to the acceptance of the drug rep's pitch as the last word without further study. Waud had the temerity to write that every kind of gift from the medical industry to physicians was a bribe, an inducement for doctors to buy instruments, contraptions, and medications that someone else finally gets billed for.[10] This is known in the Middle East as baksheesh, to anyone traveling in the Mideast, a word sharing its etymological root with nebbish, an insult describing moral character so craven that it can be easily manipulated by bribes.

The next item on the list of ethical compromises are the paid pseudo-consultancies, and "marketing research" payments.[9] Pharmaceutical and medical device manufacturers regularly pour millions into legitimate product research but somewhere along the way the manufacturers' marketing departments shouldered their way into the process, and introduced the techniques of advertising and salesmanship to what medical professionals had been led to believe was a relationship built on their scientific and clinical expertise. Though led to believe otherwise, it was no longer just the doctor's expert opinions and research programs that were sought, it was his or her influence as a sales broker for expensive products ordered for patients. Industrial money, disguised as research support, can easily be slipped into the marketing department, as the subject of the New York Times exposé appears to have done.[3] A paid medical consultant necessarily becomes the functional equivalent of a company employee, and companies, not surprisingly, expect their employees' loyalty, the thorny rose of commercialization.

But why bring the matter of physician/industrial conflicts of interest forward once again? Because the formation of tax-free charitable foundations is the latest, perhaps greatest, conflict of interest blemish on professionalism yet devised. Payments to such foundations create conflicts of interest, though not in the direct form that payments to physicians as consultants or members of speakers' bureaus do. The emergence of such foundations can easily metastasize into a subterfuge conceived of by physicians, not industry, that could lead to the rats' nest of unethical behaviors just described, touching every aspect of a physician's professional life. In this scenario, the physician's economic self-interest in the foundation is substantial if she is receiving research support from it. Her relationship with the company in question is thus an indirect conflict of interest, but no less substantial as a result. Foundations can become legal vehicles for transferring industry money to physicians that flies beneath moral radar by posing as a charitable undertaking. When receiving funds from a "foundation" one may delude themselves to believe that the intermediary eliminates the conflict of interest, but only a psychosis could permit one to forget who funded the "foundation" and who could withdrawal future funding if "research" results were not to their liking.

There have been numerous examples of gross distortions when scientific objectivity has not been scrupulously maintained. To prevent this problem, academic health centers have established conflict of interest policies, but these usually do not address indirect conflicts of interest that are created when payments are laundered through parties or entities other than the investigator.[11] The newly emerging forms of indirect conflicts of interest should be disclosed to professional organizations and hospitals and responsibly managed, so that they do not distort the decision-making processes of health care organizations.

The operative syllogism for option (A) would read: All humans have biases and must make decisions regardless. All physicians are humans. Therefore, physicians must make biased decisions. This assumes that conflicts of interest are both unavoidable and that they cannot be responsibly managed. The conflict of interest in this case is avoidable; other conflict-free cardiologists could be asked to advise the committee. Important institutional decisions should be made by individuals who are unbiased on the specific matter being discussed.

Option (B) is what used to be done when cost-plus reimbursement was in vogue. Then the hospital administrators spared no expense in having huge inventories of different types of prosthetic joints, heart valves, vascular grafts, and other supplies, but we live in a different world today. Provided there is no evidence-based clinical advantage of one therapy over another, cost merits enough consideration to be mentioned first in the American College of Surgeons Task Force on Professionalism's recommendations.[12]

Science's foundation is not democratic. It is unlikely that evidence-based consensus would be reached by taking a vote. Furthermore, polls do not responsibly manage conflicts of interest; depending upon the conflicts of interest of those polled, associated politicking might lead to less effective management of conflicts of interest.

Option (D) assumes that conflicts of interest are indirectly proportional to clinical competence when in fact "human nature" may make it just the opposite. The more professional acclaim one achieves the more infallible one may actually believe oneself to be. The fatuousness of this reasoning undermines it as a responsible strategy for managing conflicts of interest.

Option (E) is premature. There is no actual evidence of the cardiologist behaving improperly. Anyone who serves on institutional advisory committees has the obligation to contribute their expertise and advice toward questions in their sphere of knowledge. Serious conflicts of interest are morally wrong without proof of wrongdoing, but are not censurable per se.

Financial conflicts of interest disrupt scientific objectivity, and they abound.[9] Some knowledgeable sociologists describe the current societal state as a "creed of greed," and from the incessant trials of top level corporate crooks, doubt of this resides only with the most naive and uninformed.[13] Whatever, retention of medicine's exalted professional status, inherited from physician's collective efforts across the previous centuries, simple disclosure is inadequate to resolve problems inherent in serious conflicts of interest. Even simple disclosure seems too much to ask of many contributors to some of our most prestigious American journals.[14] The editor of the Journal of the American Medical Association, Dr. DeAngelis, publishes names of nondisclosing violators, when discovered, and notifies deans at their medical schools. But continued failures of authors to disclose have led to criticisms of her efforts. Perhaps, a special journal for publishing conflicted data is needed, with the articles available for citation only after nonconflicted articles confirming their findings are published.

To protect the scientific and ethical integrity of the committee's deliberations and recommendations, and the hospital's purchasing practices and policies, this cardiologist should recuse himself from participation in deliberations and recommendations concerning products manufactured by the company with which he has a relationship. There is surely expertise in his specialty from colleagues without direct or indirect conflicts of interest. If no such expertise is available within the medical staff of the hospital, it should be obtained on a consultancy basis. Option (C), rarely chosen in practice, is our selection.

References

1. Abelson R. Possible conflicts for doctors are seen on medical devices. *New York Times*. 2005.
2. Abelson R. Charities tied to doctors get drug industry gifts. *New York Times*. 2006.
3. Meier B. Implant program for heart device was a sales spur. *New York Times*. 2005.
4. Bloche M. Physician, turn thyself in. *New York Times*. 2004.
5. National Hospital Discharge Survey: 2003 Annual Summary with Diagnosis and Procedure Data. Washington D.C.: U.S. Department of Health and Human Services, Center for Disease Control and Prevention, 2006:Series 13, Number 160.
6. Jones JW. Ethics of rapid surgical technological advancement. *Ann Thorac Surg*. 2000; 69:676–677.
7. Jones JW, McCullough LB. Surgeon-industry relationships: ethically responsible management of conflicts of interest. *J Vasc Surg*. 2002; 35:825–826.
8. Jones JW, McCullough LB, Richman BW. Ethics of patenting surgical procedures. *J Vasc Surg*. 2003; 37:235–236.
9. Jones JW, McCullough LB, Richman BW. Consultation or corruption? The ethics of signing on to the medical-industrial complex. *J Vasc Surg*. 2006; 43:192–195.
10. Waud DR. Pharmaceutical promotions—a free lunch? *N Engl J Med*. 1992; 327: 351–353.
11. McCrary SV, Anderson CB, Jakovljevic J, Khan T, McCullough LB, Wray NP, et al. A national survey of policies on disclosure of conflicts of interest in biomedical research. *N Engl J Med*. 2000; 343:1621–1626.
12. Barry L, Blair PG, Cosgrove EM, Cruess RL, Cruess SR, Eastman AB, et al. One year, and counting, after publication of our ACS "Code of Professional Conduct." *J Am Coll Surg*. 2004; 199:736–740.
13. McLaughlin N. End the creed of greed. Actions, not words, are the only way to put an end to conflicts of interest, abuses. *Mod Healthc*. 2006; 36:21.
14. McNeil D, Jr. Tough-talking journal editor faces accusations of leniency. *New York Times*. 2006.

• CASE 40 •

When to Refer to Another Surgeon

Incompetents invariably make trouble for people other than themselves.
Captain Augustus "Gus" McCrae, Lonesome Dove

You are located in a large community hospital 2 miles from a world-renowned cardiovascular center specializing in complex aortic surgery. A patient whom you have previously treated just presented in your ER with a tender but hemo-dynamically stable 10 centimeter thoraco-abdominal aortic aneurysm. A CT scan shows extravascular blood. The patient and his family trust you and insist that they want the patient to remain under your care. You are an excellent technical surgeon, but you haven't repaired a thoraco-abdominal aneurysm since residency. What is the most ethical course of action?

(A) Send the patient directly to the specialty center.
(B) If you believe that the outcome will be satisfactory, take the patient to the operating room.
(C) Explain the situation to the patient, and let him choose where he wishes to have his surgery.
(D) You must understand your limits, and you base your decision accordingly.
(E) Recommend that a more qualified surgeon perform the operation and, with the patient's consent, arrange transfer to the specialty center.

During the first part of the last century, it was well recognized that many new operations should be done by only a few highly skilled and specially trained surgeons. In the last part of the last century, surgeons became creden-tialed to do everything their conscience would allow. A certain cavalierness about even the most difficult procedures developed, and even the rarest cases were liberally managed up by multiple specialties. This freebooting attitude has created the great danger of exposing patients needing unusual and complex procedures to surgeons in a perpetual learning curve.

Option (A), immediate direct transfer, would not be appropriate without careful clinical evaluation to insure that the patient was sufficiently stable to insure that transportation to another center would not aggravate his condition. The patient's consent to transfer must be sought and obtained, and the refer-ring surgeon should personally insure that a duly qualified surgeon is available and willing to treat the emergent condition before the patient leaves your center. Option (B) places the patient at undue risk, when you are not current in the skills required to perform a highly difficult operation.

Option (C) places an unfair burden upon the patient. Clinical studies have shown that patients are excessively trusting of the surgeon's skills, particularly in life-threatening situations.[1] This patient has been treated successfully by you in the past, and is likely to believe that you will be equally capable in treating any surgical situation. Although you have done your best to fully explain all elements of the current situation to him, his judgment may be adversely affected by the duress of acute illness. Many patients cannot appreciate enough about the subtleties of treating a complex condition to make an informed distinction between variously capable surgeons. Recommending, rather than simply offering, transfer is a more appropriate approach to the management of this problem.

Evaluation of one's limitations, option (D), should not be performed at the expense of patients requiring urgent care. When outcomes cannot be reasonably predicted, the independent surgeon's efforts to expand his armamentarium can be rightly considered reckless experimentation.[2] Furthermore, the emergent nature of the patient's condition does not permit the quiet reflection on alternatives typically available before elective operations.

Option (E), recommending referral, obtaining the patient's consent, and arranging transfer to a surgeon with the current skills and knowledge to treat the condition, meets the ethical and clinical needs of this situation. When a dangerous condition requiring special skills presents, and a better qualified surgeon is readily available, a referral should be strongly urged if transfer will not increase the patient's risk. This reflects the physician's obligation in the process of informed consent: when evidence supports one alternative as clearly superior, it should be recommended.[3] In 1996, the Wisconsin Supreme Court (in *Johnson v. Kokemoor*) was asked whether the reasonable person standard of disclosure for the informed consent process includes disclosure to patients of information about the availability of other physicians with better outcomes.[4] The court answered affirmatively for cases in which "different physicians have substantially different success rates with the same procedure and a reasonable person in the patient's position would consider such information material." Material information is what a lay person of average sophistication should not be expected to know and which a person in the patient's situation needs to know to make an informed decision.

The transfer of care must be surgeon to surgeon to insure that the exchange of pertinent information is timely and complete, to confirm that the specialized care required is available, and to confirm that another surgeon accepts responsibility for the patient.

References

1. McKneally MF, Martin DK. An entrustment model of consent for surgical treatment of life-threatening illness: Perspective of patients requiring esophagectomy. *J Thorac Cardiovasc Surg.* 2000; 120:264–269.
2. Jones JW. Ethics of rapid surgical technological advancement. *Ann Thorac Surg.* 2000; 69:676–677.
3. McCullough LB, Jones JW, Brody BA. Informed consent: Autonomous decision making of the surgical patient. In McCullough LB, Jones JW, Brody BA, eds. *Surgical Ethics.* New York: Oxford University Press, 1998:15–37.
4. Icenogle DL. Update on informed consent law: The Johnson v. Kokemoor decision. *Wis Med J.* 1997; 96:58–61.

• CASE 41 •

HIV Infection, Professional Responsibility, and Self-Interest

Life is a sexually transmitted terminal disease.
Anonymous

You are a successful 38-year-old surgeon who has applied for a large life insurance policy to secure your family's future. The insurance company ordered a complete physical exam, including blood work, as a condition of enrollment. Your HIV test has come back positive, and the finding has been confirmed on repeat testing. Your immune system remains intact. You inquire about medications and prognosis, and are advised that you have a 10- to 20-year life expectancy. You study the literature and find that the incidence of HIV positive surgeons infecting patients is very low. The large group practice you are affiliated with has been planning to make you a partner within the year. Your most ethically responsible action is:

(A) Double glove and take every possible precaution in the OR, but do not disclose your condition to anyone and continue your surgical practice.

(B) Maintain secrecy about your HIV status until your partnership in the group is formalized.

(C) Inform your group, your hospital, and your patients of your condition, and continue to practice surgery.

(D) Retire from surgical practice and seek patient care opportunities in a specialty that does not involve invasive procedures. Cooperate in notification of recent patients.

(E) Ignore the laboratory results and carry on as before; the condition is not transmittable unless you become symptomatic.

With improved pharmacologic management of HIV-associated complications, this once uniformly lethal infection has been transformed into a chronic disease with which patients can live and function for many years. Public perceptions of HIV infection have begun to track this change in clinical reality. When HIV infection was first documented in the mid-'80s, the public reaction was fear, ostracism, and rage toward those infected. The sympathy usually afforded the terminally ill was regularly denied the HIV patient, who was furthermore made to bear the burdens of blame and shame on withering shoulders. These reactions are now far less common, and they have become socially unacceptable. But kindness and empathy are not the only ethical issues at play when the practice of an HIV positive physician is under consideration. Questions about contagion, financial liability of associates, the obligation to control iatrogenic risk, and the responsibility to disclose clinically relevant information during the informed consent process are legitimate ethical concerns, and exist well beyond the realm of social prejudices.

Physicians have an obligation, under the long-established ethical principle of beneficence, not to subject their patients to unnecessary, preventable iatrogenic risk. This obligation includes protecting patients from oneself should one become a vector for infection of patients. Although Centers for Disease Control estimates that risk of patient infection by an HIV infected surgeon may be as low as between 1 in 40,000 to 400,000 surgeries,[1,2] the American Medical Association contends that "physicians who are HIV positive have an ethical obligation not to engage in any professional activity which has an identifiable risk of transmission of the infection to patients,"[2] and even 1 in 400,000 is "identifiable." Confirmed cases of surgeon-to-patient transmission of HIV have been reported.[1,3] Although recent improvements in pharmacologic management of HIV infection are clearly effective in extending life and functionality, they do nothing to lower the risk of disease transmission. HIV remains a virulently contagious disease, transmitted through the mucosal tissues and vital fluids which are the surgeon's working environment.

Surgeons are further obligated by ethical considerations of the informed consent process to disclose information to patients about the benefits and risks of surgical procedures.[4] This disclosure should be guided by the reasonable person standard, which requires the surgeon to provide patients with clinically significant information that a layperson of average sophistication in the patient's circumstances cannot be expected to know.[5] The layperson of average sophistication should not be expected to know that he is at risk of HIV infection from his surgeon. The patient providing legitimately informed consent for performance of an operative procedure by you must first be made aware that you are infected with a life-threatening communicable disease, and that any added risk can be eliminated by seeking the services of another capable surgeon.

The ethical dilemma is further complicated by your relationship to the organizations and institutions with whom you are necessarily affiliated. Most hospitals reprivilege physicians annually, and the process typically includes inquiry about any recent changes in health status that would affect one's ability to care for patients. The practice group which intends to offer you partnership on the basis of your outstanding record of professional achievement, and with it some significant guarantees of salary and benefits, will do so in the expectation that you will continue to be a clinically productive and economically profitable contributor. Both the privileging hospitals and the practice group will bear substantial liability should your disease manifest itself in a patient's illness or injury.

Option (D) is, regrettably, the only answer that satisfies all the associated ethical issues. This difficult course is the least satisfactory to your immediate self-interest, and will very likely require retraining and substantial interim sacrifices in income and lifestyle.

Option (A) is ethically problematic because even the most scrupulously-observed infection control precautions are not always effective in protecting surgical patients from transmission of infectious disease by an HIV–positive physician. Every surgeon knows that breaches in infection control technique occur routinely in the OR, and that needle sticks, glove tears, and fingers cut by sutures and sharp instruments place both surgeon and patient at risk.

Option (B) involves intentionally misleading one's closest colleagues in the service of one's financial interest and at the expense of theirs. Because reporting the infection is likely to affect their decision to offer you partnership, withholding the information is tantamount to financial fraud, for which there is no ethical support.

Option (C) fulfills one's obligations to the process of informed consent and to your responsibility to notify your affiliated organizations, but does not satisfy the beneficence-based obligation to prevent unnecessary and avoidable patient risk. In a practical sense, the surgeon who attempts to continue his surgical practice under these conditions is likely to find painfully few patients willing to proceed under his care once they are made aware of his condition.

Option (E) is scientifically erroneous and denies the immediate gravity of the situation to one's self as well as to the potentially affected patients, colleagues, and organizations places at unconsenting risk.

References

1. Orentlicher D, American Medical Association. Office of the General Counsel. HIV-infected surgeons: Behringer v. Medical Center. *JAMA*. 1991; 266:1134–1137.
2. Daniels N. HIV-infected professionals, patient rights, and the "switching dilemma." *JAMA*. 1992; 267:1368–1371.
3. Lot F, Seguier J-C, Fegueux S, Astagneau P, Simon P, Aggoune M, et al. Probable transmission of HIV from an orthopedic surgeon to a patient in France. *Ann Intern Med*. 1999; 130:1–6.
4. Faden R, Beauchamp T. *A History and Theory of Informed Consent*. New York: Oxford University Press, 1986.
5. Wear S, Milch R, Weaver W. Care of dying patients. In: McCullough LB, Jones JW, Brody BA, eds. *Surgical Ethics*. New York: Oxford University Press, 1998:171–198.

· CASE 42 ·

Ethics of Combining Romance with Medical Practice

Multi famam, conscientiam pauci verentur. (Many fear their reputation, few their conscience.)

Gaius Plinius Caecilius Secundus (Pliny the Younger) (63–113 AD), Letters

An elderly, widowed man with early dementia has required several surgical procedures for treatment of his regional ileitis over the years. Each of the operations has been performed by a single surgeon, for whom the patient and his family have developed enormous respect and admiration. The patient is quite wealthy, and, at the urging of his unmarried adult daughter, his guardian, he has endowed a professorship and directed that this surgeon be the first appointment to the new position. The surgeon has recently divorced. Soon after he accepts the medical school's offer, the daughter invites him to dinner alone at her apartment. What should he do?

(A) Prohibitions against practice-related romantic involvement refer to patients only. He should accept the invitation.

(B) Physicians are not legally permitted to socialize with relatives of patients. He must decline.

(C) He should graciously accept a harmless dinner invitation from one of his sponsors.

(D) There are no legal or professional prohibitions against social or romantic relationships with relatives of patients. Accept gladly.

(E) Entangling professional influence with social and potentially romantic involvement is imprudent. He should tactfully decline.

At least as long ago as the time of Hippocrates, it was understood that the physician's special influence could be misused in relationships with patients, their relatives, and servants.[1] The Hippocratic Oath clearly anticipates and prohibits physicians from transforming the gratitude and respect of patients and their families into predatory sex: "Into as many houses as I may enter, I will go for the benefit of the ill, while being far from all voluntary and destructive injustice, especially from sexual acts both upon women's bodies and upon mens', both of the free and of the slaves."[2] Sexual relations with anyone remotely associated with patients were considered important enough to be mentioned in the same breath as the importance of confidentiality and the prohibition against administering poisons. Any manipulation of the physician's special status to seduce or otherwise obtain sex was considered intentional injustice and mischief. Designating this behavior as mischief suggests that it damages all participants in addition to distracting from the provision of medical care. In this day and age, sexual relations with patients are everywhere considered professional misconduct, punishable by the legal and professional sanctions of medical boards and professional societies. Most workplaces acknowledge the potential harm of combining business and romance, even at the nonprofessional level, because it may reflect uneven distributions of power and "infringe on the proper conduct of business."[3] Any nonscientific influence on the physician's clinical judgment, decision making, or behavior is potentially much more serious than infringements on the conduct of business.

In a survey of almost 1,900 family physicians, internists, obstetrician-gynecologists, and surgeons, 9% admitted that they had sexual relations with one or more patients, and 23% reported being told by a patient that they had sex with another of their physicians.[4] Contradicting the notion that the problem was primarily one of the psychiatric specialty, a nationwide survey of psychiatrists showed that 6.1%, comparable to the general physician population, had been involved sexually with current patients.[5] Attitudes varied among specialists regarding appropriateness of relationships with patients during treatment. While only 3% of internists and obstetrician-gynecologists considered concurrent relationships to be acceptable, 9% of family practitioners, and 12% of ophthalmologists saw nothing ethically wrong with the behavior. More than half the respondents would permit a relationship after the end of treatment.

Throughout history, the morality of sexual behavior has been paramount among societal concerns. Most notably, incest avoidance to the point of being a taboo is the norm among all human societies, primate troops, and other advanced wild animals because "close inbreeding would be disadvantageous to sexually reproducing organisms who live in a changing environment, since loss of genetic variation, and thus loss of flexibility in adaptation, would result."[6] Higher animals force maturing males to leave the family pack, while humans control incest with criminalization of sexual relations and marriage between close relatives, by religious prohibitions, and through societal customs which communicate an attitude of group revulsion toward the behavior. Severe prohibitions toward forcible sexual relations and sex with children are strongly enforced in all cultures. While discouragement of sexual activities such as adultery and homosexuality has been moderated, opposition to sexual harassment and child pornography has been sharpened. Acknowledgment and expansion of respect for personal autonomy in the later part of the last century has made safeguards a necessary part of professional behaviors in all of the workplace. Despite periodic claims to the contrary, no society has ever really considered sex to be private. Every culture senses a deep investment and seeks control of its membership's sexual behavior.

But our hypothetical surgeon is only considering having dinner with the relative of a patient whom he has known and respected for years. Why should anything be considered wrong? In 1998, the American Medical Association adopted opinion E-8.145, entitled "Sexual or Romantic Relations Between

Physicians and Key Third Parties." The published opinion suggested that physicians refrain from sexual or romantic interactions with key third parties when there may be an appearance that the trust, knowledge, influence, or emotions emerging from a professional relationship have been exploited. The nature of the patient's medical problem, the duration of the professional relationship, the degree of the third party's emotional dependence on the physician, and the importance of the clinical encounter to the third party and the patient are the probative factors to be evaluated when determining whether a relationship with a significant third party is ethically appropriate for the physician.[7]

The Federation of State Medical Boards considers sexual relations with a patient's surrogate to be "an exploitation of the physician-patient relationship because it may influence the medical judgment of the physician and the decision making process of the patient's decision maker." The Federation concludes, "The Committee proposes that the definition of sexual misconduct include any sexual contact with patient surrogates that occurs concurrent with the physician-patient relationship."[7]

These professional prohibitions are intended to protect patients, their families, and their physicians from potentially terrible entanglements. Attendance at a dinner party with many other guests will not be within their purview, but a private dinner between an unattached physician and an admiring single family member is an obvious prelude to the organization's concerns. Option (A) is therefore eliminated. Legal opinion is thus far silent on such matters, and therefore provides no guidance, removing option (B) as factually incorrect. Option (D) is mistaken about professional prohibitions; we have just quoted several. Option (D) is also ruled out as factually erroneous.

In this case, the patient's daughter clearly has considerable influence on the patient, and as his guardian will become his surrogate decision maker when he loses the capacity to make his own determinations. It is entirely foreseeable that close involvement with her at this juncture of the surgeon's personal life could stimulate romantic and sexual involvement. Such a relationship can improperly influence the daughter's later decisions as the patient's surrogate and guardian, or the surgeon's as his treating physician. Withdrawing as the patient's surgeon, after long-established familiarity with his treatment history, is not in the patient's best interest medically, and would furthermore demoralize him. There is a high likelihood, under the circumstances, that the daughter has become enchanted with the surgeon as a result of his masterful care of the father, and intends their private dinner to be the start of a romantic relationship. The invitation is not innocuous, as assumed by option (C), which should therefore be rejected.

Option (E) emerges as the most ethically appropriate response to this problem. It is the only course among those offered which fully resolves the physician's ethical conflicts, actual and potential, and maintains the integrity of his ancient responsibility in whatever houses he may visit.

References

1. Prioreschi, P. The Hippocratic Oath: A code for physicians, not a Pythagorean mani- festo. *Med Hypotheses*. 1995; 44:447–462.

2. Hippocrates. Oath. Trans. Von Staden H. In von Staden, H. 'In a pure and holy way': personal and professional conduct in the Hippocratic Oath?" *J Hist Medi Allied Sci*. 1996; 51(4):404–437.

3. Gregg, RE. Restrictions on workplace romance and consensual relationship policies. *J Med Pract Manage*. 2004; 19:314316.

3. Gartrell NK, Milliken N, Goodson WH, III, Thiemann S, Lo B. Physician-patient sexual contact: Prevalence and problems. *West J Med*. 1992; 157:139–143.

4. Gartrell N, Herman J, Olarte S, Feldstein M, Localio R. Psychiatrist-patient sex- ual contact: results of a national survey. I: Prevalence. *Am J Psychiatry*. 1986; 143: 1126–1131.

5. Stone, L. *Kinship and Gender*. Boulder, Colo: Westview Press, Harper-Collins, 1997.

6. Special Committee on Professional Conduct and Ethics. Boundary Issues as Related to Patient Surrogates. 2000: Federation of State Medical Boards of the United States, Inc.

• CASE 43 •

Ethics of Operating on a Family Member

In the physician or surgeon, no quality takes rank with imperturbability.
Sir William Osler (1849–1919), Aequanimitas

You have developed an effective new surgical procedure to treat a heretofore terminal disease for which all previous therapies were perilous and substantially ineffective. The statistical data indicate that you have mastered the learning curve and can perform the operation with low morbidity and consistently good outcomes. Colleagues are beginning to visit your institution to observe your conduct of the procedure, and you plan to present your results on a small series of patients at an upcoming national meeting. You have for many years been recognized as one of the most technically skilled surgeons working in your specialty. This week you've learned that your grandfather has just been diagnosed as suffering from an advanced state of the condition for which you developed the new operation. What should you do?

(A) Legal and professional prohibitions prevent you from operating on a family member.

(B) You must accept the established ethical principle that a surgeon cannot operate on a family member under any circumstances.

(C) Have a qualified colleague at another institution do the procedure.

(D) Have a colleague do the procedure under your direct supervision.

(E) If you and your grandfather agree, you should do the procedure.

Providing medical or surgical treatment to family, friends, and close colleagues has always touched nerves that lie undisturbed in caring for all other patients. Every physician has had relatives and close friends ask for medical advice or care of one sort or another. Most respond easily with a few suggestions or prescription of a routine noncontrolled medication when the ailment is easily identified, minor, and acute. Many fewer are willing to attempt complex treatment of serious or long-term illnesses among people personally close to them. Surprisingly, one large, well-organized survey found that 9% of qualified physicians had actually operated on family members.[1] Twenty-two percent of the study's respondents said they felt uncomfortable treating family. Another study ranked physician's comfort levels in treating different relatives. Reagan found physicians were most comfortable when providing therapy for their own child and had the least comfort level when treating grandparents, which is why grandpa was chosen for our case.[2]

Emotional overlay markedly affects performance by contributing all the strengths and weaknesses we refer to when we use the term "humanity." Without these feelings we would be without the qualities of empathy, compassion, concern, and much respect for the reasons that there is a medical profession at all. Emotions filter the sensory information we receive and rank-order its importance through personalization. They augment our thoughts, exaggerating or moderating responses; otherwise identical inputs, thus reinterpreted, may yield entirely different reactions dependent upon their emotional contextual interpretation. Emotional organization of perceptual input also has a critical survival function, augmenting discriminative processes. When faced with the realization that a saber toothed tiger was on the prowl, our hominid ancestors would have had entirely different emotional reactions depending upon whether the beast was at the entry to their cave, at the periphery of their tribe's campground, or across the river in the vicinity of another hostile tribe. Great impulsive heroic acts and devotional enhancements to family, nationality, ideals, and religion are stimulated by emotional linkages.

For all the enhancements emotions add to human life, emotions are generally considered in the world's great literature to be at variance with reason. Considered with words denoting behaviors such as impulses, desires, and passions, the ancients, noted philosophers, and the Bible instructed that emotions had to be controlled.[3] Paul instructed the Lycaonians when they wished to honor Barnabas and him that, "We are men of like passions with you, and preach unto you that ye should turn from these vanities..." (Acts 14:15).

As Sir William Osler recommended a century ago, surgeons require detachment and imperturbability because the performance of major surgery is counterintuitive: in any other situation the slicing of another person with a sharp instrument and invasion of the internal organs is the gravest manifestation of aggression and ill will. Surgery harms before it heals, and the consequences of misadventure can be terrible. A clear, disciplined, and decisive mind is critical in evaluating when and how to operate, manage contingencies, and control risks.

These kinds of important considerations help us to understand the cautionary view of the American Medical Association's Council on Ethical and Judicial Affairs: "Physicians generally should not treat themselves or members of their immediate families."[4] The Council is concerned about whether the quality of care a doctor is able to provide will be adversely affected by strong emotional attachments to family members who become patients. Operating on family members can obscure objective judgments and affect the physician's ability to proceed with high-risk options, even when they are most necessary. The emotionally involved physician may misinterpret or deny data suggesting that a family member's diagnosis is more serious than expected, or worsening despite treatment. The physician so-affected may depart from his proven routine to perform an "extraordinary" operation, sometimes euphemized as a "blue plate special," behaving desperately and ill-advisedly to protect his emotional investment and perhaps ultimately doing the patient more harm than good. Relatives may themselves sense the awkwardness of a profound disruption of long-accustomed family roles and find the adaptation difficult when a spouse, child, or sibling suddenly becomes their authoritative physician. It is not unlikely that relatives may be deeply uncomfortable reporting intimate, perhaps embarrassing, personal information to a treating physician who is also a family member, and they may in fact not do so, providing an inaccurate history that ultimately confounds correct diagnosis.[5]

In most ordinary circumstances, patients understand that they must adopt a dispassionate posture toward their physician during the course of treatment, much like the physician's approach to them, so that therapy can proceed smoothly and rationally. The overlay of normal familial affections (or disaffections) upon the doctor-patient relationship risks the addition of a deadly contaminant to this critical dispassion. Issues of control, authority, and boundaries influence all physician-patient relationships, and are prominent factors in the effectiveness of care; they naturally intensify, and can take unexpected and uncontrollable turns, when physician and patient have a long-established history in an entirely different context.[6] The patient who is also your grandfather may be reluctant to accept crucial instructions for postoperative care from his grandson, and you may be unable to invoke the voice of medical authority necessary to insure that your grandfather/patient will act in his own best interest. Your obligation to patient confidentiality will become complicated as other family members begin to impose their own expectations and emotional demands upon you. As the treating physician, you will surely learn things about your grandfather and his medical condition that would normally be far out of bounds to his grandson, and may even pique your nonprofessional interest. You'll have to be prepared to compartmentalize that information and wall it off from your future affectionate relationship with him.

It will be ethically and clinically vital that you do not permit fantasies of heroism to intrude upon your decisions; your grandfather should receive exactly the same preoperative evaluation that you would give any other patient, and you should proceed to operate only after establishing reasonable certainty that his advanced condition will be susceptible to your surgical intervention. Among the additional, and profound, considerations in treating a relative, particularly surgically, will be the potential damage that a bad outcome might have upon your own emotional well-being, and your future interpersonal family relationships.[7] In our fictitious scenario, application of a novel procedure that has been neither extensively tested nor peer reviewed is heavily laden with risk despite early successes.

The ethical principles involved in implementing a new surgical technology demand a sound scientific basis, careful development and refinement, and close training and supervision of newly minted surgical adherents.[8] The surgical learning curve is real. Even relatively minor procedural changes in a center renowned for its surgeons' technical skills required a period of accommodation and refinement among experienced thoracic surgeons who began to use bilateral rather than single internal thoracic artery grafts for coronary bypass.[9] The pattern is consistently replicated with every technical or technological innovation in surgery.[10,11]

Despite published opinions urging special caution, there are in fact no legal or professional prohibitions against operating on family members, eliminating option (A) as a reason for rejecting the concept. The AMA's position specifies exceptions:

> It would not always be inappropriate to undertake self-treatment or treatment of immediate family members. In emergency settings or isolated settings where there is no other qualified physician available, physicians should not hesitate to treat themselves or family members until another physician becomes available.[7]

These considerations reject the absolutist posture of option (B) as well. Refusing to provide essential care to a person in need solely on the basis of relativity places an arguable intellectual principle before relief of acute human suffering, and cannot be defended. Option (C) must be dismissed because there is as yet no surgeon qualified to perform the necessary procedure available at another institution.

Option (D) at first appears to be ethically acceptable. Having a colleague under your direct supervision at the operating table would allow your expertise to benefit your grandfather and would buffer the emotional constraints. Most surgical expertise is transferred to inexperienced surgeons in just such a manner during surgical residencies and fellowships. Nevertheless, even a very skilled and adept colleague will still be low on the learning curve, with an added increment of risk to the patient. To manage such risk, the possibility that you may have to step in and take over the operation cannot be ruled out.

Option (E) is ethically acceptable, provided that you frankly acknowledge and prospectively manage the sort of personal and professional conflicts we've just described. The advantage of accepting option (E) is of course that you are the only surgeon qualified to perform this operation. You can help to minimize the disadvantages by fully adopting your medical persona during the course of treatment. Think of and refer to your grandfather in clinical reflection and in discussion with colleagues as "the patient" and not as "my grandfather." The words you use will help to frame and discipline your judgment and behavior. You would be well advised to thoroughly review the patient's case with an experienced colleague, accept the dispassionate authority of his recommendations, and ask him to join the case as second surgeon. You should assure the patient that he can speak freely about his health and other concerns, and describe to him how the usual rules for managing confidential information will be rigorously followed: only information that he specifically authorizes will be disclosed to family. You should not abbreviate the consent process or otherwise permit an atmosphere of familiarity to alter your standard patient procedures. Fully explain both the benefits and risks of the proposed operation, neither shielding the patient from such information nor protecting yourself by hanging crepe. You must anticipate, and discuss with a thoughtful and disciplined colleague, the possibility that the patient could experience major, potentially unmanageable complications. Finally, you should have a frank and detailed conversation with the patient about end-of-life care in the event that the operation leaves him dependent on a ventilator in the SICU or otherwise dysfunctional.

You should present options (D) and (E) to the patient, as well as information about their benefits and risks. You should make it clear to your grandfather that you will implement the alternative that he prefers. Your grandfather has probably lived long enough to have encountered complicated emotions and contending imperatives before, and may even be able to lend you some of his own wisdom to untangle the problem, as so many patients do.

References

1. La Puma J, Stocking CB, La Voie D, Darling CA. When physicians treat members of their own families: Practices in a community hospital. *N Engl J Med*. 1991; 325:1290–1294.

2. Reagan B, Reagan P, Sinclair A. "Common sense and a thick hide": Physicians providing care to their own family members. *Arch Fam Med*. 1994; 3:599–604.

3. Editorial Staff of the Great Books. Emotion. In: Adler M, ed. *The Great Ideas: A Syntopicon*. Chicago: Encyclopedia Britannica, Inc., 1952.

4. American Medical Association. *Council on Ethical and Judicial Affairs, Code of Medical Ethics: Current Opinions with Annotations*. Chicago: AMA Press, 1996.

5. Moreno J, Lucente F. Patients who are family members, friends, colleagues, family members of colleagues. In: McCullough LB, Jones JW, Brody BA, eds. *Surgical Ethics*. New York: Oxford University Press, 1998:198–215.

6. Street R Jr, Krupat R, Bell RA, Kravitz RL, Haidet P. Beliefs about control in the physician-patient relationship: Effect on communication in medical encounters. *J Gen Int Med*. 2003; 18:609–622.

7. American Medical Association. Council on Ethical and Judicial Affairs. American Medical Association. Opinion 8:19: Self-treatment of treatment of Immediate Family. Code of Medical Ethics. Chicago: AMA Press, 2002.

8. Jones JW. Ethics of rapid surgical technological advancement. *Ann Thorac Surg*. 2000; 69:676–677.

9. Lytle BW, Cosgrove DM, Loop FD, Borsh J, Goormastic M, Taylor PC. Perioperative risk of bilateral internal mammary artery grafting: Analysis of 500 cases from 1971 to 1984. *Circulation*. 1986; 74(Pt 2):III 37–41.

10. Dagash H, Chowdhury M, Pierro A. When can I be proficient in laparoscopic surgery? A systematic review of the evidence. *J Pediatr Surg*. 2003; 38:720–724.

11. Gates EA New surgical procedures: Can our patients benefit while we learn? *Am J Obstet Gynecol*. 1997; 176:1293–1298.

· 6 ·

THE ETHICS OF SURGERY

AS A BUSINESS

Somehow, calling medicine a business strikes a wrong chord, one that might even suggest a pejorative association. "Profession" seems at first more appropriate, implying that physicians are specially educated and reliably conform to ethical standards of behavior. But don't we apply these terms to the oldest profession, or to "professional" athletes? Perhaps medicine can better be thought of as a calling, a calling to a well-compensated secular priesthood of health.

When relieved of the lay public's idealistic fantasies about what we do for a living, the practice of medicine is in fact both a profession and a business. Dealing, usually honorably and skillfully, in the near-priceless commodity of health and life it is an honored calling, but it nevertheless remains a business. The practice of medicine is unique in its ethical complexities because it is founded in the instincts of altruism, yet exchanges its services for money. Altruism always has limits. The witch's brew of lengthy specialized preparation, human frailty, human mortality, ethical commitment, high overhead, generous impulses, complex finances, third-party payers, government regulations, and the various benefits and corruptions of the medical-industrial complex, comprise what economists consider the most complicated micro-economic model in existence.[1]

There are many ways for Mammon to tempt the modern physician; some have been around for centuries, and some have been more recently concocted. The oldest and still prominent way in which physicians are paid is the fee-for-service. Before the introduction of third-party private insurance and national payment systems, most medical and surgical services were available only to the well-to-do, who could afford the physician's fees. Over two centuries ago, Dr. John Gregory made a strong distinction between medicine as an "art" and medicine as a "trade." As an "art," the practice of medicine involved the application of scientific knowledge and clinical skills in the management of disease and injury, and could be considered a "profession." As a "trade," medical practice was a source of income, an activity deeply embedded in self-interest.

Gregory was among the first to address the potential for conflict between medicine as art or profession, and medicine as a vehicle for financial self-interest. He wrote that:

> Physicians, considered as a body of men, who live by medicine as a profession, have an interest separate and distinct from the honor of the science. In pursuit of this interest, some have acted with candor, with honor, with the ingenuous

and liberal manners of gentlemen. Conscious of their own worth, they disdained every artifice, and depended for success on their real merit. But such men are not the most numerous in any profession. Some impelled by necessity, some stimulated by vanity, and others anxious to conceal ignorance, have had recourse to various mean and unworthy arts, to raise their importance among the ignorant, who are always the most numerous part of mankind.[2]

Here Gregory refers to the then-common practices of advertising one's practice through pamphlets, or establishing one's favorable reputation by publishing a book touting one's secret remedies. He believed that putting economic self-interest first would distort the scientific practice of medicine and thereby put patients' health and lives at unnecessary risk. He argues further that such behavior is antithetical to scientific integrity and the physician's life of service to patients. In modern terms, we can say that properly managing the inherent conflict of interest between the physician's skilled and compassionate care of the sick and the physician's legitimate entitlement to make a living requires constant vigilance and sensitivity to one's ethical responsibilities. The physician whose primary interest is the generation of income will practice medicine badly; the physician who in his or her zeal for altruism pays no attention to his or her means of personal sustenance will not be able to care for the sick for long.

Foremost in the contemporary nonsalaried practice of medicine is the conflicted situation of supplier-induced-demand (SID) that inescapably structures fee-for-service practice: physicians recommend patient therapy and thereby determine their own rate of income; the more therapy prescribed, the greater the income. This arrangement obviously presents a danger to patients of being placed at risk for overtreatment and iatrogenic disorders. Although rarely acknowledged, the SID aspect of practice places the most demand on the physician's fiduciary role. We will explore this profound ethical dilemma more deeply in one of the cases you will soon be reading.

Personal practice choices can create additional ethical paradoxes. Should one advertise as respectable businesses do? After long condemnation of the practice as inherently unethical and beneath the dignity of proper professionals, recent years have seen our most august professional organizations and the federal government itself approving the practice of physician marketing. Drug companies pepper the airways with images of smiling, happy people romping amid butterflies and tail-wagging doggies. What about reorienting a practice to serve only a select prepaid membership group, as in boutique practices, providing better service for higher fees? Isn't commercialization about giving people what they want? And what of the ancient tradition of professional courtesy, banned from medical practice not by physicians, but by insurance companies? Was the elimination of unbilled care to colleagues, who could be expected to reciprocate, ethically justified? Was the practice itself ever ethically wrong?

Surgeons in teaching institutions work with trainees, who, as part of their training, do substantial parts of the work that faculty physicians get paid to do. What is a reasonable approach to compensation for a medical teacher?

Insurers, especially managed care organizations, and the hospitals where we practice, have become more adversarial than any of us could have imagined late in the last century. What should we do when we disagree with their marketing of our medical services? Administrative, and especially economic, credentialing are big departures from the cost-plus era.

As noted in the concluding pages of the previous chapter, the medical-industrial complex has begun intrusions with research grants that exceed government research spending and are far easier to obtain. They may offer lavish consultancies, gifts, banquets, and exotic trips that can distort the fiduciary obligations of a surgical practice. In many instances, industry's thinly veiled altruism is attempting to commandeer our credentials and convert them into billboards for their products and practices. Who owns the rights to our credentials and our profession's reputation for ethical behavior? How much are you willing to sell yours for? We should not forget that our moral value is worth precisely what we will sell it for. In the pages ahead, we have tried to select case studies that explore these boundaries and suggest some direction an ethical surgeon might take upon reaching the confluence of surgical professionalism and the business of surgery.

References

1. Folland S, Goodman AC, Stano, M. *The Economics of Health and Health Care*. 3rd ed. Upper Saddle River, NJ: Prentice Hall, 2001.
2. Gregory J. Lectures on the duties and qualifications of a physician. In McCullough LB, ed. *John Gregory's Writings on Medical Ethics and Philosophy of Medicine*. Dordrecht, The Netherlands: Kluwer Academic Publishers, 1998.

· CASE 44 ·

Show Me the Money: The Ethics of Physicians' Income

Money was never a big motivation for me, except as a way to keep score.
Donald Trump, *Trump: Art of the Deal*

Starting from the middle of the last century with enactment of the first Medicare legislation, followed two decades thereafter with the concept of Diagnostic Related Groups, and then the advent of the euphemistically-named Health Maintenance Organization (HMO), the financial complexion of medical practice changed for the foreseeable future. Since then, reductions and delays in reimbursement by third party payers, ever-rising copays, and an unending proliferation of costly regulations and pressures by accrediting bodies and government agencies have rained down on us like plagues upon Egypt. Are we right to object, and how should we ethically respond to the effect these measures have had on physicians' incomes?

(A) Society is trying to ratchet down the cost of medical care while expecting constant improvement in medical science, technology, procedures, and life expectancy. Tell your patients that this is unfair to physicians.

(B) Political promises of low-cost medical care cannot be met. Influence the political system by opposing all candidates unsympathetic to physician interests.

(C) Stop accepting Medicare and Medicaid patients and don't enter preferred provider contracts with private insurers who will fix your rates at discounted prices.

(D) Continue to base your practice on the best available clinical evidence, and strictly limit your interventions to indicated treatment.

(E) Compensate for lost revenue by performing more billable procedures and scheduling more appointments for your patients to increase your total charges to Medicare and private insurers.

The physician's fiduciary relationship with patients is one of the major foundations of medical ethics. The fiduciary relationship compels the physician to place the patient's clinical needs before the physician's self-interest in professional advancement, convenience, or personal compensation. The ethical requirement that the patient must come first does not, however, mean that the physician's individual needs cannot come next, or that the physician has no legitimate entitlement to the fruit of his or her labor. Only a relatively few in any culture can satisfy the rigorous requirements essential to the physician's function. Few indeed have endured as long or as rigorous a period of preparation or are expected to contribute as much to their societies as physicians, and it is just and proper that their compensation is calculated accordingly. Medicine remains a relatively lucrative profession for most practitioners despite recent annoyances, and most of us earn everything we make.

For almost three decades after the conclusion of World War II, the United States experienced unprecedented annual economic growth rates, primarily because the industrial capacities of our potential European and Asian competitors had been destroyed by more than half a decade of total war. With the reconstitution of foreign industry and development of a global market economy following the end of the Cold War, the U.S. growth rate returned to a solid but less robust annual pace. Business became increasingly cost-conscious, and wage expansion slowed. American corporate and individual tax payers put increasing pressure on government to contain and reduce taxes. First the Medicare system and then private health insurance plans and HMOs put downward pressure on physician reimbursement. Physicians responded to the reductions with a variety of strategies to maintain a status quo that had traditionally been very friendly to them.

Predictably, medical economists began to interpret the medical profession's defensive maneuvers as lapses in financial integrity.[1] There certainly was, and perhaps remains, enough verifiable fraud in Medicare billing by physicians to keep the economists' suspicions boiling, but, more than that, two kinds of large-scale medical economic studies lay at the base of their doubts about how doctors behaved, and became major influences in the drive to lower physician reimbursements. One of them operated from a thoroughly false premise and naturally reached faulty conclusions, and the other entangled itself in a paralyzing paradox.

The first of these two study methods is the Small Area Variation (SAV). Economic studies of SAV tended to look skeptically upon geographic differences in units of care per population, which, as a matter of convenience, usually counted easily numerated medical procedures as their units of measure. Economists were shocked to find that in some areas in the United States markedly more medical procedures of a particular type were performed than others. Studies in New England over three decades ago, showing twice the number of hysterectomies done from one town to the next, introduced the methodology.[2] Later investigators often found, after adjusting for age, disease prevalence, gender, and economic status, that some regions showed persistent variations in procedural incidence. A study of 44,000 myocardial infarction patients in 95 selected regions found statistically significant SAVs in the number of patients in each area who had received angiograms.[3] One geographic region had a ten-fold incidence of tympanostomy tube insertion over other supposedly matched regions.[4] Hundreds of other papers by medical economists over the years confirmed patterns of geographic variation in the incidence of medical procedures per population. The economists controlled for many demographic variables, but they missed the most important ones, and of course the resultant conclusion was deeply flawed.

The conclusion that the economists reached and passed on to governmental and private third-party payers was that the frequency of SAVs indicated prescription by doctors of excessive, expensive, unindicated treatment in the high-frequency procedure areas. They further concluded that the data proved that procedural medicine, of which the surgical specialties were the most prominent practitioners, was fat and ripe for cutting. Their premises and conclusions were wrong because their adjusted variables made inadequate distinctions between areas like rural counties with a single bare-bones hospital, and major urban centers. In a study of 19,000 patients having knee replacements, counties with more medical school affiliated beds had significantly higher rates.[5] The economists' main parameter was only the number of adjusted procedures per capita, without much allowance for the local ease of access to the procedures being considered or the likelihood of referral to another county having greater expertise. All these and the other complex cases were of course referred to the fully-equipped private clinics or medical schools, and the increased procedural workload in their counties was then interpreted as irresponsible wastefulness.

The second of the medical economists' major areas of study was Supplier (Physician)-Induced Demand (PID). Procedurally, much like the auto mechanic, whom we all suspect of black-hearted corruption, the physician advises a substantially naïve and anxious clientele of what's wrong and then what the physician will do to fix it. Since the physician effectively controls both the demand and the supply side of the economic equation, the environment fairly invites an expansive interpretation of the problem.

Economists developed and studied the target-income model of Physician-Induced-Demand early in Medicare's fee regulation era. As fees were decreased by Medicare managers, physicians did in fact compensate by increasing their services to Medicare patients, enough to replace from 40%[6] to 70%[7] of lost income. Medical care consumption in the more lucrative private insurance sector was also increased during this period, perhaps to an even greater degree, as doctors scrambled to catch up.[6] When physicians weren't making additional interventions to compensate for the lowered profitability of some Medicare-targeted procedures, they made up the difference by applying their time to something else. A 10% decrease in Medicare's physician payments for cataract removal caused a 5% increase in the incidence of noncataract procedures.[8] In a community which fluoridated its water, dentists compensated for the reduction in corrective dental services by increasing their restorative work.[9] Correctly reading the implications of continued reductions in Medicare fees in a PID market, economists advised Medicare governors that if physicians' fees fell too low, doctors would react by increasing the number of procedures and other billable encounters among all their patients, and ultimately, because of increased hospital bills, raise the overall national cost of medical care.[10]

When increased utilization of angiography was examined according to guidelines proposed by the American College of Cardiology, the investigators found that the increase occurred in the group for which angiography was clinically indicated and effective, not in the unindicated group.[11] As medicine becomes more successful in prolonging life, the general population increases, grows older, and requires continuing care. A significant rise in the number of patients treated does a lot more to increase the total cost of medical care than an increase in physicians' fees would by itself. Improved screening methods like mammography, advanced imaging, colonoscopy, and various batched screening laboratory tests all create new costs, in and of themselves, and by identifying disease processes which then require treatment. Public education programs encourage people to ask their doctors for these studies. Preventive care has been shown to be effective in reducing subsequent high cost morbidities, ranging from dental care to vascular procedures.[12,13] Early in the 21st century, preventive medical care is neither well scripted nor universalized. Medical care utilization obeys ancient economic laws of consumption: it rises as insurance makes its cost to the patient fall,[13] providing patients little incentive for limiting their requests.

The sum of the available evidence is that physicians and surgeons committed to preserving their elevated financial status have responded creatively at times with questionable ethics to reduced reimbursements from third-party payers. When physicians permit economic self-interest to eclipse fiduciary responsibility and professional integrity, they become more likely to offer, recommend, and perform diagnostic and therapeutic services for which clinical indications are marginal. Surgical overtreatment in particular is not benign. As costly and painful as it is to patients, it is deadly to professional integrity and public trust in our profession. As early as the mid-18th century, the medical ethicist John Gregory foresaw that unscrupulous physicians could enrich themselves by exploiting the worried well, indulging their anxieties with frequent office visits and abundant medical procedures, and ultimately create an actual threat rather than a benefit to their patients' health, as well as to doctors' professionalism. Gregory urged physicians to understand that their best long-term personal and professional interest lay in honoring their fiduciary responsibility, observing an ethical standard of care in treating patients, and building community trust in the profession's knowledge, effectiveness, and integrity.[14]

Option (A) invites patients to respond sympathetically to their doctors' complaints of reduced economic circumstances, and perhaps to gladly take a greater proportion of the physician's compensation upon themselves. There is a subtly coercive element in such an approach, an implication that the patient's stated agreement is required if he is to continue to receive the doctor's best effort in treating him. Patients are unlikely to spontaneously respond sympathetically to the personal financial worries of physicians whom they rightly believe are in most cases far more affluent than themselves. Option (A) should be rejected as potentially unethical at worst and unseemly at best.

As the data we've cited support, physicians do indeed bear considerable responsibility for the amount of medical care they provide. Asking the political system alone to save physicians denies their own poor practice, ultimately shifting the burdens of these costs to others in the society. It evades responsibility for correcting problems internal to the medical profession, and does nothing to improve the quality or availability of care. Option (B) should be rejected.

Option (C) must be rejected as unethical because if widespread, it would deprive needy elderly and poor patients of access to technically superior care. As a business decision, it would surely be disastrous; many of the surgical disciplines are substantially geriatric specialties supported by Medicare. The greatest proportion of coronary bypasses, carotid endarterectomies, aneurysmectomies, joint replacements, and major intestinal procedures that are the bread and butter of thoracic, vascular, orthopedic, and general surgical practices are performed on elderly patients who rely on Medicare to cover their costs. Private insurers with whom you decline discounted contracts simply advise their patients that they should seek other providers to maximize their coverage.

Option (E) subjects patients to the serious risks of overtreatment, diminishes the physician's professionalism, and is in many cases grossly illegal. It is to be rejected as the most unethical of the choices offered.

Option (D), continuing to practice surgery on the basis of scientific evidence, clinical indications, fiduciary responsibility, and empathic regard for the genuine needs of patients, remains the best response to the forces that have buffeted medicine. Your long and difficult years of training, the knowledge and skill you have acquired through hard and dedicated work, and the enormous good that you do within your community have indeed earned you the opportunity to make a comfortable and secure living. They have not earned any of us the right to game the system, mistreat patients, or take more than we've earned. The culture continues to hold us in high esteem and compensate us well, substantially because it still trusts us to behave ethically, empathically, and to serve our patients' interests before our own. When any members of our profession overtreat and sicken their patients to feather their own nests, we are all put at risk for losing the trust of our fellow humans.

References

1. Folland S, Goodman A, Stano M. *The Economics of Health and Health Care*. 3rd ed. Upper Saddle River, NJ: Prentice Hall, 2001.
2. Wennberg J, Gittelsohn M. Small area variations in health care delivery. *Science*. 1973; 182:1102–1108.
3. Wright JG, Hawker GA, Bombardier C, Croxford R, Dittus RS, Freund D, A, Coyte PC. Physician enthusiasm as an explanation for area variation in the utilization of knee replacement surgery. *Med Care*. 1999; 37:946–956.
4. Coyte PC, Croxford R, Asche CV, To T, Feldman W, Friedberg, J. Physician and population determinants of rates of middle-ear surgery in Ontario. *Jama*. 2001; 286:2128–2135.
5. Guadagnoli E, Landrum MB, Normand SL, Ayanian JZ, Garg P, Hauptman PJ, et. al. Impact of underuse, overuse, and discretionary use on geographic variation in the use of coronary angiography after acute myocardial infarction. *Med Care*. 2001; 39:446–458.

6. Rice T, Stearns SC, Pathman DE, DesHarnais S, Brasure M, Tai-Seale M, A tale of two bounties: the impact of competing fees on physician behavior. *J Health Polit Policy Law*. 1999; 24:1307–1330.

7 Yip W. Physician response to Medicare fee reductions: changes in the volume of coronary artery bypass graft (CABG) surgeries in the Medicare and private sectors. *J Health Econ*. 1998; 17:675–699.

8. Mitchell JM, Hadley J, Gaskin DJ. Spillover effects of Medicare fee reductions: Evidence from ophthalmology. *Int J Health Care Finance Econ*. 2002; 2:171–188.

9. Grembowski D, Fiset L, Milgrom P, Conrad D, Spadafora A. Does fluoridation reduce the use of dental services among adults? *Med Care*. 1997; 35:454–471.

10. Bernstein J., Policy implications of physician income homeostasis. *J Health Care Finance*. 1998; 24:80–86.

11. Litzelman DK, Slemenda CW, Langefeld CD, Hays LM, Welch MA, Bild DE, et al. Reduction of lower extremity clinical abnormalities in patients with non-insulin-dependent diabetes mellitus: A randomized, controlled trial. *Ann Intern Med*. 1993; 119:36–41.

12. Guadagnoli E, Landrum MB, Peterson EA, Gahart MT, Ryan TJ, McNeil BJ. Appropriateness of coronary angiography after myocardial infarction among Medicare beneficiaries. Managed care versus fee for service. *N Engl J Med*. 2000; 343:1460–1466.

13. Anderson G.M., R. Brook, and A. Williams, A comparison of cost-sharing versus free care in children: Effects on the demand for office-based medical care. *Med Care*. 1991; 29:890–898.

14. McCullough LB *John Gregory and the Invention of Professional Medical Ethics and the Profession of Medicine*. 1998, Dordrecht, the Netherlands: Klwuer Academic Publisher.

• CASE 45 •

Ethics of Institutional Marketing: The Role of Physicians

Advertising is the rattling of a stick inside a swill bucket.
Eric Arthur Blair (George Orwell) (1903–1950)

You are a senior surgeon practicing at a private academically unaffiliated urban hospital. The program enjoys a reputation for excellent clinical care. While driving in to work this morning, you heard a radio advertisement extolling your hospital's status as the most technologically advanced surgery program in the country. As proud as you are of your hospital's genuine good work, you know this claim to be excessive and misleading. While you don't believe that anyone is obligated buy commercial air time to advertise their shortcomings, you're troubled that in this case your hospital is actually be misrepresenting itself to the community. When you approach the chief of staff with your concerns later in the day, he replied, "This is the institution's marketing policy, it is a necessary evil, and has nothing to do with you." What should you do?

(A) Complain to the hospital administration.
(B) Forget the whole thing before you get into trouble; you are not responsible.
(C) Call a newspaper reporter and tell him your story.
(D) Request a written statement of support for your objection at the next surgical staff meeting.
(E) Inform the administration that you will leave the staff if the radio ads are not withdrawn.

Most American hospitals have entered the 21st century in an intensely competitive market environment. Words like downsizing, acquisition, and even bankruptcy have entered the daily healthcare lexicon, particularly within hospitals that fail to compete successfully for patients. Some hospitals have felt the need to put survival first among their institutional goals, the position traditionally occupied by excellence in patient care. In a field where advertising was once considered unseemly, unprofessional, and unethical, "marketing" came to be viewed first as tolerable, then as normative, then as important, and ultimately as a necessary evil. The advertising industry methods that have sold so many cigarettes, patent medicines, and vacation timeshares were soon to find their way into the healthcare professions.

The prospective patients who select one hospital over another at some of the most critical and terrifying moments of their lives are not just buying products like tobacco and condominiums, though. They are very consciously paying for and relying upon the professional integrity of the hospital and the physicians who practice there. If that breaks down, no hospital can just order a new one from the manufacturer. The institution's reputation for integrity is at least as important to its survival as its medical technology. Everyone working within the organization is responsible for creating, sustaining, and nurturing the image and the reality of that integrity.

Consistent with the medical profession in which they function, hospitals must share and support the physician's core ethical principles of beneficence, fiduciary responsibility, respect for autonomy, and nonmaleficence.[1,2] Physicians, notably surgeons, and the hospitals in which they practice, are mutual trustees of one another's reputations for honesty, competence, and integrity. Mishandling or disregard of any of these precious principles by either member of the physician-hospital partnership reflects upon the other. The hospital establishes and enforces physician compliance with its professional standards by granting or withholding clinical privileges. Physicians are equivalently entitled to expect hospitals to comply and cooperate with the central ethical ideals of the medical profession. Just as the hospital's credentialing process requires the physician to document his or her claims of education, training, certification, and practice experience, the medical staff should insist that the hospital's marketers make no claim that cannot be supported by the facts.

McKneally has written that, "like electricity, which can be used for torture or illumination, medical advertising is intrinsically value neutral; its application determines its ethical standing."[3] The institution or surgeon that deals in inflated claims of clinical effectiveness becomes the ethical equivalent of the charlatan, pitching useless nostrums, preying upon the special gullibilities of the sick and desperate, and standing between patients and their true best interests. Both will justify their methods as necessary to their livelihood. Judiciously considered and applied, hospital advertising should be designed as the opening steps in the process of informed consent. Claims intended to persuade prospective patients to select one hospital and not another should share the medical profession's obligation to present factually accurate information to treatment candidates. Overstating probable benefits and minimizing disclosure of therapeutic risk is inconsistent with the principles of informed consent, and should be considered equivalently unacceptable in institutional marketing. As much as such claims misrepresent individual hospital services, they more deeply undermine the professional culture of integrity and fiduciary responsibility that patients most value when entrusting themselves to the care of a medical institution.

Option (A), protesting the false advertisement to your hospital's administration, may be like complaining to the local fox that someone has raided your henhouse. The germ for exaggerated claims about the internationally renowned surgery program probably originated in your in-house PR department before it was suggested to the advertising agency that crafted the radio spot. Although your objection is ethically sound, the chief of staff's annoyed response is a likely indication of how your lone protest will be received in the hospital's executive suite.

Option (B) is offensive to your ethical sensibility. The way your hospital conducts its business reflects upon you and your integrity. The hospital is intensely interested in the quality of your practice. You are entitled to be equally concerned about the manner in which it conducts itself.

Option (C) violates the essential spirit of professional collegiality by allowing no opportunity for reasoned internal debate among those best-suited to address these issues. Public disclosure as a first step is divisive and is likely to unfairly damage everyone connected with the hospital. Regardless of its effectiveness in creating and emphasizing public outrage, the news media rarely improves the practice of medicine. Option (E) may serve to articulate your own integrity, but is unlikely to affect the institution's failure to acknowledge its shared obligation to accept the role of patient fiduciary.

Your fellow surgeons probably share your sense of embarrassment and dismay over the hospital's exaggerated claims of technological superiority, particularly because the advertising message imposes upon them a series of expectations that the institution has not equipped them to meet. Your surgical colleagues can be expected to support you in pursuing option (D), our choice. The surgical service's united voice of alarm is likely to persuade hospital executives to resolve the advertising dilemma in one of two ways. They must refrain from advertising the institution's technological superiority until they can legitimize their claims by purchasing the advanced equipment they claim to have and ensuring that their staff is fully trained in its use. If presenting a united front fails, the legitimate ethical concerns of the hospital's physicians can be taken all the way to the board of trustees or board of directors if necessary. Conformation and validation of the ethical breeches can be obtained by appealing to your institutional ethics committee or the Ethics Committee of the American College of Surgeons. If such a concerted effort fails, the surgeon and all of his colleagues must consider whether they want to continue to associate themselves with an organization that knowingly violates the standards of intellectual and moral excellence required of a medical cofiduciary.

Eventually, all hospitals will have to conform to the ethical principles of honesty, integrity, and fiduciary responsibility which guide physicians in every element of their practice. A true cofiduciary relationship should be achieved and prized in every medical care institution.

References

1. McCullough LB. A basic concept in the clinical ethics of managed care: Physicians and institutions as economically disciplined moral co-fiduciaries of populations of patients. *J Med Philos.* 1999; 24:77–97.
2. Chervenak FA, McCullough LB. Physicians and hospitals as co-fiduciaries of patients: rhetoric or reality. *J Healthc Manag.* 2003; 48:172–179.
3. McKneally MF. Controversies in cardiothoracic surgery: is it ethical to advertise surgical results to increase referrals? *J Thorac Cardiovasc Surg.* 2002; 123:839–841.

• CASE 46 •

Ethics of Boutique Medical Practice

The higher the buildings, the lower the morals.
Noel Coward (1889–1973)

You are a surgeon sitting on the board of directors of a large private clinic. The group is considering offering a premium healthcare option to patients. For a direct monthly retainer of $150 over and above fees covered by the enrollee's insurance plan, patients will receive unhurried visits, same day appointments, regular comprehensive physical exams, house calls, and complete direct access to the physicians providing their care every day around the clock. Staff physicians will accompany patients requiring emergency care to the ER. Patients who do not choose the high-option plan will continue to receive the same excellent care for which the clinic is well-known, but without preferential access. The VP for marketing strongly advocates the proposed program because it will draw an affluent patient population, and most likely one that requires a higher than usual frequency and complexity of care, broadening the clinic's revenue base with enrollment and a substantially higher volume of third-party billing. What is your position on the question of whether to adopt such a program?

(A) Boutique practice reduces medicine to a commodity, unacceptably diminishing professionalism. You vote "No."
(B) There is no ethical compromise if the marketing and quality assurance programs observe adequate standard safeguards.
(C) The clinic should separately incorporate physicians serving the high option patient group from those who do not, and limit their practices to their respective groups.
(D) The additional funds must be dedicated to indigent care.
(E) Each physician is entitled to structure his practice as he sees fit within the regulations of the presiding state medical board.

Because the intrinsic value of life is considered in Western culture to be equivalent among all individuals and not economically quantifiable, the quality of medical care upon which life often depends cannot ethically be negotiable based on the patient's ability to pay the physician more or less. The physician's best efforts and the resources required to implement them are expected to be made available to every patient in need of care. Despite this ideal, the world's best care is available in the world's richest countries, and the distribution of quality care manages to follow this pattern to the level of the individual patient. The thoroughness of evaluation and admission of patients with head injuries is associated with insurance coverage.[1] Receipt of coronary bypass and other costly therapies is highly correlated with the ability to pay.[2] Socioeconomically disadvantaged myocardial infarction patients were less likely to receive appropriate diagnostic and treatment services than affluent cohorts.[3] A number of studies confirm that adequate pain management is more readily available to the affluent than to those who are not.[4]

Economic pressures on surgeons exist and are mounting. Medicare and Medicaid reimbursements are adjusted ever-downward, internists broaden their practices to include invasive procedures, and we graduate more new competitors from our residency programs than the profession can provide for. In such an environment, it is entirely sensible for surgeons to survey the landscape for new revenue sources. If the practice of medicine were nothing more than another entrepreneurial scheme, few could object to the proposal that this physician group add a boutique option to its practice. The only ethical constraints would be those of honest business practice in maintaining good quality care for all.[5] Option (B) would therefore be entirely acceptable.

Our profession is not, however, understood in either medical law or medical ethics to be an entrepreneurial undertaking. Instead, medicine is understood to be a profession characterized by fiduciary responsibilities not expected of entrepreneurs. This concept was developed in the 18th century by physicians John Gregory[6] and Thomas Percival,[7] the foundational medical ethicists to whom we have regularly referred throughout this volume as authoritative voices in untangling many of the dilemmas we evaluate.

The ethical concept of physician as patient fiduciary has three components. First, the physician should be scientifically and clinical competent. Percival both understood competence in terms of applied scientific knowledge, and introduced the nascent concept of what we now call evidence-based medicine.[7] He wrote that physicians should use their knowledge and skills primarily to benefit their patients and not primarily to advance the physician's self-interest. The physician's self-interest, even including his or her right to an income and personal security, should be a secondary consideration in the practice of medicine. Third, the medical profession should be considered a public trust, to be protected and advanced primarily for the benefit of patients, both present and future. To be sure, physicians and surgeons work hard to acquire and improve their clinical knowledge and skills, but they do not create such knowledge and skills using only their own resources: they rely very much on the past achievements of physicians and surgeons and the huge expenditures of societal resources invested in medical education, research, and patient care to learn and refine their craft.

Gregory in particular was concerned that physicians gave better treatment to those who could better afford their services than to the working sick poor. These patients were typically seen in the Royal Infirmary of Edinburgh, newly founded by Scotland's major industrial employers to insure the health and regular work attendance of their labor pool. Physicians and surgeons who were publicly paid to care for Infirmary patients were considered unworthy of professional status, while those serving the carriage trade were afforded high status. Gregory was offended by the resulting hypocrisy.

It might be said that patients opting for boutique medical treatment are merely purchasing convenience. By buying additional increments of the physician's time and attention, they likely believe they are investing in superior care. There is, however, no evidence that boutique medicine and surgery improves or does not improve outcomes. Either result would be ethically unacceptable, and on that basis alone the concept violates the ethical principle of care unrelated to physician self-interest. The bargain offers better access and the illusion of better care, but actually provides only better access.

The alleged standard of care—including prompt scheduling, continuity of care, rapid response to urgent needs—that boutique practices offer should already be the standard of care for all patients, as a matter of strict fiduciary responsibility. The provision of improved accessibility for one group necessarily diminishes accessibility for the have-nots.

A two-tiered system of medicine is inconsistent with intellectual integrity because it lacks any support in evidence-based medicine, and with moral integrity, because its ultimate goal is to advance the financial self-interest of physicians, not to improve therapeutic outcomes. Option (A) is therefore the only ethically justified response to this proposal. The acceptability of boutique practice by the American Medical Association's House of Delegates represents intellectually and morally disordered thinking and should not be regarded as authoritative.[8] The AMA's euphemism of "retainer medicine" suggests the world of divorce attorneys and private detective agencies, to whose ethical principles physicians cannot proudly aspire.

There are no established standards in boutique practice, so option (B) is unacceptable. Option (C) produces a two-tiered system of medical practice and is *a fortiori* unacceptable. Option (D) will not do, because charitable application of income obtained unethically cannot excuse the ethical breach. If shortening time spent with regular patients to increase time with higher-paying patients is robbing from the poor to give to the rich, robbing from the rich to give to the poor is no less unethical. The accumulated authority of medical ethics contradicts the proposition of option (E).

Rewarding increased convenience with increased revenue in an amount chosen by recipients is widely practiced in the nonprofessional service industry as tipping ("to ensure promptness"); its resemblance to boutique medical practice suggests a degree of abasement unworthy of our profession.

References

1. Svenson JE, Spurlock CW, Insurance status and admission to hospital for head injuries: Are we part of a two-tiered medical system? *Am J Emerg Med.* 2001; 19:19–24.
2. Jones JW. The question of racial bias in thoracic surgery: Appearances and realities. *Ann Thorac Surg.* 2001; 72:6–8.
3. Haywood LJ, Ell, K, deGuman EK, M, Norris M, S, Blumfield S, Sobel D, E, Chest pain admissions: Characteristics of black, Latino, and white patients in low- and mid-socioeconomic strata. *J Natl Med Assoc.* 1993; 85:749–757.

4. Cleeland CS. Gonin R, Baez L, Loehrer P,,Pandya KJ, Pain and treatment of pain in minority patients with cancer. The Eastern Cooperative Oncology Group Minority Outpatient Pain Study. *Ann Intern Med.* 1997; 127:813–816.
5. Brody BA. The physician as professional and the physician as honest businessman. *Arch Otolaryngol Head Neck Surg.* 1993; 119:495–497.
6. McCullough LB, ed. *John Gregory's Writings on Medical Ethics and Philosophy of Medicine.* Dordrecht, The Netherlands: Kluwer Academic Publishers, 1998:170.
7. Percival T. *Medical Ethics, or a Code of Institutes and Precepts, Adapted to the Professional Conduct of Physicians and Surgeons.* London: Johnson and Bickerstaff, 1803.
8. Fraser R. *AMA Delegates Adopt Ethical Guidelines for Retainer Practices (Boutique Care).* Chicago: American Medical Association House of Delegates, 2003.

• CASE 47 •

Ethics and Commercial Insurance

All men are frauds. The only difference between them is that some admit it.
I myself deny it.
H.L. Mencken (1880–1956)

You have just seen a 59-year-old diabetic lady with a several year history of debilitating claudication which has recently progressed to rest pain. She has just changed employers, and her new health insurance plan specifically excludes preexisting conditions. She explains that she did not specify her peripheral vascular disease on her enrollment form because she thought her symptoms were just muscle spasms. To obtain treatment approval from the insurer, your billing clerk needs to know whether or not the condition preexisted. Your response?

(A) Get the approval by whatever means necessary. It is ethical to skirt insurer's restrictions to help your patient.

(B) Call the insurer and formally appeal on the patient's behalf

(C) Tell the patient to call an attorney.

(D) Petition your congressional representatives to enact laws prohibiting preexisting condition clauses in private plans.

(E) Tell your patient to quit her job and apply for Medicaid.

Many complex ethical and economic problems are directly entangled with management of commercial health insurance.[1] Our culture is ambivalent about whether health care is a right or a privilege, with opinions varying dependent upon the population segments in question and the providing institution. The custom of employer-supported commercial health insurance began in the United States during the Great Depression, when hospitals were unable to collect reimbursements and a few large organizations wanted their employees to be quickly returned to health and to work.[2] Employer-provided health insurance expanded during World War II, when the imposition of wage and price controls on a wartime economy resulted in nonwage benefits becoming an important management tool in the recruitment and retention of scarce, skilled labor. After the War, with strong unions and a strong American economy, nonwage benefits, like health insurance, pensions, and life insurance, became even more common methods for recruiting and retaining valued employees and improving their productivity. The private health insurance that is now a regular feature of full-time permanent jobs in the United States reached that status through a series of self-interested business decisions and historical accidents rather than as a result of deliberate public policy decisions to create a right to health care.[3] Although the expansion of government subsidized Medicare and Medicaid programs strains the boundaries of the question, commercial health insurance has never become an individual right in American law, and whether it ever becomes so in the future has been the subject of often acrimonious political debate for at least the last two decades.

Third party support for health care has nevertheless been not only widespread, but ever-widening in America for nearly three-quarters of a century, about a third of our national history. It has affected nearly every living person in the country in one way or another, and what began as an innovation and grew to be a custom has by now come to be considered normative, and assumed to be an entitlement of every worker. From this perspective, the failure of this patient's new employer to provide coverage for the management of her claudication seems pitiless and morally reprehensible, self-serving capitalism in one of its worst aspects. Seen this way, option (A) would be the clearly justified response to this patient's plight.

Implementing this option might make a surgeon feel like a crusader for social justice, but doing so and feeling so would involve serious ethical errors. Surgeons surely have fiduciary relationships with their patients. Surgeons are to be competent in their fund of knowledge and clinical skills and use them to the primary benefit of their patients.[4] Fiduciary responsibility for patients, however, does not create a moral authority to consume resources that neither the surgeon nor the patient owns, and which in this case belong to the insurance company contracted by the patient's employer.[5] From her response, one can assume that this patient's employer and the insurer, as part of her employment, explained the nature and limits of the health benefits package. The exclusion of preexisting conditions on a new hire is not uncommon, and is permitted by law. In a society that is committed to the rule of law, the law commands our moral respect and compliance.

If we think that a law is ethically unjustified, we may work to change it through the political or judicial process. A judicial challenge would involve open disobedience to the law with the intention of provoking criminal or civil litigation, and a willingness to accept attendant consequences. A recent survey found that 56% of physicians would falsify insurance claims to allow their therapy for peripheral vascular disease to be paid.[6] However nobly considered, this behavior qualifies as neither political activism, civil disobedience, nor proper beneficence. It is merely criminal deception having as its intent a guarantee that some one will pay the physician. Option (A) is therefore ruled out altogether. Option (D) surely fulfills one's obligation as a citizen of conscience, and would therefore be a good thing to do in this case, but it does nothing to address your patient's immediate problem.

On the assumption that this patient reported her symptoms as muscle spasms without knowing the cause of them, it is still the case that she has a preexisting condition. Reliable clinical judgment cannot place her claudication in any other category, given that it is a chronic condition with chronic symptoms. As a matter of professional integrity, which requires the surgeon to practice to standards of intellectual and moral excellence, the surgeon must be honest with both the patient and with her insurer. The surgeon in this case should respond to the billing clerk's query with a clear statement that the patient has a preexisting condition. The surgeon should then explain to the patient that this is what he has done.

The surgeon should also explain, however, that this is not the end of the matter. Fiduciary responsibility clearly directs the surgeon in this case to offer and implement clinical management appropriate to the patient's diagnosis. Fiduciary responsibility includes an obligation to undertake reasonable advocacy on behalf of the patient, especially to arrange payment for the management of a painful and increasingly debilitating condition.[5,7] Option (B) emerges on this account as the most ethically appropriate next step, after honest reporting through the billing clerk. This option of refraining from deception and fulfilling patient fiduciary obligations through an appeal process is the recommended policy of the American Medical Association's Council on Ethical and Judicial Affairs.[8] Options (C) and (E) are not acceptable because they assume that the surgeon has no fiduciary responsibility for reasonable advocacy on behalf of this patient; they also amount to a kind of moral abandonment that itself would be insupportable.

Although the short term results of deceiving third-party payers has benefits for both patients and surgeons, Sade notes several undesirable long-term effects: (1) The fraud may be detected with legal or social consequences; (2) The physician's own integrity is compromised and virtue is eroded; (3) The physician-patient relationship is compromised ("If this physician lies to them, will he lie to me?"); (4) A potential for future diagnostic confusion is created; and (5) Systemic problems with health care remain unaddressed and unresolved.[9]

Delivery of medical care requires knowledge and resources. As long as physicians decline to acknowledge their partnership and mutual responsibilities with insurance carriers, some obligations will go unmet. Physicians are the initiators and principals in our health care system, but the other participants, including commercial third party insurers, are essential as well. Provision of medical care could not proceed without the cooperation and mutual integrity of each these major participants.

References

1. Bondeson W, Jones JW. *The Ethics of Managed Care: Professional Integrity and Patient Rights.* Boston: Kluwer Academic Publishers, 2002.
2. Kovner A, Jonas S, eds. *Health Care Delivery in the United States.* 6th ed. New York: Springer Publishing Company, 1999.
3. Starr P. *The Social Transformation of American Medicine.* New York: Basic Books, 1982.
4. McCullough LB, Jones JW, Brody BA. Principles and practice of surgical ethics. In: McCullough LB, Jones JW, Brody BA, eds. *Surgical Ethics.* New York: Oxford University Press, 1998: 3–14.
5. Morreim E. *Balancing Act: The New Medical Ethics of Medicine's New Economics.* Dordrecht, The Netherlands: Kluwer Academic Publishers, 1991.

6. Freeman VG et al., Lying for patients: Physician deception of third-party payers [see comments]. *Arch Intern Med.* 1999; 159:2263–2270.

7. Wildes K, Wallace R. Relationships with payers and institutions that manage and deliver patient services. In: McCullough LB, Jones JW, Brody BA, eds. *Surgical Ethics.* New York: Oxford University Press, 1998:367–383.

8. American Medical Association. Ethical issues in managed care. *JAMA.* 1995; 273: 330–335.

9. Sade RM. Deceiving insurance companies: New expression of an ancient tradition. *Ann Thorac Surg.* 2001; 72:1449–1453.

• CASE 48 •

Ethics of Clinical Pathways and Cost Control

Lack of money is the root of all evil.
George Bernard Shaw (1856–1950)

You are the chief of surgery in a large community hospital that has been experiencing financial difficulties. Your department has been cited by the Utilization Review Committee for excessive lengths of stay in the ICU and hospital wards. After weeks of deliberations, with minimal input from surgeons, you are directed by the hospital Executive Committee to implement a Fast-Track clinical pathway for all patients undergoing major surgical procedures. Your staff surgeons believe the data suggesting excessive lengths of stay is flawed, and that the new directive may significantly increase postoperative morbidity and mortality. Your most responsible ethical action is:

(A) Resign from the hospital staff.
(B) Direct your surgeons to implement the administration's policy.
(C) Inform the administration that you consider Fast-Tracking unethical and will not cooperate.
(D) Insist that the policy mandating Fast-Tracking be rewritten, with input of surgeons.
(E) Leak the story to the press.

Like physicians in all specialties, surgeons are increasingly answerable for the cost of patient care. Demand for accountability comes from many of the most powerful blocs in our society, including government and insurance interests, who are responding to evidence of surging increases in the cost of care. Private payers are trying to control costs to remain profitable and competitive. Public payers, such as Medicare and Medicaid, are responding to determined resistance to additional taxes.

Most surgeons believe that their responsibility to practice medicine economically is secondary to their responsibility to practice medicine effectively.[1] Surgeons can take no satisfaction from minimizing hospital costs if they have done so by minimizing the quality of patient care. The professional virtue of integrity informs our professional standards of moral and intellectual excellence, and ethically compels us to be guided in our decisions by clinical evidence.[2] This means attention to clinical outcome as well as to clinical process.

The Clinical Pathways program originated as a quality improvement process based on disease-specific algorithms. These algorithms are designed to promote standardization of diagnostic and therapeutic procedures and limit the kinds of variations that have historically been associated with errors, complications, longer hospital and ICU stays, and associated higher per-patient costs. Clinical Pathways were intended to insure that patients are treated in an efficient manner with methods long-established as effective for particular conditions. Pathways were also designed to discourage expensive and potentially dangerous idiosyncratic forays off the beaten track by overly adventurous individual practitioners. Despite these many virtues, the Clinical Pathways program has sometimes found itself calcified into a rigid Fast-Track system designed to cut costs by mandating rapid hospital discharge once each step in the Pathways process has been implemented. Advocates claim quality improvement by citing early discharge as evidence of rapid recovery, but often without reference to whether some patients *should* be discharged when they are. Though Fast-Tracking is sometimes effective in reducing such significant complications as nosocomial pneumonia, and some patients are delighted to return home earlier, not all patients respond well clinically to the Clinical Pathways-Fast-Track process, and for a few, early discharge is frightening and even dangerous. Ethical and responsible operative care requires surgeons to be instrumental in the design, practice, and surveillance of Fast-Tracking when it is applied to the patients they treat.

Evidence-based surgery evaluates clinical care comprehensively, studying the outcomes as well as the processes of treatment. Neither measure alone yields comprehensive clinical information, and neither measure alone will insure that the hospital will remain financially solvent and prepared to treat future patients. The claim that your department's patients have excessive lengths of stay is based on a process measure which has not been informed by the context of clinical outcome. Worse still, it ignores such other process measures as severity, procedural complexity, comorbidities, and individual patient histories. Isolating a process of care as a goal of care, and overlooking the health of the patient as the goal of care, will likely be a fast route to the hospital's financial demise as well as its patients' clinical demise. Concentration first upon clinical outcome and then clinical processes to achieve the primary goal honors the hospital's legitimate concern for financial strength because it subsumes it; the healthiest possible patients have fewer complications, will be the least expensive to treat, will refer friends and family, file fewer tort claims, and return for additional episodes of care when the need arises.

Option (A), resigning your hospital position to protest the mandatory Fast-Track policy, is precipitous. It displays an abundance of personal rigidity, an unwillingness to negotiate in good faith, and ultimately deprives needy patients and the hospital which sustains your community of your rare and valuable services. It violates the virtues of courage, and fortitude.

By electing option (B) and directing your surgical staff to accept and implement the mandatory Fast-Track policy, you abrogate your responsibility to patients to see that their care is your primary professional goal. You also fail in your leadership role as the department chief by not making your professional staff's clinical concerns known to the hospital administration. Although it is not inherently unethical to support your administration's efforts to contain costs and insure the hospital's function within the community, it is inconsistent with your role as an ethical surgeon to knowingly do so at the expense of good clinical care.

Although Fast-Tracking may be entirely consistent with good care for many patients, its mandatory implementation for all patients will certainly deprive some who respond more slowly, or who encounter postoperative complications, of essential inpatient services. Option (C) is inappropriate because the clinical pathways Fast-Track model is not in and of itself unethical; it becomes so only when it is indiscriminately applied as a cost-saving measure without regard to each patient's individual clinical response.

Option (D), insisting that the administration renegotiate the fast-track policy with significant input from the surgeons whose patients it affects, is the most clinically and ethically responsible position. This provides the professional staff with an opportunity to educate the administrators about significant clinical consequences of their ill-advised decision, to assume the surgeon's proper ethical role as patient fiduciary, and to provide the hospital with a defensible policy for containing costs in appropriate cases while continuing to serve the legitimate health-care interests of patients.

Option (E), taking the issue to the press, virtually insures that any subsequent negotiations between the surgeons and the administration will be acrimonious, defensive, and based more in a desire to preserve reputations and image than in guaranteeing good care. It is furthermore likely that a complex issue will be reduced to fit a headline and brief column, and thereby distorted. Most importantly, a misunderstanding of methods among people of mutual good will and common motives is likely to be mischaracterized as a morality tale, and the public's trust in your local hospital maybe seriously damaged. In that event, financial ruin will become more likely, there will be one less place to practice high quality surgery, and the entire community will suffer.

This case presents an ethical obligation frequently disregarded by surgeons. The staff surgeons should have been attentive and proactive concerning cost-control much earlier. It is common for hospital management committees with minimal surgical representation to issue edicts affecting surgical practice. Non-surgical specialists commonly complain that surgeons are in the OR all day and don't make themselves available for multi-specialty committee meetings, even when they've been appointed. It is a preventive ethical duty for surgeons to interact organizationally outside the operating room in matters of this sort. Externally imposed policies and procedures usually occur after repeated attempts to overcome appeals to professional autonomy and the resistance to change and accountability that such appeals often generate. Professional autonomy should never be the fundamental ethical concern of physicians in response to cost-control; assumption of cofiduciary responsibility, in the absence of which professional autonomy is stripped of its moral authority, should be.

References

1. McCullough LB, Jones JW, Brody BA. Principles and practice of surgical ethics. In: McCullough LB, Jones JW, Brody BA, eds. *Surgical Ethics*. New York; Oxford, 1998:3–14.
2. Gordon TA, Cameron JL eds. *Evidence-Based Surgery*. Hamilton, Ontario, Canada: BC Decker, 2000.

• CASE 49 •

Ethics of Professional Courtesy

One of the serious obstacles to the improvement of our race
is indiscriminate charity.
Andrew Carnegie (1835–1919)

A senior physician whose wife you treated surgically has called your office, irate over receiving a bill for your services. The procedure was a complex resection of a hepatoma. The patient did very well and experienced no complications following surgery. You approved the invoice your business office sent to her for the standard 15% copay specified in her health insurance coverage. Her husband is a prominent local internist who has regularly referred cases to you over the years. How should you respond?

(A) The copay should be waived as a professional courtesy.
(B) Explain that your billing clerk made a mistake and write it off.
(C) Write it off in consideration of past and future referrals from her husband.
(D) Write it off for the good will you will gain in the medical community.
(E) Cite your contractual responsibility to the insurer and explain that the charge cannot be waived.

The origin of professional cohesion expressed through dismissal of professional fees dates back to ancient codices of medicine originating in the time of Hippocrates.[1] Thomas Percival's classic 1803 treatise on medical ethics enthusiastically endorsed complimentary professional care: "All members of the profession, including apothecaries as well as physicians and surgeons, together with their wives and children, should be attended gratuitously…" The 1847 and 1949 editions of the American Medical Association's Code of Ethics endorse what has come to be known as professional courtesy in withholding charges for treatment of medical colleagues and their families, largely to discourage self-treatment.[1]

Professional medical courtesy has not been just an ideal or abstract moral norm; it has long been a practice standard. As recently as a decade ago, 96% of physicians polled reported that they gave professional courtesy to other physicians and their families through free or discounted care.[2] Further, the number of nonpsychiatrist physicians giving professional courtesy was noted to have changed little over the years.

The ethical justification for this practice in the histories of medicine and of medical ethics is obscure. One historical aspect of the justification is quite practical: physicians' and surgeons' fees were often beyond the economic reach of all but the very well-to-do, and physicians, with just a few exceptions, were not within that group until relatively recently. Indeed, physicians often came from lower social classes and struggled in a mercilessly competitive profession for market share and economic survival. Only in the last half of the 20th century have physicians in developed countries routinely achieved upper middle class economic status.[3] Professional courtesy served to keep physicians from treating themselves and their families with the associated moral and clinical problems.

This practical justification had an added ethical dimension: professional courtesy was a form of charity. This interpretation is supported by Percival's assertion that professional courtesy should be further extended to the clergy and their families, because, like physicians, their work was characterized by benevolence and they lived in economically straitened circumstances. Physicians might have been more economically secure than the clergy, but not by much.

With the advent of professional licensure, which granted allopathic and osteopathic physicians monopoly control over medicine, and with the introduction of third-party private insurance and government direct payment programs like Medicaid and Medicare, physicians now enjoy an enviable and often affluent level of prosperity and economic security. Professional courtesy can no longer be justified as aid to economically strapped colleagues.

It has been suggested that professional courtesy promotes professional solidarity,[1] but this claim stimulates some skepticism. Although the custom of professional courtesy emerged from guild practices of charitable interest in one another's welfare, our professional affiliations no longer take the form of extended families, nor is our profession widely beset by those who do not practice it. Protecting self-interest by promoting the good will of colleagues may be a shrewd business practice, but it is quite removed from the sense of solidarity that has substantive ethical content, namely the nurturance of professional integrity in the care of patients. Claims that professional courtesy maintains and strengthens professionalism seem to imbue the practice with an unearned virtue.

Moreno and Lucente also note that professional courtesy may not be without clinical consequence, in the sense that it may result in physicians and their families being overtreated. They further note that professional courtesy insulates physicians from the realities of medical care costs, desensitizing them to a major societal concern affecting access to care and compliance with treatment plans.[1]

Many health insurance contracts moot the entire question of professional courtesy by simply prohibiting the waiver of copayments and fees. In the presence of such provisions, courtesy becomes not only an ethical issue between physician and patient/colleague, but a legal and ethical issue between physician and the contracting third party payer. Insurers hope that the mandatory copay will serve as a slight disincentive to frivolous overuse of the medical care system. Although physicians are not in the business of discouraging patients from seeking care, we all understand the risks of overtreatment and the burdens that the worried well can place upon our time and effectiveness. Furthermore, we should all be fully familiar with the legal and ethical responsibilities entailed in any contract we sign. Having agreed to participate in plans which prohibit waiver of prescribed copayments, we surrender our discretion to provide professional courtesy.

However, there appears to not be much of a case for professional courtesy, as a practical or legal matter. At the very least, its advocates bear the burden of proving an ethical justification for it. Options (A), (B), and (C) are all forms of professional courtesy that ignore safeguards the copayment system is intended to defend, and may constitute insurance fraud. Option (B) first abandons a legitimate principle and compounds the error by being deceptive about it. Option (C) disregards the ethical consideration entirely in the service of financial self-interest. Option (D) represents the obsolete guild rationalization and violates contracts.

Option (E) is the ethically justified response to this case, to which a preventive ethical approach should be added. Physicians should make clear to their colleagues and to family members of colleagues that, while professional courtesy may have had a rationale in the distant past, especially to relieve economic burdens that could be quite real, it no longer does so. Colleagues will also understand the ethical obligation to abide by the terms of insurance contracts and the quite legitimate self-interest in not committing criminal fraud. Such a preventive ethics approach is crucial because it helps to control the potential economic conflict of interest associated with this patient's husband as a referral source for the surgeon. Pursuit of such economic self-interest as the surgeon's primary motivation undermines professional integrity from within. Percival taught that medicine is a public trust that physicians are obligated to maintain; it is an obligation inconsistent with referral preservation and income as prime considerations in determining the physician's choices.

References

1. Moreno J, Lucente F. Patients who are family members, colleagues, and family members of colleagues. In: McCullough LB, Jones JW, Brody BA, eds. *Surgical Ethics.* New York: Oxford University Press, 1998:198–215.
2. Levy MA et al. Professional courtesy—current practices and attitudes. *N Engl J Med.* 1993; 329:1627–1631.
3. Wear A, Geyer-Kordesch J, French R, eds. *Doctors and Ethics: The Earlier Historical Setting of Professional Ethics.* Amsterdam, The Netherlands: Rodopi Editions, 1993.

• CASE 50 •

Ethics of Administrative Credentialing

Do good with what thou hast; or it will do thee no good.
William Penn (1644–1718)

A pediatric surgeon has practiced in the same community for more than 20 years, holding privileges at the two largest local general hospitals. She is widely respected and admired by patients and fellow physicians in all specialties, and her results are consistently good. Recently, the Board of Directors at the hospital which has been the source of 80% of her case referrals has hired a notorious slash-and-burn management firm to improve their balance sheet. The new CEO installed an information technology system that can provide management with physician-specific figures on costs and reimbursements. The management consultants have identified the 10% of physicians with the worst hospital cost/reimbursement ratios over the preceding 5 years and persuaded the Board of Directors to order their clinical privileges withdrawn. Our seasoned surgeon learns that she is among the targeted group. Is there an ethical issue here, and, if so, how should she respond?

- (A) Move her practice and hope for more referrals.
- (B) Insist that sole control of the credentialing process be returned to the medical staff.
- (C) Contact the accrediting authorities and governmental agencies with relevant jurisdiction.
- (D) Hire an attorney.
- (E) Ask the AMA for support.

Hospitals have been adjusting to an intensely competitive marketplace in the decade since withdrawal of cost-plus reimbursements. Hospital administrators are painfully aware that the management model within which they must function is defective and precarious. Third party payers limit revenue by basing reimbursement on disease categories instead of actual costs incurred by hospitals. Powerful insurers, operating in a seller's market, negotiate ever-lower payments, and then contest charges with delaying tactics[1] seldom seen in ethical nonmedical businesses. The complex difficulty of controlling hospital costs just compounds the problem of keeping a positive revenue stream running for a vital community resource.

Physicians, historically independent of hospital business management in virtually all elements of their medical practice, have come to be seen as the hospital's uncontrolled cost-drivers, a problem administrators have been addressing with increasing aggressiveness. Acting through Boards of Directors, hospital business managers seek to contain costs and maximize revenues. Certainly all other businesses do so as well, but in the hospital industry the specter of cost-cutting must be monitored by medical staff to assure no reduction in the quality of medical and surgical care. The administrative authority to decide which physicians will practice at a given institution would permit hospital managers to retain only the most cost-effective physicians and eliminate those who regularly utilize more hospital resources in caring for patients than their case reimbursements replace. Economic credentialing—and decredentialing—thus emerge as powerfully seductive management tools that can imperil a physician's livelihood and ability to practice medicine without encumbrance.

Economic credentialing assumes heterogeneous efficiency among physicians. Data supporting this assumption are readily available. In a recent study of physicians' economic practice patterns, oncologists treating lung cancer were divided into high-charge and low-charge groups. Patients treated by high-chargers received significantly more chemotherapy cycles, more second-line and third-line drugs, and suffered greater associated morbidity. High-chargers had the same patient survival rates as low chargers, but with 100% higher costs and morbidity.[2] The average hospital cost for carotid endarterectomies done by one group in the same town was 43.5% higher than another, with the less expensive surgeons reporting superior clinical results.[3] Another similar study of vascular surgery practices found that individual surgeons utilizing fewer hospital resources for carotid procedures had the same or better clinical results than those costing more.[3] Still another study reported that 46% of "variability" in hospital charges for surgical procedures was attributable to neither patient characteristics nor category of procedure, but to the individual surgeon's practice style.[4]

Most sophisticated hospitals have been able to generate physician- specific financial data for more than a decade.[5] One's initial reaction might be that a medical business, a hospital, should be entitled to protect itself from wasteful staff physicians. Historically, at least in theory, the criteria for appointment and continuation as a hospital medical staff member have concentrated exclusively on a physician's conformity with institutional quality care standards for clinical outcomes. There has seldom before been a protracted frontal assault upon the concept of medical peer review as the sole arbiter of clinical quality. Established hospital accreditation bodies have certified that only fully trained and licensed physicians constituting the hospital medical staff, not the hospital's lay administrators, may suitably evaluate the performance of fellow physicians and thereby govern the credentialing process. We have nevertheless seen the definition of quality in clinical care slowly melt over the last two decades into combined considerations of what constitutes acceptable processes of care, clinical outcomes, and costs.

Clinical quality of surgical care includes mortality and morbidity relative to some standard. Clinical outcomes are associated with patient demographics, concurrent disease, and complications. Complications are independently associated with both cost and mortality of surgical care, and patient variability explains only part of the complication rate variances.[6]

No organization, however beneficently disposed, is obligated to drive itself out of business by persistently incurring more cost than it can replace. In the particular case of a hospital, neglecting its balance sheet to the extent that it cannot survive to continue providing services to the sick and injured of its community would constitute gross irresponsibility, an ethical outrage in its breach of a critical social contract. Physicians and hospital administrators share a cofiduciary responsibility for the welfare of patients who require the institution's care,[7,8] and that duty includes making sure that the hospital is financially intact and operational when patients need it. The other essential responsibility shared by physicians and the institutions they practice in is satisfaction of the public expectation, long fostered by both doctors and hospitals, that medical decisions will be made solely by trained, licensed, and experienced medical professionals, and that the sole intent of those decisions will be the provision of the best available care to each individual patient. The most basic of these medical decisions is of course the evaluation and selection of physicians properly trained and experienced to take good care of patients in the hospital. Intrusion into this process by laymen, and timid acquiescence by physicians in decisions based solely on economic consideration, deceives a trusting public.

As cofiduciaries, hospitals and the physicians who are privileged to practice in them are obligated to be technically competent in patient care, to use their competence primarily for the benefit of patients, and to systematically place their own self-interest, as organizations and as individuals, secondary to the welfare of their patients. Among its important ethical implications, the concept of cofiduciary responsibility means that hospital administrations should, as a rule, subordinate institutional economic self-interest to the well-being of patients, just as physicians should. Economic stability is surely a legitimate interest of hospitals, because it is a necessary condition for their having the resources necessary to meet their cofiduciary obligations to their patients. That is, economic stability may be seen as a means to the ethically significant end of fulfilling clinical responsibilities, not as an end in itself.

Many hospitals manage costs using continuous quality improvement techniques, through their medical staffs. Modified from industry for hospital application, CQI employs evidence-based processes of care intended to improve and preserve patients' health and functional status. Happily, and not coincidentally, most patients treated in this manner not only get over their illnesses quickly, but they routinely cost hospitals the least, with fewer complications, shorter lengths of hospital stay, and fewer unreimbursed posthospital clinic visits. CQI, properly implemented, doesn't aim to reduce costs by cutting corners, but by recognizing that the faster patients get well, the fewer resources they consume. Using this model, good care can be legitimately equated with inexpensive care without violating cofiduciary responsibility.

The studies cited here suggest that not all physicians provide the best patient care. Geographic and individual variations in practice styles are sometimes inconsistent with physicians' fiduciary obligations, and those responsibilities they share with the institutions in which they practice. Physicians are not only ethically obligated to participate in those institutional CQI activities that improve the quality of patient care and contribute to the continued stability and viability of their hospitals, they should take the lead in them.

Management decisions that affect patient care and that are made solely on an economic basis violate lay administrators' cofiduciary responsibility, which requires that the effect of such decisions on patient care must not be left to chance. Physicians are the authorities in patient care determinations, especially in determination of the composition of the medical staff; the physician leadership should review the economic data objectively and decide whether or not privileges should be withdrawn. Decisions about credentialing by lay administrators based solely on economic considerations systematically put the hospital's economic self-interest before fiduciary responsibility and undermine the physician's essential role in CQI. Such decisions are completely incompatible with cofiduciary responsibility, and are therefore unethical.

Our embattled surgeon is ethically fully justified in asking her hospital's Chief of Staff to convene a medical staff meeting, suggesting that the hospital CEO be invited to attend and explain whether the hospital's new credentialing policy has been formulated upon evidence-based standards of quality and cofiduciary responsibility, or on the basis solely of the hospital's economic self-interest. If the policy is directed toward improving care, the administration might be firmly reminded that such matters properly and exclusively reside with the medical staff. The medical staff should take the lay administration's views into consideration as it ponders the question of whether efficient practice is essential to a determination of high quality practice when it, and it alone, deliberates questions of recredentialing individual physicians.

If the new policy is not directed toward improving clinical quality as a means of containing costs, but rather toward cost reduction as an end in itself, then it is correctly interpreted to mean that the hospital administration has made financial success its primary goal. In doing so, the hospital administrative leadership has disconnected cost management from cofiduciary responsibility. If so, it can not consider its medical staff ethically obligated to follow its lead or honor its intent. The medical staff might honorably seek the resignation of an administration so clearly anathema to the basic ethical principles of the medical profession and hospital management.

Option (D) is not a good first response because it fails to address the ethical issues at the heart of the matter and would probably disintegrate into the surgeon's sole pursuit of personal interest as she fought to maintain her own privileges. The core issue here is the medical staff's responsibility for maintaining its informed control of medical care, including those elements of care that may intersect with hospital finance. Physicians properly defend their prerogative in these matters not in their own interest, but as the otherwise unheard voice of their patients. Hospital care determined by lay administrators solely on the basis of economic considerations is not medical care; it is also irresponsible management.

Option (E) must fail in all respects, because although a national association of physicians can provide support it has no regulatory authority in such matters. As suggested, option (B) is an appropriate first step, perhaps best introduced in the context of a medical staff meeting of the sort described. If this option meets with failure, option (C) becomes the physician's ethical responsibility; the major hospital accreditation organizations in the United States support independent medical staff control of its membership. Option (A), dissociation from an untrustworthy and dysfunctional organization, becomes the third and last line of moral defense of our surgeon's professional integrity.

As the practice of medicine evolves in the 21st century, medical staffs must retain leadership in assuring that the goals of hospital managers and trustees remain focused on improved patient care. This retention of professional power must be deserved by placing guild mentalities and personal finances secondary to professionalism.

References

1. Pallarito K. Falling behind in the payment game: Providers are feeling squeezed by HMOs that don't pay on time and keep changing the rules. *Mod Healthc.* 1999; 29:104–106, 108.
2. Hoverman JR, Robertson SM. Lung cancer: A cost and outcome study based on physician practice patterns. *Dis Manag.* 2004; 7:112–123.
3. Luna G, Adye B. Cost-effective carotid endarterectomy. *Am J Surg.* 1995; 169: 516–518.
4. Lester DK, Linn LS. Variation in hospital charges for total joint arthroplasty: an investigation of physician efficiency. *Orthopedics.* 2000; 23:137–140.
5. Riley D. Economic credentialing survey of university teaching hospitals. *Healthc Financ Manage.* 1993; 47:42, 44–48.
6. Pronovost P, Garrett E, Dorman T, Jenckes M, Webb III TH, Breslow M, Rosenfeld B, Bass E. Variations in complication rates and opportunities for improvement in quality of care for patients having abdominal aortic surgery. *Langenbecks Arch Surg.* 2001; 386:249–256.
7. McCullough LB. A basic concept in the clinical ethics of managed care: Physicians and institutions as economically disciplined moral co-fiduciaries of populations of patients. *J Med Philos.* 1999; 24:77–97.
8. Chervenak FA, McCullough LB. Physicians and hospital managers as cofiduciaries of patients: Rhetoric or reality? *J Healthc Manag.* 2003; 48:172–179; discussion 180.

• CASE 51 •

Ethics of the New Economic Credentialing: Conflicted Leadership Roles

A hospital is a living organism, made up of many different parts having different functions, but all these must be in due proportion and relation to each other, and to the environment to produce the desired results.

John Shaw Billings (1883–1913), Address upon the opening of Johns Hopkins Hospital, 1889

For many years, Dr. M. Idas, the chief of surgical services, has been the only credentialed vascular surgeon in a midsized, seriously underfunded private hospital in a small city. He now also serves on the hospital's board of directors. An opportunity has arisen for him to join several professional friends in founding a local physician-owned ambulatory surgery center (ASC). He planned to pursue this project while maintaining his positions at the hospital, but when the hospital administration learned of his plans the board of directors asked him and his partners to resign their hospital staff memberships. This would of course require surrender of his other hospital positions as well. He could do outpatient procedures like AV fistulas at the ASC, but would require continuing access to inpatient services. The nearest other hospital suitably equipped for major inpatient vascular procedures is fifty miles away. What should he do?

(A) Withdraw from the ambulatory surgery center project.
(B) Refuse to resign any of his hospital positions.
(C) Resign from the hospital and accept the associated inconveniences imposed.
(D) Resign from the board of directors but refuse to resign his medical staff privileges or position as chief of surgery.
(E) Resign as board member and chief of surgery, but refuse to leave the medical staff.

Modern medicine is an altruistic business with a complex organizational structure, inviting a tangle of knotty financial conflicts. As long as the cost-plus payment system was in effect, these conflicts were considered trivial because the pool of resources was deep enough to accommodate everyone very nicely. Since every medical doctor, regardless of efficiency, turned a handsome profit for the hospital, conflicts were usually resolved in the physician's favor. As third party payers' business strategies squeezed hospitals and physicians by raising financial risks, economic conflicts began to be taken more seriously.

The authorization to practice medicine at a particular hospital is clearly understood as a privilege, not a right. Medical staff privileging stresses the physician's responsibilities and restrictions upon their scope of practice. Almost every hospital's privileging documents specify the institution's authority to rescind hospital access for violations of the medical staff bylaws. Because physicians are considered to be the only legitimate judges of their colleagues' practices, the institutional responsibility guaranteeing the quality of care within its domain is assigned to peer review. Historically, at least in theory, the criteria for appointment and continuation on a medical staff member have exclusively been those used for determining whether a physician meets institutional quality standards in patient care.

The peer review system in credentialing works fairly well, when it is permitted to. Sometimes occult criteria with territorial financial undercurrents are permitted to influence and even determine where some otherwise qualified physicians practice. Physician's interests in limiting competition, and hospital executives' recruitment through economic incentives, have accompanied the process for some time without drawing much objection. Whether that is a good or a bad thing in the life of a hospital can become a complicated question. Hospital administrators are always concerned about the fiscal well-being of the institution, and carefully scrutinize the efficiency of the doctors who practice there. Nevertheless, the lay administration's overt role in deciding which physicians practice in its hospital has typically been secondary to the process of peer evaluation.

Both the hospital administration and medical leadership are interested in clinical quality and in economics when they consider their medical staffs. Historically, quality was exclusively the concern of the medical staff, and finance was left to the administration. This longstanding tradition faded when cost-plus reimbursement systems were replaced by diagnostic-related groups (DRGs) and other schemes designed to reduce hospital reimbursements. Inefficient medical practices like redundant lab tests and lengthy inpatient stays were once gold mines for hospitals, but have become intolerable liabilities. Quality of care, once measured only by clinical outcome, began to be evaluated by financial variables like average hospital or ICU days, OR cost, total cost of hospitalization by diagnosis, or even the time it takes a particular surgeon to do a procedure. Rightly or wrongly, physicians have been made to feel unmistakable and ever-increasing pressure from cost-conscious hospital administrators to reduce expenses by closely monitoring resource utilization. Though recredentialing decisions are properly reserved to the medical staff, most administrators quietly believe they can veto the reappointment of physicians whose practice styles, or even practice groups, appear to lose money for the hospital. Only relatively recently have hospital boards begun unilaterally revoking the privileges of physicians they believe practice inefficiently. The practice is termed "economic credentialing," and it has become a regular event.

The physician's milieu is necessarily a public trust, with the most restrictive moral obligations upon personal-professional relationships of any human endeavor in which money is exchanged for service.[1] There is a significant difference between the ethical standards required of a medical professional and those expected of an honest businessman.[2] The virtues, values, goals, and their applications are distinct: the physician's interests are voluntarily subordinated to the patient's best interest. Fundamentally, business decisions are made with consideration of how the business will benefit most; fiduciary decisions are made to ensure that purchasers will be the beneficiaries of the most good. Commercial ethics promote the concept that each party is justified in acting to protect and advance its self-interest. Medical ethics are directed toward the advancement and protection of the patient, with the self interest of the provider, or seller, of services sublimated to a secondary position.

Medicine nowadays commingles professional and commercial ethics. The activities required in managing an office, negotiating with third party payers, teaching trainees, and interacting with hospital administrations reflect both value systems, but the physician's primary responsibility is always to care for the sick, the injured, and the helpless. How should a conscientious physician determine which element of a given relationship should be governed by a professional medical ethic that sublimates self-interest, and which by the business ethic that places primary value upon self-interest?

Physicians do not have the same fiduciary obligations toward their office landlords, their hospital administrators, or their investment companies that they have toward their patients. Nor do these nonpatients owe the same respect and deference to physicians during business dealings.

The test to be applied is straightforward. The professional fiduciary role applies to all decisions which affect patient care of the medical "community" served, directly or indirectly. The ethical constructs of business apply to wholly financial decisions which do not affect the quality of patient care. As used herein, the word "quality" is understood in the clinical outcomes context of patient therapy rather than cost of outcome. Although modern doublespeak has conjoined cost and quality, and they often parallel each other, they are not identical. The cheapest way to treat a disease is to have the patient die early in the course of therapy.

Is our well-established, successful surgeon, serving in multiple leadership roles at the hospital, within his rights to form new business allegiances without reproach? Will his division of loyalties affect patient care? Ownership of a competing medical facility clearly conflicts with the hospital leadership positions this surgeon holds. His seat on the board of directors is especially conflicted. The position's conferral of extraordinary influence upon institutional decisions and special access to its most sensitive information is based on a trust that he will never favor a competitor, an assurance he can no longer make. This eliminates option (B) as an ethical response. Likewise, the position of chief of surgery reflects a trust endowed with substantial influence over the practices of the institution's largest profit centers. His duty to honor the integrity of the position with undivided loyalty eliminates the propriety of option (D).

The struggle between the surgeon's right to retain medical staff privileges on the basis of his sound practice and compliance with medical staff rules, and the hospital's right to decredential a practitioner solely on the basis of commercial competition is, therefore, more ethically indistinct, more complex, and very context dependent. If our surgeon resigns his leadership positions and becomes a member of the general medical staff, he will no longer exercise special influence, receive privileged information, or affect hospital business policies. He will control his own practice by deciding where patients will have their operations, at the hospital or at the ambulatory surgery center in which he has invested. Selection of sites will be determined less by financial than by resource requirements, with the nature of the procedure effectively dictating whether it is to be done on an inpatient or an outpatient basis. Lost revenue from the highly profitable outpatient surgery business may nevertheless seriously affect the hospital's ability to continue providing the community with some loss leader services like geriatric and burn units, or its emergency center.

Option (E) appears initially attractive, because it eliminates the ethical dilemmas associated with retaining his leadership roles in the hospital. This option remains problematic, however, when we consider the fiduciary obligation to patients and the community at large the surgeon shares with the hospital.[4] As a hospital staff member, the physician is entitled to expect his hospital to conduct its business to the benefit of its patients. The physician must join the hospital in recognizing cofiduciary obligations, not only to his own patients but to the entire patient population served by the hospital. Our surgeon's transfer of his patients—and the transfers of his colleagues and co-owners—to his proposed outpatient program would threaten the legitimate economic self-interest of the already struggling hospital. Indeed, its financial stability could be undermined, denying it resources that it needs to serve all of its patients, and perhaps even survive as an essential community resource. The surgeon's primary motivation in planning to invest in the surgery center is not fulfillment of fiduciary responsibility to his patients—he's already doing that at the hospital—but economic self-interest. Among those privileged to be physicians, financial self-interest should always be secondary to more ethically demanding patient responsibilities. Option (E) thus lacks ethical justification.

Option (C) does not violate the fiduciary obligation the surgeon shares with the hospital because it eliminates the hospital role that incurs this joint responsibility. By resigning all his hospital affiliations, though, our surgeon will jeopardize any patients who need emergency inpatient vascular surgery or emergency transfer to the hospital from the ambulatory surgery center.

Option (A) is the ethically justified alternative. By planning to invest in the surgery center to advance his self-interest at substantial risk to the hospital, our surgeon would violate his ethical obligations. He should instead sublimate his own interests to the needs of people whom he has accepted an obligation to serve. These sacrifices are routinely made by ethical physicians.

Assertions of individual autonomy and protection of economic self-interest should not be the fundamental responses of physicians to hospital restrictions and cost-controls. Assumption of shared fiduciary responsibility, in the absence of which professional autonomy is stripped of its moral authority, should be.[5] Insisting that hospital leadership accept the principles of professional cofiduciary responsibility confirms the physician's equivalent obligations. The building of a competitive surgical facility in a small market would harm the hospital's patient population and should be abandoned.

This hypothetical construct is intended to illustrate the physician's institutional cofiduciary responsibility and the need to consider the consequences of entrepreneurial activities upon the community. Some other types of administrative infringement upon the privileging process, such as those discussed in the preceding case, are not to be tolerated, but the hospital's harsh response to this case of potentially damaging economic competition emerging from within its own leadership is a legitimate defense of its clinical care programs.

References

1. Jones JW, McCullough LB, Richman, BW. An impaired surgeon, a conflict of interest, and supervisory responsibilities. *Surgery*. 2004; 135:449–451.
2. Brody BA. The physician as professional and the physician as honest businessman. *Arch Otolaryngol Head Neck Surg*. 1993; 119:495–497.
3. McCullough LB. A basic concept in the clinical ethics of managed care: physicians and institutions as economically disciplined moral co-fiduciaries of populations of patients. *J Med Philos*. 1999; 24:77–97.
4. Jones JW, McCullough LB, Richman BW. The ethics of clinical pathways and cost control. *J Vasc Surg*. 2003; 37:1341–42.

• CASE 52 •

Whodunit? Ghost Surgery and Ethical Billing

Once integrity goes, the rest is a piece of cake.
J. R. Ewing, *Dallas*

A senior surgery resident started a percutaneous dilatational tracheotomy on a comatose patient in the surgical intensive care unit (SICU), expecting you to arrive momentarily to supervise him. You were nevertheless unexpectedly detained establishing hemostasis in the main operating suite. You arrived in the SICU as the dressing was being applied. There were no operative complications. The resident who began and finally completed the case was highly skilled and in the final month of his training; you had supervised his satisfactory performance of many similar procedures. The patient's elderly wife had consented to the procedure, which she was told you would be directly supervising while the resident performed the surgery. When the operation was over you met with her to explain your emergency conflict and assure her that you checked the resident's work and found it entirely satisfactory. She accepted your explanation. The patient's multiple comorbidities nevertheless necessitated an extended postoperative stay in the SICU, where you personally cared for him. The resident had dictated routinely that you attended the procedure, and your billing clerk had no reason to doubt the operative report's accuracy when she submitted your surgical fees to Medicare and the patient's private insurer, which paid to their contractual limits without challenge. On many occasions you have had your billings shorted by both. The resident since has graduated. What should you do?

(A) Keep the money. The patient received the appropriate care.
(B) Keep the money. The insurers owe you plenty.
(C) Return the money and bill in the resident's name.
(D) Return the money and bill for your SICU care only.
(E) Return the Medicare money and keep the commercial insurance money.

In Book II of Plato's *Republic*, Socrates tells the story of Gyges of Lydia, a shepherd who finds a magic ring with the power to make its wearer invisible.[1] Socrates explains that Gyges might now, "With impunity take what he wished even from the market place, and enter into houses and lie with whom he pleased, and slay and loose from bonds whomsoever he would." (*Republic* 360c) The shepherd has become unaccountable to anyone but himself in his invisibility and, though he might still act rightly, anyone in his position who did so "would be regarded as most pitiable and a great fool by all who took note of it." Socrates goes on to argue, however, that the just man would refrain from such behavior, voluntarily surrendering himself to the constraints of moral integrity that justice requires of men.

As the surgeon in this case, you are wearing a latter-day Ring of Gyges. You have become invisible to your unconscious patient, his anxious wife in the waiting room, and the people who pay your bills. You are accountable only to the court of individual conscience. Because of the resident's entry error, there is no mismatch between the operative and the billing records, and no other surgeon, administrator, or Medicare auditor will likely ever be aware that you have billed for an operation you didn't take part in.

"Ghost surgery" is an old and scalding term in medicine, referring originally to operations performed by an itinerant surgeon employed by a general practitioner or family doctor who signed the records, sent the bill, and otherwise led the reawakened patient to believe that he had competently done the procedure himself.[2] With development of modern institutional training methods, the term mutated to cast a sly leer toward faculty surgeons who still delighted in the shroud of invisibility wrapped around them by general anesthesia, and surreptitiously dealt their operative duties to residents or junior associates without their patients' knowledge or consent, never neglecting to collect the fees. Defenders have protested that having residents and fellows perform surgery is an obviously necessary element of any surgical training program, and that an incremental relaxation of faculty supervision is the accepted method for promoting the resident's level of responsibility and progress toward independent practice.[3] In busy academic surgical practices there has long been a tendency, and sometimes a perceived necessity, for using trainees to extend the faculty surgeon's productivity, most visibly in tedious routines like night call, clinic coverage, pre-op workups, and bed rounds, but prominently in the operating room as well. Clinical experience is an important part of the trainee's education, but faculty surgeons can let themselves become overreliant upon it when duties cluster and caseloads expand beyond the comfort level. The bargain developed in surgical residency programs provides the surgeons-in-training with an educational experience in exchange for work which increases the earning power of the institution and its faculty. Because the arrangement fairly begs for exploitation, planned and especially accidental, all the participants must constantly assess its effects upon the quality of care, informed consent, and professional integrity.

Faculty surgeons try to balance the increasing independence they afford residents as they progress through the training program with their own mature knowledge and skill to ensure safe and effective patient care in a good educational atmosphere. In the operating room, the trainee's role in the procedure is expanded as knowledge, technical skill, judgment, and confidence are developed over the course of the residency. As residents master individual procedures and approach the time for graduation into independent practice and board eligibility, the temptation to relax faculty supervision and devote one's time to other duties can become stronger. Faculty with sizeable caseloads may even find themselves slipping into Tom Sawyer's ruse, slyly seducing overeager residents into doing their routine cases on their own while they do the big ones in another room and bill for them all. When this occurs, we have crossed the line from resident education to ghost surgery.

Still, some observers protest that the cynicism reflected in the term "ghost surgery" is inappropriate to what happens in large academic medical centers,[3] where the complexity of supervisory relationships and methods can create mistaken impressions. Some senior orthopedic surgeons have been known to use video cameras and intercoms in their offices to guide residents at work in the operating room. The U.S. military commissioned development of the surgical robotics which now are finding their way into our major training centers so that in the future an absent surgeon could perform an operation on a wounded soldier on a battlefield half a world away. Many of our most renowned and sought-after surgeons operate high volume practices which can be sustained only through use of associates; their patients generally believe that the senior surgeon is at least present during the operation, and perhaps he or she is.

But room for slippage is not necessarily an invitation to slip. Although there was no deliberate intention in our case to either exploit the resident, deceive the patient, or bilk the third party payers, billing the insurers as if the surgeon had been involved in the resident's unsupervised procedure is "ghost surgery" in the commonly used sense of the term. In the hurly-burly of a sometimes frantic medical practice, conflicting imperatives regularly arise, and no one can be in two places at once no matter how grave the crisis. The conflict between procedures in the operating room and the SICU in this case couldn't be either anticipated or avoided, and was no one's fault. Even in the violation of protocol it precipitated, the patient was not harmed, his wife finally not deceived, and there weren't an abundance of better ways available to manage the problem. Nor was the error by the billing clerk an ethical failure. It will, however, surely become one if you fail to correct it now that the reimbursements have arrived and the slip-up has come to your attention. Because the federal government provides substantial financial support to accredited residency training programs, Medicare rejects charges for work done by trainees, effectively declining to pay twice for the same service. Those funds go to the hospital rather than the surgeon. Private insurers typically follow Medicare's lead. The third party payers require that faculty surgeons be present at the operating table during the major parts of each surgical procedure for which they'll accept charges (Medicare Benefit Policy Manual, Ch. 15, 30.2). Most medical schools and their affiliated hospitals impose the same demands upon the faculty to insure the adequacy of residency training and the quality of patient care; although allowances are sometimes made for emergency interventions by unsupervised residents, Medicare doesn't provide any special dispensations based on a trainee's individual talent or proximity to graduation if a faculty member never shows up for the operation.

In this case, there is no paper trail or witness to challenge what has become your claim to have done this operation. The patient received a good operation and came through satisfactorily. It would be entirely appropriate for the third party payers to cover the charges if you had done nothing more than stand at the SICU bedside with the resident while he operated. Your unintentional claim is nevertheless false, and as such violates standards of moral excellence and professional integrity, the foundations of the physician's unique relationship with the culture in which he or she functions. The legitimacy of the physician's morality and integrity is what distinguishes us from the medicine show charlatan who exploits the public's ancient trust in our profession for personal enrichment and self-aggrandizement. The only way to prove and perpetuate that legitimacy is to practice it, even when no one is looking.[4] Circumstances may make us invisible to others, but never to ourselves. We must be certain of our own integrity if we expect to receive the trust of others, without which we cannot function as physicians.

Option (A) is essentially irrelevant to the question at hand. The patient may have received appropriate care, but you didn't provide it. Should you be entitled to compensation for having trained the resident to provide the good care that he did? You already have been, when the medical school provided you with a teaching stipend, when you took satisfaction in working with him and seeing him develop during his time in the program, when he relieved you of the tedious chores that are essential to the functions of a hospital, and when you became able to pass the reins of responsibility on to him so that your children and theirs would be cared for by surgeons who will be at least as competent as you.

Most of us have at one time or another felt irritated about levels of reimbursement, which seem to be ever-falling, and by the petty equivocations with which third party payers seem to routinely delay or reduce our receipts. There are few among us, however, who have not realized an enormous net economic gain from operation of the government-supported medical reimbursement programs and private insurance plans. Every day, people who would not otherwise have come to us at all are treated and generate revenue because public and for-profit plans give them access. The attitude reflected in option (B) would ultimately kill the golden goose, but that is only the utilitarian reason for rejecting it, not the ethical one. Each of us has agreed to participate in these programs, the terms of which are perhaps overabundant but nevertheless clear, and protocols for appeal of individual grievances are in place. The contractual agreements we make with Medicare and the private carriers are sustained by the legitimate expectation that all parties will behave with honesty and integrity to sustain the system and ensure that sick people will receive care from competent doctors. No one of us is entitled to poison the integrity of our profession by enforcing an individual interpretation of vigilante justice over perceived slights. Option (B) is a poor choice.

Option (C) is not available because Medicare disqualifies charges for trainees' service. However important this procedure may have been to the patient's ultimate survival, it cannot properly claim an exception as an emergency that could not await the arrival of a supervisory faculty member.

The Office of the Inspector General in the Department of Health and Human Services studies Medicare billings with a vengeance. The United States Attorney General's Office has a full array of laws with which to prosecute malfeasants, including the False Claims Act (fines up to $10,000, treble damages, and up to 5 years in prison), the anti-kickback provisions of the Social Security Act (fines of up to $25,000, and up to 5 years in prison), civil monetary penalties (fines up to $50,000 and treble damages), the Racketeering Influenced and Corrupt Organization Act (RICO, offering prison terms of up to 20 years and civil liability with asset forfeiture), the Health Insurance Portability and Accountability Act (up to 10 years in prison, or up to 20 years if serious bodily injury results, or up to life in prison if death occurs), and, if prosecutors just feel the need for lighter armaments, the Department of Health Services can merely exclude a health care provider from the Medicare system. Federal lawyers decide which of these legal cannons to fire depending on whether the breach is considered fraud or abuse. Were you to accept and keep the Medicare payment for an operation you did not attend, the offense would be classified as fraud. The private insurance companies seldom audit closed billings the way Medicare does, and would typically only require repayment if they did discover the sort of discrepancy we've described, though the behavior is no less ethically defensible than claiming Medicare's money. Option (E) is another wrong choice, confirming intent to defraud.

Option (C) is legitimately available to you. Withdraw the surgical charges, explain that an error has been made, return the money, and submit charges for the care you actually provided postoperatively in the SICU. This will necessarily mean that there will be no charge rendered to Medicare, the private insurer, or to the patient for the operation performed by the resident.

Surgeons do function with a great deal of invisibility, not because they wear a magic ring, but because the culture in which they function has come to trust their professional integrity. Certainly no one would permit an automobile dealer to put them to sleep and invade their bodies, no matter how much good the dealer claims it will do them. None of us have gone through the long and arduous process of becoming surgeons with the intention of deceiving the sick, evading responsibility, and absconding with vast and unearned funds. No one expects this kind of behavior from us, and if we are to be able to pursue our genuine intention of contributing to the general welfare of the human race, we must make sure that we never give them reason to. Our integrity is not all we have as surgeons, but without it we don't have much.

Note: The late Dr. Francis D. Moore, a beloved friend, suggested several years ago that one of the most serious surgical ethical infringements was faculty surgeons who failed to properly supervise their residents and claimed the undeserved rewards. He suggested the title of "Whodunit" for a paper decrying the practice.

References

1. Plato. *The Republic of Plato. Translated into English with Introduction, Analysis, Marginal Analysis, and Index*. 3rd ed. London: Oxford University Press at the Clarendon Press, 1888.
2. Foster JH. Who does an operation? *Arch Surg*. 1981; 116:743.
3. Holmes MK. Ghost surgery. *Bull NY Acad Med*. 1980; 56:412–419.
4. McCullough LB, Jones JW, Brody BA. Principles and practice of surgical Ethics. In: McCullough LB, Jones JW, Brody BA, eds. *Surgical Ethics*. New York: Oxford University Press, 1998:3–14.

• CASE 53 •

Other People's Money: Ethics, Finances, and Bad Outcomes

It costs a lot of money to die comfortably, unless one goes off pretty quickly.
Samuel Butler (1835–1902), *Notebooks*, "A Luxurious Death," 1912

You performed a straightforward radical gastrectomy on a middle-aged, otherwise healthy patient 6 months ago. He succumbed four weeks after surgery following one of the most turbulent, complication-laden postoperative courses you have seen in your entire career. He had an excellent commercial medical insurance plan, with 85% coverage of hospital and medical expenses. Today, his wife, a practicing tax attorney, visits your office carrying a cardboard carton of accumulated unpaid medical and hospital bills and letters from the insurance company notifying her that payment has been denied and inquiry sent to the hospital for such things as "exorbitant charges," "failures to code properly," "failures to bill promptly," and "failure to precertify." She is highly agitated and is grieving deeply for her husband. She demands to know why she has received such extensive charges, and why she has been charged so much by physicians whose names and functions she doesn't know. She insists that you as her husband's attending surgeon explain, "Why I am being charged so much to watch my husband suffer and die?" How should you respond?

(A) Tell her how terribly you have been tormented by her husband's death, what you might have done differently to prevent it, and agree to waive your copay in consolation.

(B) Refer her to the hospital billing office.

(C) Call the hospital's Risk Management Office.

(D) Tell her that medical care is expensive and unfortunate complications occur from time to time despite the best possible care.

(E) Offer to review with her the details of her husband's hospital course and the care that was provided.

None of the options offered will fully resolve the grief and frustration the widow is expressing in her complaints about the high cost of her husband's futile care, and no accounting for the accuracy of the invoices she's received will replace the one priceless thing she has irretrievably lost on your watch. The enormity of her financial burden is real nonetheless. Even though most high-quality commercial insurance plans cover all but about 15% of hospital charges and cap catastrophic expenses, the thousands left due on a half-million-dollar hospitalization would be an almost unbearable blow to nearly anyone, the more so when it just happens to fall at the same time as funeral expenses and the loss of the patient's regular income. Can the value of what we do as surgeons possibly be equal when we discharge a preoperatively functional patient to a mortuary or long-term care facility and when we release him for return to work and full activities? Should adjustments be made accordingly?

Most patients and their families pay the amount due on their medical bills without question, so much so that many hospitals no longer itemize the statement of copay charges they send home after insurance settles unless they are specifically asked to do so. Even if they did, the patients would understand little of what went on and whether most listed items were reasonable. Certainly few patients make distinctions between the surgeon's charges, the anesthesiologist's charges, consultant charges, and hospital charges. Most don't understand why they receive several different statements for a single episode of surgical care, but they pay them all, trusting to the integrity of the medical care system, even when the outcome of treatment has been disappointing.

Likewise, many surgeons are relatively naïve about the sometimes complex finances of the care we provide because office or hospital business staff handle this work for us. The price of our surgical procedures is effectively fixed by Medicare and the insurance companies that follow its lead, and our fees are unbundled from other charges associated with a patient's care, including those posted by other physicians working in support of our care during a patient's hospitalization for surgery. Many of us have been further insulated from confronting the high cost of copayment by the ancient customs of professional courtesy (now taboo but sometimes still quietly practiced) when we need care ourselves.[1] Resultantly, we are poorly prepared to decipher the vagaries of 20 page invoices for the few patients who want explanations.

In many functions of Western culture, determination of compensation is closely associated with the buyer's degree of satisfaction with what is provided. Low-cost disposable goods like groceries, clothing, and small household articles have well-defined criteria for acceptability. Meat must be unspoiled, clothing must fit, and toasters must toast. When these standards are not met, merchandise is typically replaced or the cost refunded without loss to the customer. Refunds or replacement of larger, more expensive products like automobiles or new homes are less likely, but there is an expectation that suitable repairs will be provided to a dissatisfied buyer.

Customer dissatisfaction is necessarily managed differently by providers of custom services or products that are individually rather than mass produced. A cabinet maker's product should not only be of the correct size, shape, and ornamentation, it should also satisfy the aesthetic expectations of the buyer. But if the cabinet maker met the terms of their premanufacturing agreement, the buyer must accept the product and the dissatisfaction. If the buyer did not specify the finished cabinet's appearance, the negotiation may involve some cosmetic carpentry, but full payment will still be required.

Compensation in other service industries is based variously on time spent, piecework, competitive bidding, fixed salary, or achievement of milestones and goals. The customs influencing professional compensation are different still. When not working on contingency, trial attorneys bill and are typically paid the same hourly rate whether the client goes home or is hung. Because the final arbiter is a judge or jury, the attorney bears responsibility only for the technical and intellectual quality of the advocacy. Only the contingency lawyer guarantees a favorable outcome or no pay, and does so in exchange for hugely inflated compensation if the case is won. Otherwise, the trial attorney's fee is based upon the training, experience, time, effort and physical resources invested on each client's behalf, with the understanding that the case's resolution may be heavily influenced, but not wholly determined, by the work of the professional. Likewise, physicians.

Because surgical fees are essentially charged at a flat rate per specified OR procedure, postoperative care is bundled with payment for the operation. The more difficult cases require more, sometimes immensely more, effort and time, but payment is the same as for routine cases. Nevertheless, surgeons characteristically take pride in their mastery of complexity, and the differential between effort and compensation has generally not resulted in difficult cases being turned away. Complex cases may be transferred to tertiary care centers, but the referral is usually made because superior expertise or facilities are required, not over grievances about the reimbursement per unit of time.

People come to us for good outcomes and we prepare very hard, work very hard, and expend enormous resources in trying to provide them. Every surgeon, every physician, grieves the loss of every patient we have watched spin out of our control and die. Although it is fully appropriate to empathize with the widow's loss, it is unseemly to ask her to feel the additional weight of our own emotional burden, or to attempt consolation by outdoing the depth of her sorrow. Although a copayment waiver may seem like the best redeeming gift you can make in these sad circumstances, it isn't. Furthermore, such a waiver unethically violates the terms of the contract you signed with the patient's insurers, and unfairly imposes upon others who provided care an expectation that they should do so as well. Option (A) should be rejected on all counts.

The insurer's notification of billing errors is certainly the responsibility of the hospital's billing office to resolve, but it is unnecessary to direct the poor widow with her box of invoices there or elsewhere around the hospital like a prep school freshman sent to retrieve 50 feet of shoreline. As a matter of gentility and kindness, you might more reasonably ask your own administrative support staff to call the billers and make certain that they have received the insurer's notices and have initiated routine steps to resolve them. You may then reassure the widow accordingly. Coding errors and other filing mistakes are ordinary events in the tortuous communication between care providers and insurers, and are routinely resolved with amended filings, but unless someone tells them otherwise, they can seem like yet one more catastrophe to a patient's family. Option (B) can be set aside, for the time being at least.

Hospital Risk Management offices ask providers to advise them if they have reason to believe that a malpractice claim or other lawsuit may be impending.

Although you might feel a little extra wariness because the widow is an attorney, she has made no such threat, asking only for explanation of some complex material that could well bear explanation. It would be an act of bad faith to adopt an adversarial posture toward a lost patient's family member who has come seeking your guidance. Option (C) should be rejected.

As a practicing attorney, the patient's widow normally understands the concept that professionals are paid on the basis of the services they provide, that it costs you a great deal to provide that care, and that you must be fully compensated, irrespective of unforeseen complications or an ultimately unhappy outcome. Although it would not be factually inaccurate to remind her of this, it would clearly be heard as callous and unfeeling were you to recite it so baldly under the circumstances, and would certainly deepen her current sense of disaffection for the medical profession. Option (D) would be a poor choice.

The widow's anguished question about why such a bitter disappointment comes at so high a price can be accepted as an entirely appropriate opportunity to pursue option (E), which may be ethically viewed as part of an ongoing process of informed consent. Reviewing with her the changes in her husband's condition and what responses were made, then inviting her to ask detailed questions about his hospital course and all the measures that were taken to arrest the heartbreaking process of his decline, will give her a better sense than she came in with of "Why." You may make it clear that while you do not determine the charges submitted by critical care and infectious disease specialists, radiologists, and pathologists, it was you who sought their consultation in your husband's care, just as it was you as the attending surgeon who referred him to the Intensive Care Unit, which has accounted for so much of her charges, in the interest of saving his life. You may reassure her that the acumen and performance of all these professionals in your husband's care was entirely consistent with what you asked and expected of them. You may explain in more or less detail what services her husband's care required from each. Such a discussion may in fact repeat things she was told on a day-by-day basis during the hospitalization, but a consolidated retrospective is likely to give her a better grasp of what occurred, help her to come to terms with her loss, and effectively help her to understand what it is that she is now being asked to pay for, which is what she came to you to ask. You may be inclined to articulate what you both acutely feel in different ways, a sense of helplessness when the abilities of medicine make hard contact with their limitations.

The concept of variable fees based on patient outcome has a glimmer of rational attraction, even justice, to it. Almost everyone tries harder when the rewards are increased, so might such a system not insure better patient care from harder working surgeons?

Upon first reading the harsh retributive strictures upon surgeons in the ancient Babylonian Code of Hammurabi, most medical students ask, "Who would want to be a surgeon if it means risking the loss of your hand?" It's a good question. The glimmer quickly fades from a system of outcome-based payment upon recognition that it could mean enormous outlays of money and energy with no payment at all for care of complex or high-risk patients. Surgeons would necessarily protect the basic financial interests of themselves and their families by declining to operate on diabetic, geriatric, far-advanced, or otherwise increased-risk patients, who could find themselves totally without access to surgical treatment. The masters at the pinnacle of our craft who accept referral of the most difficult patients might no longer do so. Surgeons might elect to withhold referral to ICU or decide not to seek consultation when patients develop postoperative complications, lest they run up expenses that won't be reimbursed. In short, the patients who need us most could be systematically shut out of our practices if we depended upon guaranteed good outcomes to replace our spent resources and provide us with a livelihood. With our current fixed-price system, surgeons are already disproportionately underpaid for managing the most complicated and work-intensive cases. We are proportionately best-paid in caring for the easiest and least complicated cases, and for the patient who is so terribly ill that he dies quickly after surgery. A revised compensation system that demands the modern equivalent of a sacrificed hand when our ministrations fail could ultimately incite us to less, not more, effort.

Modern surgeons have never offered to work on contingency, with a very high fee if the patient lives and no fee if he doesn't. None of us took the hard road into this profession with the intention of doing anything but good for the people who come to us, and we know that we cannot function at all without the absolute trust of our patients. To maintain that intent and that trust, almost all of us work at consistently full effort, with no sliding scales. It is in everyone's interest that we continue to do so.

References

1. Jones JW, McCullough LB, Richman BW. Ethics of professional courtesy. *J Vasc Surg.* 2004; 39:1140–1141.

• CASE 54 •

Consultation or Corruption? The Ethics of Signing on to the Medical-Industrial Complex

So one elephant with a trunk was odd, but all elephants having trunks looked like a plot.

G. K. Chesterton (1874–1936), *The Ethics of Elfland*

A prominent vascular surgeon is approached by a representative of a large medical device company with a proposal to implant a new self-sealing patch for closing open carotid endarterectomies. The patch is made of a new synthetic material that established immediate hemostasis and inhibited restenosis in animal studies. It has just been approved for human use by the FDA. The cost of the new patch is much higher than for well-established comparable products, even when potential long-term benefits are considered, but using it would reduce the operative time required for achieving hemostasis. The manufacturer's representative tells you that the company will pay a selected group of vascular surgeons $500 apiece each time they insert the patch on their patients and complete a one page report. Surgeons with the highest volume of cases utilizing the patch will be offered a paid clinical consultancy with the company. You've used another company's product for several years and found it entirely satisfactory, but have followed development of the new patch with interest and considered trying it in your carotid endarterectomies. What should you do?

(A) Join the study. You probably would have used the new patch on your patients anyway.

(B) If the early data warrant, implant the patch on a trial basis without enrolling in the project, and finally decide whether to continue using it based on your clinical experience and additional published reports.

(C) Call some of the other investigators who have already enrolled in the project and ask them about their experience.

(D) Decline the invitation immediately. Refuse to ever speak to the representative again.

(E) Estimate the ability of your patients to sustain the high cost of the new product and decide accordingly whether to use it.

It may be that the recent felony convictions of some high-profile corporate scoundrels will herald a new era of ethical practice in our high-stakes market places. The last several years have seen all sorts of traditional winners and icons become suspect. For juiced athletes, high-rolling TV preachers, and business over-friendly politicians, the lure of money, and more money, now and as ever, turns trust into a negotiable commodity and ethical boundaries into moving targets.

Has medicine remained pure amid this seemingly pervasive culture of corruption and rapacious self-interest? More and more the effluvium arising from the halls of the medical-industrial complex has taken on an insidiously purulent quality. An assistant professor of orthopedic surgery was fined $10,000 for implanting an expensive knee prosthesis without telling his patients that the device was made by a company that paid him a $175,000 annual consulting fee.[1] Maybe the choice of the company's prosthesis was appropriate to the patient's condition, and maybe the surgeon's failure to report his paid consultancy was an unintentional oversight, but his state ethics board felt like the whole thing didn't pass its smell test. That case wasn't the only source of the peculiar odor that's been in the air. Not long ago the New York Times reported that Guidant Corporation paid 80 cardiologists $1,000 each to implant 3 of the company's new leads in their patients and fill out some forms, ostensibly to see how the $29,000 product worked.[2] A Guidant executive, advocating the physician payment program in an in-house memo, wrote, "Let's say that just 25% were incremental...that yields more than $2 million in new sales with physicians who are not necessarily Guidant-friendly. We paid each physician who completed the surveys $1,000, so our total cost was $80,000." The company appears to have made the honoraria to promote sales, not, as one of the participating cardiologists said in justifying his role, "To get feedback on how well the system worked."

Accepting consultancies, honoraria, or gifts from medical equipment manufacturers creates the potential for conflicts of interest regardless of the arrangements or exculpatory terminology.[3] Financial conflicts of interest create a competitive relationship between the physician's fiduciary obligations to the patient and the physician's economic self-interest. Fiduciary obligations are founded in professional integrity, the essential professional virtue that obligates us to practice medicine and conduct research consistent with standards of intellectual and moral excellence. The patients who permit us to practice our invasive procedures upon them when they are most vulnerable need to believe that we always exercise professional integrity, and that our clinical judgments about what is best for them are always made on the basis of our hard-won knowledge and experience. Giving primacy to financial self-interest in one's practice, or permitting personal financial interests to influence clinical judgment and decisions, clearly violates that trust, without which we cannot function as a profession. For us, as with wayward athletes, clergymen, politicians, or industrialists, money coming in over the transom distorts professional integrity. For us alone it can imperil the lives and health of patients.

With the exception of radiology, no medical specialty is more dependent upon advanced technology than surgery. The cooperation of physician expertise and industrial capital is almost always beneficial, and even critical, to development of the ever-more complex and imaginative tools we use to broaden our ability to soothe and to heal. Certainly no one could sensibly advocate the development of medical and pharmaceutical technology unguided by the expertise of practicing clinicians. The effectiveness as well as the integrity of intellectual partnerships between doctors and medical product manufacturers can only be assured, however, when physicians disinterestedly observe scientific principles uncontaminated by business principles, and businessmen do not permit their profit motives to impinge upon the scientific process. Famed economic philosopher Adam Smith (1723–1790) called the process "enlightened self-interest," recognizing that everyone liked the idea of self-interest, but that it could only be durably achieved, and achieve the societal benefit which would ensure its durability, when people took the trouble to become enlightened about all its implications. The system of communication between physicians and the manufacturers of products they use in their practices certainly originated in the context of scientific collaboration, and that legitimate and valuable kind of partnership continues to this day. The medical industry funds an enormous amount of important basic and clinical science in academic research centers around the Western world. Somewhere along the way, though, the medical manufacturers' marketing departments shouldered their way into the process, and introduced the techniques of advertising and salesmanship to what medical professionals had been led to believe was a relationship built on their scientific and clinical expertise. Though told otherwise, it was no longer just the doctor's expert opinions and research programs that were sought, it was his or her influence as a sales broker for expensive products he or she ordered at his patients' expense. And the cost to the company of the doctor's confidence in the usefulness of the product was often only a "consultancy" fee, or travel expenses to a "scientific meeting," or maybe even just dinner at the elegant restaurant where detail reps supervised an "educational presentation." Acquaintances were warmed, good feelings generated, and obligations gently accumulated. If anyone saw through the thin disguises, nobody had the poor taste to mention it, and everyone went home comfortable. Waud had the audacity to reveal that gifts from the medical industry to physicians were in fact bribes, inducements for doctors to buy instruments, contraptions, and medications that someone else finally gets billed for.[4]

Financial conflicts of interest aren't rare in medicine. They're encouraged by the medical industry's marketing divisions, and are epidemic. Topol recently estimated that 10% of physicians had consulting relationships with the investment industry,[5] but the actual incidence of some sort of potentially compromising entanglement between doctors, particularly academic physicians, and medical product manufacturers appears to be much higher. 96% of respondents in a 2004 study had received some kind of gift or other inducement from the medical equipment or pharmaceutical industry.[6] Most of the physicians who accepted gifts from pharmaceutical companies acknowledged that the company's intent was to influence their practice, but still believed that it was not inappropriate for them to accept what was offered. They nevertheless did not want their acceptances made public.[7] Patients generally disapproved of physician gifts like restaurant meals that were unrelated to their medical practice (48.4%), but were less critical of free medical books.[8] Most significantly, 70% of patients believed that physicians' practices were influenced by gifts, and 64% thought that gifts to physicians from medical companies added to the cost of their medical care.

Innovation and technology, inseparable necessities of the surgeon's armamentarium, produce most of the major advances in surgery. Most of the surgical device technology originates in industry R&D sections, not merit review grant-supported research in academic clinical and basic science labs. Even when generated peripherally, the commercial rights to medical devices are typically sold to industries that proceed to patent, test, and put them into production. Industry is an essential component of medical practice, and physicians are an essential component of the medical industry. But roses always have thorns. Industrial money, disguised as research support, can easily be slipped into the marketing department, as the subject of the New York Times expose' appears to have done.

Appointing lots of physicians as "investigators" to curry favor on behalf of medical products and thus stimulate sales is becoming painfully common, but, because industry still supports so much legitimate science, physicians must learn to distinguish the two activities from one another when industry comes calling.[9] The absence of a research protocol, generation of unpublishable data, inappropriately high compensation, lavish travel perks, inclusion of inexperienced investigators, appointment of an excessive contingent of investigators, and token oversight are tip-offs that the physician is probably being approached by a company's marketing division rather than its research arm, and that the plan is ultimately to generate loyalties and boost sales rather than develop reproducible scientific data.

Spurred by a congressional investigation, a flurry of indignant articles condemning industry's unethical marketing forays appeared in the early 1990s, but the indignation cooled with the election of administrations more sympathetic and beholden to big business, and the compromising practices have crept back to where they were, with fewer complaints. A good deal of the public outrage stemmed from an intuition that the medical industry should observe the same ethical principles that guide the medical profession. The industries that manufacture our instruments, therapeutic devices, and nostrums have taken some pains to argue that they share and abide by the principles of medical ethics, but they are most pious in these protestations only when the lights are on. Guardianship of medical ethics is finally the responsibility of physicians, and if we leave the job to others we will inevitably see medical ethics in ashes. The American College of Surgeons' position on collaboration with industry appears to be limited to the College's own role in managing money it receives from medically-related industries, without much concern for the responsibilities of individual surgeons in handling their potential conflicts of interest when big business comes around waving fists full of money. The College's statement suggests that an ethical line is crossed when patient care is improperly influenced: "The primary objective of professional interactions between surgeons or surgical organizations and industry should be the improvement of patient care. It is the responsibility of surgeons to ensure that this care is not inappropriately affected by collaboration with industry."[9] England's Royal College of Surgeons is only a little more helpful. It suggests that, "If you have financial or commercial interests in organisations providing health care or in pharmaceutical or other biomedical companies, these must not affect the way you prescribe for, treat or refer patients."[10] These torpid positions seem to be about as much as our professional leaders have been willing to commit to on the subject of industry contamination of the surgeon's practice. The other major international surgical organizations have been content to lie suspiciously mute in the matter; their annual meetings are of course generously subsidized and their journals lavishly supported by manufacturers' advertising dollars.

The United Kingdom's Royal College of Physicians' position statement is more direct than its surgical counterpart on the subject of physicians' financial relations with industry. It advises that, "Doctors should avoid accepting any pecuniary or material inducement that might compromise, or be regarded by others as likely to compromise, the independent exercise of their professional judgment and practice."[11] The Royal College of Physicians suggests that physicians not place themselves in a compromised position. All their meeker surgical colleagues seem able to manage by contrast is a recommendation that we accept what industry offers us and then somehow summon the ethical fortitude to deny our gentle benefactors the influence they've purchased when we make our patient care decisions. One statement keeps the fox out of the henhouse, the other throws open the henhouse doors but expresses pious hope that the fox won't eat anything while he's in there. In the history of the world, only the Manicheans are known to have had such discriminative powers, and the Manicheans have long been gone.

The American Medical Association provides good guidance on the appropriate ethical terms for entering a financial relationship with the medical industry:

> Any financial compensation received from trial sponsors must be commensurate with the efforts of the physician performing the research. Financial compensation should be at fair market value and the rate of compensation per patient should not vary according to the volume of subjects enrolled by the physician, and should meet other existing legal requirements.[10]

Physicians interested in behaving ethically should avoid the kinds of rationalizations suggested in option (A). We can probably all think of good reasons for bad actions, particularly when low-hanging rewards are dangled before us. Are the reasons we invent sufficiently compelling to risk violating the trust our patients have in us? Are they likely to improve the quality of the care we provide? The answers to these questions are unlikely to lure the thoughtful physician into abandoning professional integrity, and the first of the options offered here should be rejected.

Option (C) may appear at first to have some virtue. We certainly consult experienced and trusted professional colleagues when we are about to do a new procedure for the first time, or when we are considering recruiting to our own staffs a surgeon with whom they have prior familiarity. But it may be too late to get an objective opinion about the new patch from a colleague who's already signed up for this questionable "study"; his loyalty to the product has already been bought and paid for. Cynical as such a view of a fellow professional might seem, the chances of a frank or critical assessment are probably slim, and it would be difficult to distinguish a carefully considered and well-supported positive report from one that has been compromised by a conflict of interest. Option (C) is ultimately not a reliable choice.

The absolutist position reflected in option (D), rejecting any sort of cooperative relationship with industry, overlooks the importance of ethically sound partnerships between surgeons and the companies that make the tools of our trade. If surgeons categorically decline to provide expert guidance to surgical instrument and supply manufacturers, who will? How responsive to our needs can they be if we never tell them what we need in the products they deliver to us? A better approach than disdainful, out-of-hand rejection would be to hear what's being proposed, remaining alert to the red flags suggesting potential exploitation and manipulation. If we have the scientific training and the resources, of course we may properly consider participating in a scientifically sound, protocol-based study that will yield reproducible publishable data and make a genuine contribution to the accumulated body of professional knowledge. Expenses incurred by your program in conducting a well-designed study should be covered by the sponsor, but assurances of personal enrichment should raise your skeptical antennae. And before agreeing to do any company-sponsored research study, you should establish in writing your entitlement to publish your findings independent of company control.

No doubt your patients will appreciate your sensitivity to the costs they incur in seeking surgical care, but it is no less odious for you to make clinical decisions on the basis of cost than it is for managed care clerks do it. Particularly when significant illnesses requiring major surgery are involved, your patients want you to provide them with outstanding care before they want you to provide them with inexpensive care. If you have legitimate reason to believe that the expensive new patch is the best choice for your patient's individual clinical condition, you are ethically obligated to use it. All your patient asks is that your decision be made on the basis of clinical indications, not marketing manipulations. Option (E) is neither an ethically nor a clinically sound approach.

Option (B) reflects the methods that thoughtful and ethical surgeons use in making virtually all their clinical decisions, without regard to the soothing assurances of manufacturers' reps, lucrative consultancies, four-color advertising brochures, or continuing education seminars in the Bahamas. It is the same process we use when none of these seductions are in the picture. It relies upon your training, your intellect, your clinical experience, your independent study of the peer-reviewed literature, and your individual assessment of your patient's unique clinical characteristics. The preservation of your judgment and integrity, and the quality of your care, is assured if you avoid unstable situations with a high risk for ethical compromise. Not every proposal you'll receive from every quarter is intended to corrupt you, but only physicians, not foxes, are bound to honor our exacting system of ethics, and those ethical principles are clearly anathema to interests that would turn us to their own purposes. We must guard our own henhouses.

References

1. Abelson R. Possible conflicts for doctors are seen on medical devices. *New York Times*. 2005.
2. Meier B. Implant program for heart device was a sales spur. *New York Times*. 2005.
3. Jones JW, McCullough LB. Surgeon-industry relationships: Ethically responsible management of conflicts of interest. *J Vasc Surg*. 2002; 35:825–826.
4. Waud DR. Pharmaceutical promotions—A free lunch? *N Engl J Med*. 1992; 327: 351–353.
5. Topol EJ, Blumenthal D. Physicians and the investment industry. *JAMA*. 2005; 293:2654–2657.
6. Halperin EC, Hutchison P, Barrier RC Jr. A population-based study of the prevalence and influence of gifts to radiation oncologists from pharmaceutical companies and medical equipment manufacturers. *Int J Radiat Oncol Biol Phys*. 2004; 59: 1477–1483.
7. Blake RL Jr, Early EK. Patients' attitudes about gifts to physicians from pharmaceutical companies. *J Am Board Fam Pract*. 1995; 8:457–464.
8. Guidelines for collaboration of industry and surgical organizations in support of research and continuing education. American College of Surgeons. 2000.
9. Financial interests in hospitals, nursing homes and other medical organisations. Royal College of Surgeons of England. 2001.
10. Bennett J, Collins J. The relationship between physicians and the biomedical industries: advice from the Royal College of Physicians. *Clin Med*. 2002; 2:320–322.
11. Morin K, Rakatansky H, Riddick FA Jr, Morse LJ, O'Bannon JM III, Goldrich MS, Ray P, et al. Managing conflicts of interest in the conduct of clinical trials. *JAMA*. 2002; 287:78–84.

CHALLENGES TO MEDICAL PROFESSIONALISM: ASSAULTS FROM WITHIN AND WITHOUT

Physicians confront challenges to their medical professionalism almost daily, emerging from inside and outside the medical establishment. Physicians' ethically effective reactions to these assaults obligate them to understand the nature of professional responsibility.

Many physicians believe that the concept of medicine as a profession was first introduced to Western culture by the authors of the Hippocratic Oath and its accompanying texts. This belief is complemented by the comforting assumption that the ideals of medical professionalism have reached contemporary physicians in an uninterrupted tradition of more than two millennia. These associated beliefs have become ritualized in the nearly universal adoption of some version of the Hippocratic Oath at medical school graduations and, more recently, at "white coat" ceremonies, where first-year medical students are solemnly inducted into their professional apprenticeship.

Scholars who have examined these historical claims have found them to be inaccurate. Baker, for example, has studied the Hippocratic texts carefully and found reason to question the concept that the history of medical ethics is just a footnote to the Hippocratic Oath, much like Alfred North Whitehead's (1861–1947) claim that all of the history of Western philosophy is but a footnote to Plato.[1] Indeed, there is no unbroken lineage of the Hippocratic or any other Oath in the history of Western medicine. Nutton has shown that the ritual swearing of the Oath is of rather recent historical vintage, asserting a link between current and ancient medical ethics that does not exist.[2] Many modern scholars of classical antiquity interpret the Hippocratic writings, and the oath in particular, as statements of guild fidelity, primarily designed to protect the monopolies of practitioners from interlopers, and to advertise their practices to those in need of them. It has been noted that the Hippocratic writings do not refer to "patients," but only to "the sick," and the concept of the special relationships physicians have toward their patients was to emerge centuries in the future.

The idea of medicine as a profession, or of physicians as moral fiduciaries of their patients, comes to us from the work of the two 18th-century British physician ethicists whom we have cited often throughout this volume. Dr. John Gregory's discussion of ethics,[3] published in 1772, became influential in the history of medical ethics in the United States primarily through the advocacy of Dr. Benjamin

Rush, a signer of the Declaration of Independence. Thomas Percival's *Medical Ethics*[4] was the primary influence on the 1847 Code of Ethics of the American Medical Association, the first modern, national code of medical ethics.[5]

Gregory and Percival wrote their works on medical ethics in response to the increasingly entrepreneurial character of medicine. They were concerned, for good reason, that medicine had become simply another trade, and that physicians and surgeons practiced primarily for financial gain. The predominance of self-interest among medical and surgical practitioners had created a crisis of confidence among the sick. They were concerned about whether these physicians knew what they were doing, and whether they had a genuine interest in the well-being of the sick over and above their interest in generating personal wealth.[5]

Gregory and Percival responded to the widespread intellectual and moral mistrust in physicians and surgeons by determining to reform medicine into a profession, probably for the first time in the history of Western medicine. Gregory and Percival built their account of medicine as a profession on the philosophy of science posited by Francis Bacon (1561–1626), and on the best moral philosophy of their own day.

Between them, Gregory and Percival forged a three-part account of the ethical concept of the physician as moral fiduciary of the patient. First, the physician should commit to becoming scientifically and clinically competent and maintaining the currency of his or her skills and knowledge through continuous study and technical improvement. Gregory and Percival had a nascent concept of what we now know as evidence-based medicine, especially the requirement that physicians be accountable for the quality of the processes and outcomes of medical and surgical care. Second, the physician should make a commitment to protecting and promoting the patient's health-related interests as the primary concern and motivation of his work, systematically sublimating self-interest to the welfare of the patient. Considerable self-sacrifice on behalf of patients remains an essential requirement of practitioners within the medical profession. Third, physicians should maintain, strengthen, and teach medicine to others as a public trust, for the benefit of future physicians and patients. These were the axes upon which the practice of medicine turned from a merchant guild, concentrating on protection and promotion of members' economic, social, and political interests, to a profession, concentrating upon the health and welfare of the patients in its care.

In the history of ideas, the ethical concept of the physician as the patient's fiduciary is young and fragile; we should not expect it to self-sustain itself like such truly ancient ideas as monotheism. Medical professionalism will be preserved and strengthened only by the self-conscious choices of physicians and surgeons to make it a reality in everyday practice, and in the culture of healthcare organizations. The cases discussed in this section, in a variety of ways, challenge medical professionalism and recommend ethically durable defenses to those challenges.

References

1. Baker RB. Medical propriety and impropriety in the English-speaking world prior to the formalization of medical ethics: Introduction. In: Baker RB, Porter R, Porter D, eds. *The Codification of Medical Morality: Historical and Philosophical Studies of the Formalization of Western Medical Morality in the Eighteenth and Nineteenth Centuries: Volume One: Medical Ethics and Etiquette in the Eighteenth Century.* Dordrecht, The Netherlands: Kluwer Academic Publishers, 1993:15–17.

2. Nutton V. The discourses of European practitioners in the tradition of the Hippocratic texts. In Baker RB, McCullough LB, eds. *The Cambridge World History of Medical Ethics.* Cambridge: Cambridge University Press, 2008.

3. Gregory J. Lectures on the Duties and Qualifications of a Physician. London: W. Strahan and T. Cadell, 1772. Reprinted in McCullough LB, ed. *John Gregory's Writings on Medical Ethics and Philosophy of Medicine.* Dordrecht, The Netherlands: Kluwer Academic Publishers, 1998:161–245.

4. Percival T. *Medical Ethics: Or a Code of Institutes and Precepts, Adapted to the Professional Conduct of Physicians and Surgeons.* London: J. Johnson & R. Bickerstaff, 1803.

5. Baker, Robert, et al., eds. *The American Medical Ethics Revolution.* Baltimore, Md: Johns Hopkins University Press, 1999.

• CASE 55 •

Going Public with Amazing Cases: Fiat or Fiasco?

Death wins! Bravo! But I laugh in his face, as he noses me out at the wire.
E. P. Baynes, *The Philosophy of Life*

Discussion in the doctors' lounge this morning concerns Dr. I.M. Dicey's elective endovascular abdominal aneurysm repair on a supercentenarian yesterday, and this morning's enthusiastic coverage in the local newspaper. The patient was asymptomatic, ambulatory, and mildly demented, but newsworthy because he was the oldest person known to have undergone and survived this major operation. A smiling Dr. Dicey was photographed by local newspaper in scrubs, with the OR lights forming a haloed backdrop. Several surgeons had declined to operate before he was consulted. Dicey commented for the press on his history of superior results with difficult cases. What should his colleagues think?

(A) Praise for extending the surgical frontier.
(B) Praise for an accomplishment if the facts of the case warrant it, but disapproval of his self-promotion.
(C) Like all medical curios, it does not merit any ethical valuation.
(D) Disapproval for operating on the extremes of survival, and for self-promotion.
(E) He should be reported to the state board of medical examiners.

As long as there have been surgical meetings, the greats and wannabes, more often the wannabes, describe truly amazing cases from the podium as a condiment to the scientific presentations. The best of these presentations are published, as retrievable literature; the rest remain as "fish stories." Whether one agrees or not with the merits of reporting individual cases, professional forums are the proper venue for medical knowledge. Other surgeons may be amused, irritated, entertained, or even awed, but are unlikely to refer their difficult cases, and they might just get a better idea of what works. On the other hand, some of the mass media coverage of surgeons' exploits seems less like reporting and more like advertising, akin at times to infomercials selling gold coins, rejuvenating creams, or stock-picking computer programs. The message is, if this surgeon operated successfully on one of the oldest people on the planet, he certainly can help a sick octogenarian. The public reporting of astonishing cases is somewhat like the stockbroker who reports only the best years and triple-bagger stock picks; it provides limited and therefore slanted information, may alter the checks and balances of the physician referral system, and may influence people who don't need operations to seek out self-promoting surgeons.

A local newspaper recently advertised an extremely low cost lease for a luxury car, but when customers visited the showroom they found the actual price doubled by hidden add-ons. The salesman lamely explained that, "We have to get people in the door." The self-aggrandizing surgeon could similarly claim, "We have to get patients into the consulting room." What he would really mean is, "We have to get patients into the operating room." But then major surgery would be the equivalent of leasing a car, ergo, a commodity, and the surgeon would become a peddler and no longer a professional with fiduciary responsibility to protect patients. This fiduciary responsibility includes the obligation of surgeons like our self-aggrandizer to protect patients from their own enthusiasm, from scientifically undisciplined thinking and impulsive behavior.

Physicians who decide to enter the public forum should remain aware that they act indirectly as spokespersons for all members of the profession, and must therefore be especially careful to display high levels of professionalism, especially since the lay audience is not qualified to make expert clinical judgments about whether a surgical procedure can be reliably expected to clinically benefit a patient. This is a matter of evidence-based clinical judgment, and therefore professional responsibility, which physicians who enter the public arena are obligated to discharge. From time to time, physicians find it necessary to raise public awareness about medical information that has been discovered through legitimate scientific research, or about public health information that should be disseminated. Their efforts are laudable.

More often of late, physicians like our posing surgeon have gone first to the lay press seeking their brief flash of celebrity. A recent front page article in a major Texas metropolitan newspaper reported on a surgeon who performed a really big procedure.[1] The patient weighed 851 pounds (BMI = 137.5, serious morbid obesity > 60), and was touted as the largest patient ever to have bariatric surgery. The surgeon told the newspaper that the patient was doing well the day after the operation. Despite the reportedly "successful" procedure, however, the patient died a few days later. The newspaper article was the surgeon's first publication on the subject, and in a follow-up article Dr. Dicey told the reporter that he "did not think the surgery . . . was a triggering event" for the patient's death. The record setting operation thus will not become a new benchmark for future surgeons to exceed: Guinness never uses the adjective almost.

Homo sapiens (knowing man) would perhaps be more accurately described as *Homo contentis* (competitive man). Competition is a compelling lifelong human instinct, from grabbing another child's rattle to "fighting" cancer at life's end. Humans look for a chance to exceed what has been done or seek to outdo someone or something else. Any measurable activity that humans can witness likely has records recorded somewhere. Ripley, Guinness, and entire libraries of athletes' top achievements testify to the interest generated by exceeding what has been done.

Robert Craig "Evel" Knievel gained fame and fortune by daredevil behaviors such as attempting to jump a quarter mile across the Snake River Canyon astride a rocket-powered motorcycle, at considerable personal cost; one of his world records in Guinness is for sustaining 40 fractures. When setting records in medicine, however, the caution bred of scientific discipline must prevail, as a strict matter of professional integrity and, above all, because the patient is the one taking the risk. Physicians, as a matter of professional responsibility, have an ethical obligation to protect patients from the unfavorable risks associated with their own enthusiasm.

In our case, the patient's extreme age is the broken barrier. As a relative contraindication, primarily to elective surgeries, age with its potential ravages has been almost counterbalanced by technology. Dr. Michael E. DeBakey became the oldest survivor of major aortic surgical procedure, of which he was actually the originator.[2] In our case, for emphasis, we have the surgeon taking extraordinary risks by operating on a member of one of the most exclusive clubs in the world—a club with a membership fewer than the 110 years required to belong. Once a supercentenarian, life expectancy is limited to 3 years, making that age presently a firm contraindication for elective repair. In *The Art*, the Hippocratic writers noted that medicine is sometimes powerless to alter the course of fatal disease, and that struggling against nature's boundaries represents hubris, and therefore a kind of madness.[3] Accepting the ethical discipline of professional integrity in the form of constant recognition of surgery's limited ability to challenge the borders of life has not been confined to medicine's prescientific era. Ethicists are at this moment embroiled in debate about our right to engage ourselves in the earliest and latest stages of human existence.[4] Realistically, mankind has firm control over only one side of the equation of life, the ability to end it, at which he excels. The concept that he gives life is a pompous distortion; he only appeases nature to delay life's inevitable ending. Only four people in all Western literature have departed earthly life without taking the fabled unidirectional boat ride; two mentioned in the Bible and two from Greek mythology.

Fiduciary responsibility to patients includes the obligation and consequent self-discipline to recognize the limits of medicine and surgery; responsibility to society includes recognition of finitude. Engelhardt believes that medicine's failure in this regard has "redefined the character of the encounter between physicians and patients…because of a reluctance [of physicians] to accept medicine's finite abilities in postponing death and curing disease."[5]

Our grandstanding surgeon rates no praise, because even an exceptionally large asymptomatic aneurysm would not have a sufficiently high incidence of rupture to result in a favorable risk/benefit ratio. The patient is over 110, and the oldest person living is barely 113. The patient has over an 80% chance not to see his next birthday, with or without the aneurysm. One cannot help but understand the surgeon's motivation as egotistical, as he sensed his destiny when scheduling this frail patient for a contraindicated procedure. Furthermore, imagine his swelling pride as the triumphant Dr. Dicey called the medical reporter, who had no way of knowing that the laudatory story should have been an exposé. Choices (A) and (B) are wrong. Furthermore, professional apathy about a colleague's bad behavior should be considered a threat to the ethical progress of our profession. Disregard option (C).

There is no evidence that there is a history of ongoing practice problems with taking excessive risk, and all of us have experienced occasional lapses in judgment. Having an articles in the newspaper, or even placing a personal advertisement is not regarded as an offense; the government made it so. Option (E) is unwarranted and premature.

Option (D) is our choice. The criticism of colleagues is a powerful stimulus to change one's behavior, especially when it comes *en masse* or from respected leadership figures. Our physician colleagues are indeed the second family of us all but the most reclusive, and as such can exert tremendous peer pressure. As Thomas P. "Tip" O'Neil, the former Speaker of the U.S. House of Representatives, succinctly summed it, "All politics is local." The best way to avoid laymen regulating surgery is for surgeons to be responsible self-regulators, locally. Apathy for self-regulation in cases like this substitutes enthusiasm for recognition and thereby replaces scientific and clinical integrity with ambition, eroding professionalism like a cancer.

Incidentally, the bariatric surgeon got unexpected results from the newspaper article. A relative of a previous patient who died was stirred to file a malpractice suit.

References

1. Ackerman T. 841-pound woman who sought a better life dies. *Houston Chronicle.* 2007:1.
2. Altman L. The Doctor's World; the Man on the Table was 97, but He Devised the Surgery. *New York Times.* 2006:1A.
3. Jones W. *Hippocrates.* Loeb Classical Library. Cambridge, Mass: Harvard University Press, 1923.
4. Gallagher P, Clark K. The ethics of surgery in the elderly demented patient with bowel obstruction. *J Med Ethics.* 2002; 28:105–108.
5. Engelhardt H. The deprofessionalization of medicine. In: Bondeson W, Jones JW eds. *The Ethics of Managed Care: Professional Integrity and Patient Rights.* Boston: Kluwer Academic Publishers, 2002.

• CASE 56 •

Ethics of Unprofessional Behavior That Disrupts: Crossing the Line

Law is necessary because men are subject to passions. If all men were reasonable, law would be superfluous.
Will Durant, *The Story of Philosophy*

As chief of surgery, you have been contacted by the managing OR nurse about Dr. Frank N. Stein's behavior earlier this morning. Dr. Stein, a senior surgeon, has long had a reputation for outlandish behavior in the operating room. He is an impeccable gentleman outside the OR, loved by patients and nonoperating personnel alike. He has an international reputation as a master technical surgeon, operates as efficiently as anyone on the planet, and has the largest practice at the medical center. He has survived beyond the generation of tolerance because he has retained the same OR crew who, over the years, have become calloused enough to regard his scurrilousness as just being Dr. S. Today, he crossed the line. Dr. Stein, known for his colorful diatribes, trounced decorum when he ordered the operative team, excepting the anesthesiologist, out of the OR and demanded that a new team be substituted. This resulted from a shouting match with a new circulator when she took issue with a personal insult. The transition was made, causing delays in both Dr. Stein's room and several other rooms from which substitute nurses were commandeered. At least one other faculty surgeon has complained about the inconvenience. Called to your office, Frank, long a colleague, insists that the nurses involved are assassins and refuses to work with them from this day forward. What should be done?

(A) Assign ex-bouncers to assist him.
(B) Give him what he needs. The support staffs are there to support, not to disrupt.
(C) Survey the nurses, physicians, administrators, and all support personnel to determine institutional relations. If the problem is part of a pattern, require Dr. Stein to accept training in professionalism as part of an institutional program.
(D) Dismiss him from the staff.
(E) Make working in difficult surgeons' ORs voluntary and give combat pay.

Aberrant outlandish behavior is part of the fading macho surgical stereotype. In the not so remote past of the last century, surgeons were given more latitude in the workplace; one classification involved whether or not surgical instruments became projectiles. Generally, one's OR behavior was not reported unless injury or the possibility of injury to coworkers was involved. Crass assertions by surgeons were commonplace, and still are in some ORs, albeit with steadily lessening frequency.

Medical professionalism has received much attention recently from the major professional organizations whose goals are to codify and improve behavioral standards.[1] Extreme behaviors that disrupt medical care are not mentioned, just as ethics treatises do not routinely discuss why murdering innocents is wrong; their ethical unacceptability is considered obvious. Formalized professionalism concentrates on dealings with patients and finances, while professional disruption is related more to interactions with professional colleagues and coworkers, typically without the patient's knowledge. According to Wilhelm, "Disruptive behaviors include repeated episodes of: sexual harassment; racial or ethnic slurs; intimidation and abusive language; and persistent lateness in responding to calls at work."[2] Although the surgeon is the captain of the team, surgical therapy is dependent on the proper functioning of all the members of the health care team. The introduction of behaviors by members of the team that disrupt the team's functioning, especially by the captain, clearly is unacceptable.[3] Disruptive behavior suggests that fulfilling the surgeon's own ego needs are his primary concerns and motivations. Tyrannical demands become the primary concerns and motivations of the other members of the surgical team. In such an environment, the patient's needs are seen only in the rear-view mirror. However, as Dr. Thomas Percival put it, when addressing the ethics of potentially disruptive relationships among consulting physicians (one of the most persistent topics in the history of medical ethics), "the good of the patient is the sole object in view."[4]

We live in an era in which we are skeptical about the connection between behavior and character. In particular, we are skeptical about whether we can reliably infer good character from good behavior. Fissell notes that at some time in the late 18th century, "medical manners and morals became unglued; no longer were codes of conduct based on courtesy functional."[5] Despite our skepticism, patterns of disruptive behavior of physicians invite the inference that bad behavior reflects bad character and deficient professionalism. Such disruptive behavior, from the perspective of the ethics of professionalism, is a very serious matter indeed, calling for serious responses by physician leaders.

Option (A) *en passant* does have possible merit. A rather famous surgeon, legendary for abusing surgical residents, would characteristically announce in the middle of a procedure that "I can whip you with one hand tied behind my back." He unknowingly had a resident assigned to his service who before medical school had been a successful professional boxer. When challenged, the ex-boxer resident replied, "No sir, it is I who could whip you using only my left hand." The abuse stopped for the remainder of that rotation but restarted with the following resident. Option (A) would not work longterm.

Option (B) permits unacceptable behavior in patient care areas to continue with administrative support. It is the least ethical of the options offered. Option

(E) is a variant of (B). It too is objectionable as well but at least attempts to compensate those most abused.

Option (D) should be chosen if remedial measures are not effective. The courts clearly support an institution's right to remove staff privileges when it can be proven that a physician's behavior disrupts the institution's ability to provide quality medical care.

Management assesses whether untoward events are unique or global and acts acccordingly. Data from a national study showed that 74% of healthcare professionals had witnessed disruptive behavior by physicians.[6] This figure climbed to 86% when only data from nurses were counted. Regarding surgeons, specifically, disruptive behaviors were more common in the peri-operative area,[7] where 97% of nurses reported witnessing surgeons behaving badly. Surgeons themselves had the thickest skins or greatest forgiveness: only 43% reporting witnessing such events. So it seems that although behavior has improved in recent years, problems remain.

The results of every published study on organizational team processes in the medical care professions finds there is need for improvement of the physician's interpersonal communicative skills. The behavior of our surgeon and others like him is just the tip of the metaphorical iceberg drawing attention to an opportunity medicine should not ignore. Since the Institute of Medicine published its findings about a high frequency of medical errors, a large body of literature has accumulated emphasizing the need for improvements in communication skills among team members in complex high-risk environments such as the operating room.[8,9] Direct observation of medical teams treating patients identified errors in 30% of emergency room cases,[10] and more than one event compromising patient safety per surgical case.[8] The main identified cause was lack of effective communication in environments with "normally behaving" surgeons.

Option (C) emerges as the preferred option. More to the point, it stands that dysfunctional surgeons captain dysfunctional operating teams and should be viewed by the profession as having incapacities that must be addressed. No surgeon would fail to take decisive action if he noticed a tray of unsterilized instruments being delivered for use to a colleague's OR. Disruptive behaviors can be just as harmful, without microorganisms to fault, and should be taken just as seriously as a threat to patient well being and therefore to medical professionalism.

References

1. Jones JW, McCullough LB, Richman BW. Ethics and professionalism: Do we need yet another surgeons' charter? *J Vasc Surg.* 2006; 44:903–906.
2. Wilhelm KA, Lapsley H. Disruptive doctors: Unprofessional interpersonal behaviour in doctors. *Med J Aust.* 2000; 173:384–386.
3. Purtilo R, Shaw B, Arnold R. Obligations of surgeons to non-physician team members and trainees. In: McCullough LB, Jones JW, Brody BA, eds. *Surgical Ethics.* New York: Oxford University Press, 1998:302–321.

4. Percival T. *Medical Ethics: Or a Code of Institutes and Precepts, Adapted to the Professional Conduct of Physicians and Surgeons.* London: J. Johnson & R. Bickerstaff, 1803.

5. Fissell ME. Innocent and honorable bribes: Medical manners in eighteenth-century Britain." In: Beker RB, Porter R, Porter D, eds. *The Codification of Medical Morality: Historical and Philosophical Studies of the Formalization of Western Medical Morality in the Eighteenth and Nineteenth Centuries: Volume One: Medical Ethics and Etiquette in the Eighteenth Century.* Dordrecht, The Netherlands: Kluwer Academic Publishers, 1993: 19–45.

6. Rosenstein AH, O'Daniel M. Disruptive behavior and clinical outcomes: perceptions of nurses and physicians. *Am J Nurs.* 2005; 105:54–64; quiz 64–65.

7. Rosenstein AH, O'Daniel M. Impact and implications of disruptive behavior in the perioperative arena. *J Am Coll Surg.* 2006; 203:96–105.

8. Christian CK, Gustafson ML, Roth EM, Sheridan TB, Gandhi TK, Dwyer K, et al. A prospective study of patient safety in the operating room. *Surgery.* 2006; 139: 159–173.

9. Espin S, Levinson W, Regehr G, Baker GR, Lingard L. Error or "act of God"? A study of patients' and operating room team members' perceptions of error definition, reporting, and disclosure. *Surgery.* 2006; 139:6–14.

10. Morey JC, Simon R, Jay GD, Wears RL, Salisbury M, Dukes KA, et al. Error reduction and performance improvement in the emergency department through formal teamwork training: Evaluation results of the MedTeams project. *Health Serv Res.* 2002; 37:1553–1581.

• CASE 57 •

My Brother's Keeper: The Ethics of Uncompensated Care for Illegal Immigrants

English was good enough for Jesus Christ and it's good enough for the children of Texas.

Miriam "Ma" Ferguson, Governor of Texas in 1924

An undocumented immigrant was brought to the emergency room with severe injuries from a traffic accident. Since his arrival in the United States from Latin America 2 years ago, he has made a bare but steady living as a brick mason for home builders who pay him a fraction of the prevailing union wage and provide him with no health insurance or other benefits. His postoperative course was complicated by infection and multiple organ system failure. After nearly six weeks in the intensive care unit, he became stable enough for transport to a hospital near his home. Hospital charges have reached the high six figures. Who should bear the financial responsibility for his care?

(A) The government of the country of his origin.

(B) The patient's wages should be garnished when he returns to work.

(C) The hospital should accept the loss. It can bill added indirect costs to patients with insurance to compensate.

(D) The patient's employers.

(E) Enact a system of mandatory universal health insurance, with workers' premiums deducted from payrolls with indigent premiums subsidized by federal and state governments.

The ongoing unabated flow of unauthorized immigrants into the United States is commanding unprecedented attention from the nation's government, news media, and citizenry. Few nations have been so intently sought as a destination by the citizens of other countries, and fewer still have been so ineffectual at compelling new arrivals to comply with its immigration laws. Since 2001, demands for better border control, and tighter accountability for landed aliens who have evaded immigration laws, have been loud and clear. Threats to national security, to the prevalence of the English language, to the country's predominant Eurocentric culture, to jobs and the economy, and to the capacity of tax-supported services to sustain the surge in demand from a large new underclass have all been perceived and articulated. These concerns have been countered on a lesser scale by pleas to insure that all immigrants, regardless of legal status, be afforded access to education, employment, and health care as basic human rights.

Political recognition of undocumented aliens, and attempts to accommodate to them, essentially began with the Bracero Agreement in 1942. The pact arranged for Mexican agricultural laborers to be granted temporary work permits to harvest crops in Texas and California to compensate for depletion of the U.S. workforce during World War II. U.S. farmers found the arrangement profitable, had the program extended until 1962, and gave the Mexican laborers continuing work. The laborers were happy to stay for much better wages than what they could earn at home, and many determined never to return to Mexico. From that time until recently, the American border patrols allowed unrestricted entry, though the Mexican authorities tried to prevent departure of their nationals.[1] When the problem boiled over as unmanageable toward the end of the last century, the Immigration Reform and Control Act of 1986 granted amnesty to almost two million aliens living in the United States, but resulted in no measurable reduction in illegal immigration.[2] President Reagan supported free movement across the borders of the United States with Mexico and Canada through a guest worker program that Congress never enacted.[1]

As it did when it adopted slavery early in the nation's history, America wanted cheap laborers to do the backbreaking jobs, but not the cultural baggage they carried, and certainly not their human needs. The large policy questions consequent to these issues are beyond the scope of a discussion of surgical ethics, but there is an important question that medical and surgical ethics must address: How should essential medical care be provided to a large population of undocumented and uninsured foreign nationals who can't pay for it?

American medical care has been deeply affected by massive immigration. Half of the cases of tuberculosis (TB) diagnosed in the United States, more than 30,000 in a recent survey, occurred in foreign-born patients who comprised less than 10% of this country's population.[3] Poverty and fear of discovery and deportation among illegal immigrants with TB invariably delays their presentation for care by months, and in the interim they can infect as many as 10 others.[4] Along sparsely populated sections of the U.S.-Mexican border, trauma surgeons have described the prevalence of a new location-specific event that produces multiply-injured victims and a 9% mortality rate: the overcrowded motor vehicle accident.[5] In a 4-year period, 663 persons, averaging 17 per vehicle, were involved in high speed rollovers of poorly maintained vehicles used to smuggle Hispanics into the United States along the Arizona border. Rural hospitals, and many major medical centers, are poorly prepared, either clinically or financially, for the sudden and simultaneous arrival of 17 severely injured indigent patients.

Is medical care a right? In 1986, the U.S. Congress enacted the Federal Emergency Medical Treatment and Active Labor Act (EMTALA), effectively declaring each individual's entitlement to emergency care. Access to nonemergent medical care, even if the uncorrected condition will become life-threatening, can be a problem for the uninsured and some cultural groups.[6] After a Dutch hospital administrator disallowed emergency care for an undocumented immigrant to the Netherlands because the injury was not life- threatening, the British Medical Journal led an international uproar by editorializing that treatment of alien patients must be equivalent to that of a nation's citizens.[7] Hospitals have historically covered the expenses of uncompensated care by cost-shifting to paying patients, and resorting to government subsidies. Dispro-portionate-Share Funds (DSH, or "Dish"), made available to hospitals by the U.S. government for indigent care, are never adequate to meet expenses, have exasperating strings attached, and often find their way to hospitals providing less, not more, indigent care. In 2005, Houston's Ben Taub General Hospi-tal spent $128 million to treat 57,000 uninsured undocumented immigrant patients. Only $31 million was reimbursed through government and other sources.[8]

Cost shifting strategies by hospitals can create additional ethical prob-lems. As the uninsured nonelderly population has grown beyond 16% of the national total, fewer hospitals have been providing indigent care, and abusive billing practices have become more common.[9] Many hospitals have strained to the limit and beyond their creative efforts to extract even more from paying patients. Private insurers and government medical programs wind up paying not only for those who have policies or eligibility, but indirectly for those who don't. Eventually, these additional costs wend their way back to the productive members of society as higher premiums and higher taxes. Medical insurance reduces the individual financial burden of treatment; it doesn't eliminate it. Premiums, copays, and deductibles are increased annually for all of us, and more and more employers are seeking ways to limit and even escape from subsidized coverage as a standard employee benefit.

Should these trends continue, only the most affluent among us will have regular access to medical care, and the strength of the culture will be mark-edly diminished. The medical profession itself could wither and weaken absent an adequate workload of compensated care. There are currently no national systems in place to prevent this eventuality, and as many as 45 million unin-sured Americans are in the same straits as 11 million poor and undocumented immigrants when they become sick or injured. In this context, Weissman's assessment is pertinent: "Until the country decides to provide health coverage for all residents, the problem of uncompensated care will not go away."[9]

How should physicians address these issues clinically when presented with individual patients like the unfortunate man in our scenario, desperately ill, destitute, and far from home? In the absence of guiding governmental policy at any level, one thing is certain in surgical ethics: Physicians and hospitals have a fiduciary responsibility to protect and promote the health-related interests of their patients.

A key element in this ethical standard is the question of when an individual becomes a patient. People become patients when they present to a physician in some manner of distress that medical interventions can be reliably expected to limit or resolve.[10] None of these qualifying conditions is dependent upon citizenship or immigration status, nor should they be. The moral condition of becoming a patient is independent of an individual's national identification, and without regard to the statutory, administrative, or bureaucratic procedures legitimizing one's presence within one national border or another. Humanity precedes nationality. And finances.

There has long been an outraged cry that undocumented immigrants place an intolerable parasitic burden upon educational, welfare, and medical systems to which they do not contribute. Many immigrants, legal and illegal, in fact pay substantially the same taxes as citizens. Although they are often stereotyped as itinerant yardmen who deal only in cash, most undocumented aliens have organizational jobs and earn wages from which state and federal income taxes, Social Security, and Medicare are withheld. They realize no return on their contributions to Social Security and Medicare, and these payments constitute a net gain to the U.S. treasury.[11] Those paying taxes have the same economic and moral claim on publicly funded services as do citizens.

It is generally conceded that undocumented foreign nationals make major contributions to local and national economies. Their lower wages may result in many commodities and services being priced lower than they otherwise would be. They provide the greatest economic advantage (about $1.5 billion annually after subtracting the lost wages to citizen laborers) to employers and owners of capital that is only partially passed on to consumers because free market pricing is based on what the market will bear.[12]

While it may seem reasonable that the nation of origin should be responsible for such expenses as public assistance, incarceration, burial, and medical care incurred by its unauthorized emigrants in another country, responsibility effectively vanishes when borders are crossed. The 1848 Treaty of Guadalupe Hidalgo, which ended the Mexican War and added almost 25% to the land mass of the young and avaricious United States, did not address economic responsibilities for emigrants traveling from one country to the other, nor has any subsequent pact between the United States and another nation. Our patient properly received the accepted standard of care for his diagnosis. No prior authorization to treat was sought or received from his native country. As a resident and an economic contributor to this country, there is no statutory assignment of responsibility for reimbursement of his medical costs to the country from which he emigrated. Option (A) is not available.

Neither ethical standards, humanitarian instincts, nor the provisions of EMTALA preclude the entitlement of surgeon and hospital to reasonable compensation for their services. Insured patients accept financial responsibility for their premiums, copayments, and deductibles. Expecting this patient to make some financial contribution toward the cost of his care is entirely reasonable. It is not, however, practicable. He is virtually penniless, and his meager living as a contract laborer is scratched from a different source with every job. Although his short-term employers make required payroll deductions, there is no steady salary to garnish, and for purposes of cost recovery his situation is identical to the uninsured indigent citizens whom most hospitals regularly treat. Option (B) is not available either.

Option (C) imposes upon the hospital sole responsibility for a cost it did not solely incur. EMTALA should not be an unfunded mandate, but in practical application it often is. DSH reimbursements are maddeningly meager. The abject failure of the United States government to enforce its own policies on immigration into this country effectively placed this patient at the hospital's doorstep. Perpetuation of the Robin Hood method currently used by hospitals to shift costs is ultimately unsustainable, and could disable the entire health care system. It is patently unfair, and therefore unethical, for the insured, their employers, heavily taxed workers, and the elderly on fixed incomes to bear an ever-increasing burden they had no hand in fashioning. Medical cost-shifting amounts to a financial deception that is falsely inflating the cost of medical care and poisoning the relationship between the at-large population and the medical profession. Hospitals that have provided enough charity care to have satisfied their tax exempt status should not be expected to bear these additional costs. Option (C) is a poor and destructive choice.

Option (D) would make support of health care the responsibility of the employers who have exploited this immigrant's undocumented status to pay him an unfair wage for his skilled labor and deny him the health insurance that is regularly available to other full-time workers in similar trades. By deflecting an employer's regular responsibility for subsidizing health insurance, the building contractors who hired our patient are effectively stealing the cost of his treatment from the societal institutions that will ultimately pay for this episode of care. Unfortunately, there is presently no statutory provision requiring these employers to support their employee's health care, and option (D) cannot be enforced.

Medical treatment for illegal immigrants is a growing problem, complicated and inflated by elements of jingoism, fear, and cultural identity. It is nevertheless just a small subset of this country's larger problem of uninsured healthcare. Despite the current political furor around them as election-year fodder, the 11 million illegal immigrants distributed around the country represent too small a sample of uninsured indigents to statistically affect the larger problem the individual states confront in caring for all the patients who can't pay their medical bills because they are uninsured.[13] Congress, and the insurance lobby, roundly rejected a detailed program for national health insurance in 1994, and no federal official has stepped forward in the years since to propose a plan that will guarantee medical coverage to everyone as a basic human right. Schroeder noted that,

> A constant feature of health care in the United States is our national willingness to tolerate having large numbers of people without health insurance. This is in stark contrast to the situation in virtually every other developed country, where guaranteed health insurance is provided either by the state or through employers, with government backup for the unemployed.

Whatever the number of uninsured people, we put the values of the entire health care system at risk by accepting their condition as inevitable.[14]

At a recent House of Delegates meeting in Chicago, the American Medical Association recommended that all Americans who can afford it be required to purchase health insurance, with premium surpluses used to support the care of indigent patients. The state of Massachusetts has recently implemented landmark legislation requiring that all state residents have medical insurance.[15] No exception for undocumented foreign nationals was written into the bill, perhaps guaranteeing their access to the same health care as legal immigrants and citizens of the state. Community leaders cited the "spirit of generosity and respect for the dignity of the person written into this bill," acknowledging its soundness as ethical policy. It is a unique and possibly definitive solution to the issues of universal coverage and indigent care without regard to extraneous conditions such as immigration documentation. Although legislation of this sort will not solve the immediate problem of assigning financial responsibility for the care of our patient, it is an excellent application of the principles described in our option (E), and we believe it is an ethical and effective choice.

References

1. Hansen LO. The political and socioeconomic context of legal and illegal Mexican migration to the United States (1942–1984). *Int Migr.* 1988; 26:95–107.

2. Orrenius PM, Zavodny M. Do amnesty programs reduce undocumented immigration? Evidence from IRCA. *Demography.* 2003; 40:437–450.

3. Kahn K, Muenning P, Behta M, Zivin J. Global drug-resistance patterns and the management of latent tuberculosis infection in immigrants to the United States. *NEJM.* 2002; 347:1850–1859.

4. Avery JK. The disaster of a suspected cover-up. *J Ark Med Soc.* 2002; 99:82–83.

5. Lumpkin MF, Judkins D, Porter JM, Latifi R, Williams MD. Overcrowded motor vehicle trauma from the smuggling of illegal immigrants in the desert of the Southwest. *Am Surg.* 2004; 70:1078–1082.

6. Jones JW. The question of racial bias in thoracic surgery: Appearances and realities. *Ann Thorac Surg.* 2001; 72:6–8.

7. Sheldon T. Dutch minister warns that illegal immigrants must receive care. *BMJ.* 1999; 318:1234.

8. Murphy B. County's cost for illegal immigrant's care soars. *Houston Chronicle.* 2006: 6.

9. Weissman JS. The trouble with uncompensated hospital care. *N Engl J Med.* 2005; 352:1171–1173.

10. McCullough L, Chervenak F. *Ethics in Obstetrics and Gynecology.* New York: Oxford University Press, 1994.

11. Weintraub S. Illegal immigrants in Texas: Impact on social services and related considerations. *Int Migr Rev.* 1984; 18:733–747.

12. Huddle DL. The net national costs of illegal immigration into the United States. *Curr World Lead.* 1995; 38:11–34.

13. Castel LD, Timbie JW, Sendersky V, Curtis LH, Feather KA, Schulman KA. Toward estimating the impact of changes in immigrants' insurance eligibility on hospital expenditures for uncompensated care. *BMC Health Serv Res.* 2003; 3:1.
14. Schroeder SA. The medically uninsured—will they always be with us? *N Engl J Med.* 1996; 334:1130–1133.
15. Steinbrook R. Health care reform in Massachusetts—a work in progress. *N Engl J Med.* 2006; 354:2095–2098.

• CASE 58 •

From Premiums to Payouts: Who's Behind the Professional Liability Crisis, Anyway?

It is now, as it was then and as it may ever be; conceptions from the past blind us to facts which almost slap us in the face.
William Stewart Halsted, *Surgical Papers*, Vol. II

With the passing of each year since the turn of the new millennium, malpractice insurance rates have risen by over 20% as your reimbursements have dropped. Your medical malpractice insurance premiums have reduced your net income more than any other single cost of practice. Most physicians have never experienced a malpractice allegation or lawsuit to account for the descent of this plague upon the medical profession. Hospital and medical school administrators report that insurance rates for institutions are advancing even more sharply than for individual physicians, and may soon affect their ability to fund charitable or marginally profitable healthcare programs. As a leader in your medical community and in your national specialty organization, and as a surgeon paying premiums at a much higher rate than many colleagues in less demanding and less critical specialties, what should you do?

(A) Insurance companies have colluded to gouge their physician customers. Target them in your professional society's political activities.

(B) Plaintiff's attorneys are responsible for 90% of the malpractice crisis and must be brought under control. Target them.

(C) Juries are awarding larger and larger verdicts. Agitate to change a judicial system which empowers lay juries to pass judgment on complex medical and scientific questions.

(D) Physicians are mostly to blame. Modify physician behavior toward patients and police renegade physicians representing themselves as expert witnesses.

(E) Patients are filing more suits. Educate the public that frivolous suits are jeopardizing the viability of a medical profession that exists to help them.

Are physicians, particularly those who work in what insurers classify and bill as "high-risk" specialties, themselves being treated ethically within the social network they help to sustain? If not, how might they most effectively direct their attention toward limiting malpractice indemnity rates and better controlling those elements of the adjudication system that most of us agree sometimes functions unjustly? Like everyone else, surgeons want to be treated ethically. No sensible person, no matter how otherwise self-interested, advocates the crippling or destruction of our profession. Many of us have nonetheless felt this threat, and some have taken such extreme measures as closing their practices, discontinuing certain procedures, or relocating to escape the terrors of the existing medical malpractice tort system in all its manifestations, from insurance premiums to jury findings. There is a widespread belief, within and without the profession, that a socially endemic ethical failure lies at the base of these problems and that everyone is placed at risk by it.

Doctors have always grumbled about the cost of malpractice insurance premiums, but early in this decade malpractice insurance rates began rising at rates steep enough to threaten disruption of the medical care system. Many have questioned the legitimacy of the steep rise in premium costs, which are generally believed to far exceed the cost of indemnity and to exceed what many specialists have calculated they can afford if they are to continue to practice in an economically sustainable fashion.

Less than a handful of fingers are necessary to do the pointing at potential causes. First, are the premium increases a response to higher costs within the insurance industry, or a deliberate profiteering conspiracy among the carriers? The National Association of Insurance Commissioners (NAIC) reports that physicians' malpractice premiums in all 50 states increased from 2000 to 2003 (the last available data year) by a whopping 67%, from $6.38 billion to $10.65 billion. Every available source indicates that the higher premiums still failed to meet the insurers' costs of coverage. In 2002, insurers paid out $1.65 for every premium dollar collected from physicians.[1] The loss ratio on premiums fell to $1.37 in 2003.[2] Data from the NAIC were in the same range, showing a 43% loss in 2002 and a 28.6% loss in 2003. Premium revenue is of course not the carriers' only income; their average total profit from all sources, primarily capital investments, in 2003 was 5.3%, not exactly a killing.

Why did the cost of doing business in the medical malpractice insurance industry escalate as it did? The absolute number of physician malpractice cases nationwide has not varied much since 1999, when 15,093 adjudicated or settled payouts were recorded in the National Practitioner Data Bank (NPDB). There were 15,289 such reports in 2003 annual entries, an increase of only 1.3%.[3]

Likewise, the data don't confirm beliefs that routinely outlandish jury awards are driving the problem. Awards of a million dollars or more per case tend to make good newspaper copy, and just a few of them can create a general impression that they are the normative outcomes of medical malpractice trials. They aren't.[4] Figures like these are almost always associated with cases involving death or permanent disability as a result of negligent or incompetent care.[5] Otherwise, the NPDB reports that the average malpractice payment in 2003 was $294,814. This compares to an inflation-adjusted average since the NPDB began to compile statistics in 1990 of $251,000, not much of a difference. Using these data in 2003, the total national payout on medical malpractice claims was $4.5 billion, not including the costs of defending cases won and lost. 67% of filed malpractice cases are dismissed or dropped without an award or cash settlement to the plaintiff.[6] Each case filed, obvious or frivolous, is a potential loss of millions of insurance company money and must be defended by top attorneys at escalating legal costs. Furthermore, when absolute dollars, unadjusted for inflation, are calculated, the effect is multiplied over time, costing the insurance industry more and more each year just to stay even, and insured physicians have those costs passed directly on to them in the form of ever-higher premiums.

Dark rumors waft about from time to time proposing bizarre manipulations of the regulatory authorities by the insurance companies. Some physician leaders believe the present malpractice rate increases are secondary to insurer's desire to avoid paying taxes on the windfall profits of the late 1990s,[4] or that they are intended to cover investment losses incurred in the dot-com bust and the bear market years that opened the 21st century. Others have postulated that insurers periodically encourage lawsuits, happily paying losses to justify a new wave of rate increases. Were these conspiratorial theories true, they would certainly reflect poorly on the business sense of people who make their livings by calculating long-term probabilities with high actuarial exactitude. More to the point, they just don't pass the sniff test.

Most physicians nevertheless resent the fact that their premiums increase every year even though they've never been sued or done anything to deserve being sued. Clearly, this reflects an insurance system in which the whole medical profession supports the extraordinary costs incurred by a few of its members so that carriers can stay in the business of indemnifying us all against allegations of medical malpractice. No individual physician can pay premiums sufficient to cover the cost to the insurer if he or she loses a major adjudicated malpractice action. The insurance company pays not only the cost of the award to the limits of coverage, but also the cost of legal defense for all insured physicians, guilty and innocent alike. Despite increasing premiums and popular mythology, the medical malpractice insurance business is really not lucrative—many carriers have discontinued medical malpractice coverage or declined to write new policies in the last several years.

It has been suggested that plaintiffs' attorneys rush to file multiple malpractice suits. Each case is a lottery ticket, one more chance to hit the big one. It follows that patients with a real or perceived grievance find their pathway into court lubricated by the contingency fee arrangement, which insures that there is usually no cost to the patient unless there is an award or settlement. The attorney collects and has the considerable expenses of prosecution reimbursed only if he wins the case for his injured client. Because the contingency arrangement requires the plaintiff's attorney to run the risk of no return and substantial losses, the prudent attorney accepts only cases he or she reliably believes can be won for a significant award. The contingency fee model actually reduces the total number of cases filed, by subjecting the patient's claims to a self-interested attorney's trained scrutiny before they are brought before a court. With his own livelihood at stake, the attorney will necessarily screen out frivolous or poorly substantiated claims by declining to represent them. In a survey of 113 plaintiffs' medical malpractice attorneys, most ranked the economic burden of the injury, physician worthiness, and potential for compensation as the factors most influencing their decisions to file suit on behalf of clients.[7] Suits were most often filed when patients were more seriously injured, when patients had higher paying jobs before injury, and when the physician's credentials were suspect. When attorneys agreed to work without fee and assume all prosecution costs in exchange for a percentage of the award or settlement, however, the essential deciding factor was the potential for winning the case.

How does an attorney contemplating contingency work decide which cases are most likely to be won at trial? Characteristics of the injury, the patient, and the physician are important. The attorney considers "evidence that relates to the validity of the overall conceptualization."[7] A physician expert is contacted and asked to review the medical record and provide an opinion based on the evidence. One quarter to one half of patients who seek counsel with the intention of suing a doctor, and more than half when an attorney actually accepted the case, were told by other health professionals that their care was not satisfactory.[8] In 100% of malpractice actions formally filed by a sensible and experienced attorney, however, a well-compensated physician expert reviewed the medical records and advised the plaintiff's attorney that his potential client was indeed a victim of medical malpractice. This is of course a conclusion the aggrieved patient/client is pleased to hear because it validates his belief. It is the conclusion the plaintiff's attorney is content to hear because therein lies a potential source of income. It is the conclusion the "expert consultant" is pleased to provide because it insures that he will be further engaged and additionally compensated on the case, and likely on subsequent cases of a similar nature. The system has an abundance of professional experts who find a comfortable supplement to their livelihoods in encouraging attorneys to pursue malpractice cases. Should the ethical consultant repeatedly advise inquiring attorneys after reviewing the medical records that insufficient cause exists for a claim of medical malpractice, he or she might begin to notice that he is receiving fewer and fewer calls from friends in the legal profession. They will become increasingly popular among plaintiffs' attorneys when regularly shading evaluations of how other physicians managed a case to support counsel's role as the complainant's advocate. Without "experts" who abandon professional integrity and pump poisoned air into the system, it is probable that medicine would see decreases rather than a steady rate of malpractice cases arriving in court, with all the associated costs receding.

Every seasoned physician knows the shameful state of medical expert witnessing; its most egregious features blacken the integrity of both the medical and the legal professions. Fair and impartial expert testimony must be available to plaintiff and defendant alike. Expert testimony should be the province of practicing physicians with extensive and demonstrable scientific or clinical experience with the problem under debate. "Professional" medical expert witnesses, for sale to the highest bidder and willing to argue either side in a malpractice case, have severely compromised the integrity of the tort system.[9] Advocacy masquerading as expert testimony is the primary cause of unjust outcomes in the trial of medical malpractice cases. It introduces scientifically false standards of care under the guise of authority. Judges, juries, and attorneys on either side of a suit are not trained or otherwise able to distinguish a genuine physician expert from a skillful charlatan. Comportment, appearance, and articulateness on the witness stand are typically the layman's only basis for assessing the actual authority of expert witnesses who are so-certified by the loose standards of the legal profession.

So long as the medical profession does not act to restore professional integrity to medical expert witnessing, these intellectually decrepit "standards" will continue to plague the only regulatory device society has left at its disposal, malpractice litigation. Only the medical profession can identify and take action against those of its own who would exaggerate their mastery of the field and falsely impugn the ability and integrity of colleagues for personal enrichment and self-aggrandizement. The American College of Surgeons and allied professional organizations acknowledged the importance of fair and just expert witness testimony in recently published criteria requiring that witnesses "uphold certain professional principles." The College of Surgeons' document disallows expert advocacy and requires its members to agree to peer review of their testimony when requested, a good start toward more honest, disinterested, evidence-based expert opinions.

Some state medical boards propose to discipline physicians proven to have given false or misleading expert witness testimony. Implementing this proposal may eventually cause the most persistent and intentional offenders to pause, but there are considerable limitations. These include the high volume of retributive claims, the limited expertise and resources available to medical boards, the difficulty of proving fraudulent testimony in complex cases, and a potential dampening effect on even the most legitimate expert testimony. Similar problems would likely be encountered if our professional specialty organizations were to attempt review of members' unethical behavior in the courtroom.

Policing the entire medical profession to eliminate false or biased expert testimony is clearly not possible. Perhaps medicine should address the problem of inept and dishonest expert witnesses acting as surreptitious advocates by providing independent experts with integrity, who are certified as such by the medical profession, rather than by the legal profession. The American Association for the Advancement of Science offers the courts independent experts as their solution to bad science.[10] The federal courts have begun to accept this approach, with the creation of "science panels" for expert testimony.[11] Physicians should take the lead in advocating a similar approach in medical malpractice cases. A profession-wide decision on the best mechanism for implementation could be led by the American Medical Association or an ad hoc committee comprised of senior representatives of the major specialty organizations. Legislative adoption of their recommendations would introduce system-wide changes that would improve justice for all. But none of these responses to the crisis in medical malpractice litigation can be initiated by patients, lawyers, judges, juries, or insurance carriers. They can only be introduced by physicians.

Although accounting practices can distort corporate balance sheets, it is unlikely that the insurance industry's consistent reports of premium income failing to meet payout expenses are fabrications undetected by state insurance regulators or the national political interests which have become intensely focused on the medical malpractice crisis. Physicians nevertheless have little leverage and diminishing choices in obtaining the insurance coverage essential to practice. A few have dared to "go bare," but hospitals, group practices, and training institutions will generally not permit this sort of bravado among practitioners with whom they share liability. Option (A), attacking the insurance industry, seems not the right choice for resolving the medical malpractice crisis.

While it is true that if there were no attorneys there would be no professional prosecution of malpractice claims, there would also be no tort justice for those harmed by bad doctors. Option (B) misdiagnoses the essential lesion and will not heal the disease which has beset us.

The judicial system has been a foundational component of societal justice. As far back as the 18th century BCE, King Hammurabi (c. 1810–1750 BCE) of Babylon established a legal code overseen by judges who were themselves jeopardized by incorrect outcomes. Guilt or innocence in Hammurabi's Code was often decided by a defendant's death or survival after being thrown in the Euphrates River at flood tide. During the 6th century BCE in Greece, public assemblies called Hliaia or heliastic courts were presided over by routinely bribed magistrates adjudicating civil and criminal cases. Roman courts used a corps of professional jurists who closely guarded the prerogatives of the privileged classes. Trial by ordeal, or even by personal combat between litigants, was normative in medieval Europe, until Ecclesial courts claiming divine guidance took control of the legal system. This process culminated in the Holy Inquisition, administered by agents of the Roman Catholic Church; its abuses, including fabricated and superstitious charges, unchallenged informants, torture, and quasi-judicial murder are well-known. The alleged infallibility of a self-proclaimed elite has disrupted the cause of justice in every age, even today. Perhaps defendants in medical malpractice cases would be more justly served by juries of their physician peers, but an argument would be surely made that a guild mentality would prejudice such jurors against complainants. Despite its obvious shortcomings, no one has yet found a judicial system more consistently incorruptible and better sensitized to the demands of justice than trial by a panel of lay jurors who, since they are citizens too, are indeed physicians' peers. Until the course of history can finally agree upon a superior alternative, option (C) is not a realistic course of action.

Only a very small percentage of patients harmed by medical malpractice go on to file lawsuits, and statistics show that the number of suits has remained remarkably constant since the National Databank was established. Very few patients seek personal enrichment through frivolous or intentionally fabricated claims of medical malpractice, and even fewer attorneys will facilitate their access to the courthouse. The rationale for option (E) is just another myth.

As painful as it is to acknowledge, option (D) is the correct choice. Rogue physicians representing themselves as medical experts do more to contaminate the medical malpractice tort system and drive up all its associated costs, from premiums to payouts, than all the accidental and intentional misbehaviors of insurance companies, plaintiffs' attorneys, malevolent patients, and clueless juries combined. The medical profession does not belong to them; it is, as Dr. Thomas Percival (1740–1804) argued two centuries ago, a public trust.[12] The available data further confirm that malpractice suits most typically follow not when physicians lack technical competence or good clinical judgment, but when they fail to display compassion for the unintended suffering their treatment has visited upon their patients. Patients who feel that their doctor is listening to them don't often feel the need to have an attorney or a jury listen to them. Once a properly-treated but aggrieved patient contacts an attorney, the necessary factor for a complaint to become a case is the unscrupulous physician "expert" who is circling the scene, looking for opportunities to provide well-compensated advocacy disguised as wisdom without regard to the principles of good medicine or justice. A terrible ethical failure lies there, among our own.

References

1. Hartwig R, Wilkinson C. *Medical Malpractice Insurance: Insurance Issue Series*. New York: Insurance Information Institute, 2003: 1–20.
2. Institute II. Hot Topics and Issues Updates. Vol. 2005: Insurance Information Institute, September 2005.
3. National Practitioners Data Bank Annual Report. Washington, DC: U.S. Department of Health and Human Services, 2003.
4. Roberts RG. Understanding the physician liability insurance crisis. *Fam Pract Manag*. 2002; 9:47–51.
5. White MJ. The value of liability in medical malpractice. *Health Aff (Millwood)*. 1994; 13:75–87.
6. Schmitt C. A medical mistake: Doctors and insurers say malpractice awards must be capped. Their diagnosis may be wrong. *US News and World Report*. 2003:67–70.
7. Penchansky R, Macnee C. Initiation of medical malpractice suits: A conceptualization and test. *Med Care*. 1994; 32:813–831.
8. Beckman HB, Markakis KM, Suchman AL, Frankel RM. The doctor-patient relationship and malpractice: Lessons from plaintiff depositions. *Arch Intern Med*. 1994; 154:1365–1370.

9. Jones JW, McCullough LB, Richman BW. The Ethics of serving as a plaintiff's expert medical witness. *Surgery*. 2004; 136:100–102.

10. Brickley P. Science v. law. A decade-old rule on scientific evidence comes under fire. *Sci Am*. 2003; 289:30–32.

11. Price JM, Rosenberg ES. The war against junk science: the use of expert panels in complex medical-legal scientific litigation. *Biomaterials*. 1998; 19:1425–1432.

12. Percival T. *Medical Ethics, or a Code of Institutes and Precepts, Adapted to the Professional Conduct of Physicians and Surgeons*. London: Johnson and Bickerstaff, 1803.

· CASE 59 ·

A Helping Hand Bitten: An Ethical Response to Medical Malpractice Suits

Expecting the world to treat you fairly because you are a good person is a little like expecting the bull not to attack you because you are a vegetarian.
Dennis Wholey (1939–)

A surgeon with a successful practice based in his city's largest private hospital regularly volunteers to cover indigent cases done by surgical residents at the university hospital. This afternoon he was served a summons notifying him that he'd been named as a defendant in a medical malpractice lawsuit associated with one of his *pro bono* teaching cases. This is only the second time that he has been sued by patients; both cases were filed this year and involved working with the same resident. The university provides adequate insurance and legal coverage, but if the case should end with a finding for the plaintiff, he will be registered in the National Practitioner Data Bank and his personal insurance rates may soar. What should he do?

(A) Indigent patients are more likely to sue. He should resign from the volunteer teaching position.

(B) The surgeon has just experienced a random misfortune. He should not make any changes in his professional life.

(C) Poor patients are more likely to sue. He should discontinue involvement in their treatment.

(D) Lawsuits are a part of the modern practice of medicine. Organized medicine forbids refusing to treat in anticipation of being sued by a particular patient or type of patient.

(E) Fewer suits are filed by poor people. The surgeon should look elsewhere for the source of his current difficulty and make adjustments accordingly.

For several years now, we have been in an intense national argument about the cause of what everyone seems to agree is the third crisis in as many decades around the issue of professional liability. There sometimes appears to be more concern about the escalating cost of medical malpractice insurance than there is about medical malpractice suits, and physicians surely have their attention directed to it more than they do toward the problem of actual medical malpractice.

Many of us know, and all of us have heard of, colleagues who have retired or simply closed their practices, citing the impossibility of making a living while paying malpractice insurance premiums at ever-rising rates. Some doctors have departed states with a history of favoring plaintiffs and granting preposterous awards, and some normally well-behaved, socially responsible physicians have gone on 1-day strikes and marched on state houses demanding relief.[1] Prominent political figures have argued that the problem has been created and perpetuated by the greed and dishonesty of plaintiffs' attorneys, provoking the public to litigiousness by working on contingency and encouraging hostile attitudes toward selfless, well-meaning physicians. Others believe that a grasping, oppositional culture, and resentful poor people in particular, are responsible for the surge in malpractice claims and spectacular awards. Some criticize the jury system, which submits complex medical and scientific questions to the judgment of sentimental and easily-manipulated lay-people. Few, indeed, have had the audacity to place the blame for our malpractice crisis on the doorstep of the medical profession itself.[2-5]

A great many physicians have succumbed to a professional persecution complex which identifies us as helpless victims of medical tort law. Surgeons are by nature intelligent, determined, self-assured individuals not otherwise disposed toward considering themselves either helpless or victimized. The problem of rocketing malpractice insurance premiums is apprehended emotionally, with anger, anxiety, and resentment. The financial impact of the professional liability crisis on physicians is experienced personally and palpably.

The common-law tort system requires that an ordered series of decisions be made before a lawsuit actualizes and compensatory damages are awarded. After a patient claiming iatrogenic injury decides to file a medical malpractice action, an attorney evaluates the claim and typically asks an independent physician consultant to determine its merit before accepting the case, which then becomes a costly, lengthy, and work-intensive process to be endured by both sides before a settlement is reached or a jury decides for or against the plaintiff. Once the claim is filed, there is almost nothing the charged physician can do to untrack it. The doctor, accused rightly or wrongly, is going to be in for a rough ride. There are things that physicians can do to limit the likelihood that things will go that far, however.

Malpractice claims against physicians are always initiated by patients or their families. The patients who file against their doctors believe the physicians have caused them to suffer by performing injudiciously, ineptly, or negligently. Injured patients make an inexpert, perhaps emotional, judgment about the cause of their misery, and some respond by seeking legal redress. A few attempt to exploit the tort system to knowingly and cynically wedge personal gain out of a minimally consequential medical error, and sometimes they find lawyers who'll throw in with them, but this is not the predominant pattern. The severity of lifestyle disruption from an injury considered to be a consequence of treatment increases the likelihood that a patient will believe that medical malpractice has occurred and seek legal counsel.[6] To study patient motivations, researchers answered calls from more than 700 disgruntled patients to medical malpractice attorneys' offices in 5 states.[7] The goals of the callers, both financial and nonfinancial in nature, and patient demographics were recorded.

Most injured patients who contacted malpractice attorneys had problematic relationships with their doctors. Many of them had high unpaid medical bills, and 27% said that they had been advised by other health care professionals to seek legal counsel.

A survey of physicians who had been sued and the patients who sued them found that the two groups had markedly different perceptions of the quality of their prior professional relationships; physicians usually were unaware of their patients' unmet emotional needs, the patients' level of dependence, and their thirst for expressions of sympathy and compassion from their doctors.[6] Physicians and patients in the study both agreed that improvement in communication could be instrumental in averting a malpractice suit. Patients sustaining severe lifestyle disruptions following treatment often feel intensely angry, and express a fervent desire to feel assured that the reasons for their injury are defensible and will not be needlessly visited upon others.[8] Postoperative physician behavior perceived as insensitive or dismissive also provoked a desire for retribution, a need to regain what was felt to be lost personal dignity, and a grinding rage to make the doctor experience misery equivalent to their own. While revenge is an immature emotional response, it is one of the most powerful personal motivations. Hollywood drama would surely collapse without it. Subjects revengefully punishing offenders while undergoing positron emission tomography showed activation of their dorsal stratum indicating they experienced intense pleasure even when the action was achieved with personal loss.[9] Resolving to file suit against one's physician seems just another way to satisfy these angry feelings.

Some litigants had received no explanation from their doctors for their injuries, and 85% of those who had been given explanations believed it was inadequate, untrue, or serving only the physician's interest.[8] Beckman and associates found after reading plaintiffs' depositions that 71% of patients who filed malpractice claims against their doctors said they did so because of bad interpersonal relationships with them.[10] The perceived failings included feelings of abandonment (32%), disrespect of patient and/or family views (29%), poorly delivered information (26%), or failure to understand the patient and/or family perspective (13%). Beckman's meticulous study confirmed earlier reports by finding that 54% of malpractice suits were encouraged by other health professionals. The evidence is pretty clear in its consistent suggestion that a failure to establish reasonable rapport with patients and their families by meeting their emotional needs during a time of crisis and apprehension stimulates resentment and an impulse to lash out. Patients, not attorneys, initiate medical malpractice actions. Poor physician communication skills are more likely than any other single factor, including actual bad medical practice, to precipitate a patient lawsuit.

There's a bit of professional folk wisdom holding that surgeons are simply not among the most sensitive of physicians, and are not well-trained to recognize their patients' emotional needs. A recent study examined whether patients dropped hints about their anxieties during routine interactions with their doctors. Surgical patients averaged 1.9 indirect suggestions per visit that they wanted to more deeply discuss some aspect of their medical condition, but in only 38% of these cases were the clues adequately recognized and followed up.[11] Researchers evaluated voice clips of surgeons and found that, "Controlling for content, ratings of higher dominance and lower concern/anxiety in their voice tones significantly identified surgeons with previous [malpractice] claims, compared with those who had no claims."[12]

Despite the few unscrupulous people who try to exploit medical complications for personal enrichment, most patients and their families are accepting, forgiving, and even consoling towards their physicians when faced with dreadful complications or death of a loved one. Many surgeons have noted that the pendulum of patients', relatives', and friends' absolution is distinctly on the side of their physician. Absent this favorable bias, no physician treating complex cases, especially those requiring major surgical care, could endure the emotional and financial battering and remain in practice. A study of 14,700 medical records found that 97% of people who were negligently injured did not sue the responsible physician.[13] The low rate of patients injured by medical errors who go on to sue is partially attributable to their not knowing how they were hurt. Most patients get satisfactory closure from the knowledge that, if a mistake occurred, it was recognized and will not be repeated among future patients. A physician's apology, when appropriate, was perceived as soothing and reassuring of integrity and beneficent intentions.[14]

There is a quiet assumption by many in medicine that poor urbanites and minorities are dangerously mistrustful and resentful of doctors, and file malpractice suits with the greatest frequency. Burstin and associates examined 31,000 records and were surprised to find that poor and uninsured patients who sustained iatrogenic injury were actually significantly less likely to sue than middle class insured patients.[15] There was no difference between ethnic groups in litigiousness. Again, this study found that the likelihood of filing a malpractice claim was highly correlated with the severity of medical injury. Medicaid patients were no more likely to file malpractice actions than privately insured patients in higher socioeconomic strata.[16] Studdert's study of 14,700 closed medical records found that poorer patients, Medicaid patients, and older patients filed fewer claims for negligent adverse medical events than younger and more affluent patients[13].

Although there was a lower frequency of lawsuits against physicians in a group of economically disadvantaged and uninsured patients, it is precisely this patient population that is at increased risk for injury from poor care, receiving much of their treatment in busy emergency centers, from trainees, with bare minimum lengths of hospital stay, and assembly line treatment with longer waits for appointments in overburdened community clinics.[17]

By choosing options (A) or (C), our surgeon would stop providing a valuable service to the needy in his community and to the trainees in the local medical school's vascular surgery residency. His volunteer work among the indigent represents one of medicine's core ethical values, the spirit of beneficence, and he properly derives personal satisfaction from its exercise, as well as from his contribution to the excellence of future vascular surgeons. Most sadly, he would be terminating these vital services for the wrong reason, an incorrect belief that poor patients often bring malpractice claims and represent a significant threat to the doctors who care for them. Option (D) is incorrect because none of the prominent medical or surgical organizations forbids refusal to treat patients considered likely to initiate malpractice actions.[18] Option (D) furthermore violates professional integrity because it, like option (C), is factually groundless. Option (B) is not factually incorrect, and the surgeon's professional life should indeed continue largely as it has, but by limiting his response to its terms our surgeon would relinquish important opportunities to consider the possibility of corrective measures which might reduce his future exposure and perhaps even improve the quality of his professional contributions.

Option (E) grasps this opportunity, and is the best of the responses available in an admittedly bad bargain. It first declines to misplace blame upon an entire social class which is already at high risk and often underserved. This being the second recent suit initiated by patients treated by one particular resident under his supervision, there is a reasonably high likelihood that the resident has much to learn about the critical interpersonal management skills that so often forestall the kind of patient rage that finds its expression in a malpractice claim. We have all seen how many a young surgeon, having born the extraordinary intellectual and physical burdens of medical school and residency, has had his pride and self-assurance metastasize into arrogance. Some of us have regrettably been that young surgeon until experience, maturity, and perhaps a strong mentor have straightened us out. When patients detect this kind of superciliousness, and they almost always do when it's there, the emotional kindling that is smoldering after a less than fully successful operation can burst into flames. Unlike many of our colleagues in specialties like psychiatry and family medicine, surgeons seldom have an opportunity to establish extended relationships with their patients, and the trust they have in us is based largely upon confidence in our credentials and their respect for our profession. We do indeed have fewer occasions than most other specialists in which to build a doctor-patient relationship, but that does not relieve us of the responsibility. The limited opportunity to know our patients personally, and for them to know us, means that we must be more sensitive, not less, to their emotional needs, and particularly because our invasive and usually painful therapies almost always mobilize more patient anxiety than the treatments offered by nonsurgical specialists. Our results are often easier to judge as well. In electing option (E) and giving deep consideration to what provoked two claims of medical malpractice against his resident and himself as supervisor, our faculty surgeon may well realize that despite good technical training, he neglected to teach the resident the interpersonal skills which might have satisfied his patients' emotional needs and provided them with an outlet other than malpractice claims to express their frustrations. Not only because it is among the best front-line defenses against claims of medical malpractice, but because it is good medical and surgical care, surgeons must indeed recognize and respond to their patients' fears and hopes. To do so does not eliminate legitimate grievances against gross technical incompetence and professional negligence, but it can help patients to appreciate a distinction between mispractice and malpractice when an outcome is not all that doctor and patient had hoped for.

References

1. Amon E, Winn HN. Review of the professional medical liability insurance crisis: lessons from Missouri. *Am J Obstet Gynecol.* 2004; 190:1534–1538.
2. Jones JW, Richman BW, McCullough LB. Professional self-regulation: eyewitness to incompetent surgery. *J Vasc Surg.* 2002; 36:1092–1093.
3. Jones JW, McCullough LB, Richman BW. What to tell patients harmed by other physicians. *J Vasc Surg.* 2003; 38:866–867.
4. Jones JW, McCullough LB, Richman BR. Ethics of serving as a plaintiff's expert medical witness. *Surgery.* 2004; 136:100–102.
5. Jones JW, McCullough LB, Richman BW. Who should protect the public against bad doctors? *J Vasc Surg.* 2005; 41:907–910.
6. Shapiro RS, Simpson DE, Lawrence SL, Talsky AM, Sobocinski KA, Schiedermayer DL. A survey of sued and nonsued physicians and suing patients. *Arch Intern Med.* 1989; 149:2190–2196.
7. Huycke LI, Huycke MM. Characteristics of potential plaintiffs in malpractice litigation. *Ann Intern Med.* 1994; 120:792–798.
8. Vincent C, Young M, Phillips A. Why do people sue doctors? A study of patients and relatives taking legal action. *Lancet.* 1994; 343:1609–1613.
9. de Quervain D, Fischbacher U, Treyer V, Schellhammer M, Schnyder U, Buck A, et al. The neural basis of altruistic punishment. *Science.* 2004; 305:1254–1258.
10. Beckman HB, Markakis KM, Suchman AL, Frankel RM. The doctor-patient relationship and malpractice: Lessons from plaintiff depositions. *Arch Intern Med.* 1994; 154:1365–1370.
11. Levinson W, Gorawara-Bhat R, Lamb J. A study of patient clues and physician responses in primary care and surgical settings. *JAMA.* 2000; 284:1021–1027.
12. Ambady N, Laplante D, Nguyen T, Rosenthal R, Chaumeton N, Levinson W. Surgeons' tone of voice: A clue to malpractice history. *Surgery.* 2002; 132:5–9.
13. Studdert DM, Thomas EJ, Burstin HR, Zbar BI, Orav EJ, Brennan TA. Negligent care and malpractice claiming behavior in Utah and Colorado. *Med Care.* 2000; 38:250–260.
14. Gallagher TH, Levinson W. Disclosing harmful medical errors to patients: a time for professional action. *Arch Intern Med.* 2005; 165:1819–1824.
15. Burstin HR, Johnson WG, Lipsitz SR, Brennan TA. Do the poor sue more? A case-control study of malpractice claims and socioeconomic status. *JAMA.* 1993; 270:1697–1701.

16. Baldwin LM, Greer T, Wu R, Hart G, Lloyd M, Rosenblatt RA. Differences in the obstetric malpractice claims filed by Medicaid and non-Medicaid patients. *J Am Board Fam Pract.* 1992; 5:623–627.

17. Burstin HR, Lipsitz SR, Brennan TA. Socioeconomic status and risk for substandard medical care. *JAMA.* 1992; 268:2383–2387.

18. Jones JW, McCullough LB, Richman BW. Ethics of refusal to treat patients as a social statement. *J Vasc Surg.* 2004; 40:1057–1059.

• CASE 60 •

Case-Load Outcome Credentialing: Taking from the Have-Nots

Not even a dog-killer can learn his trade from books, but only from experience. And how much more is this true of the physician!
Paracelsus (1493–1541)

The surgeon-in-chief at a large metropolitan hospital long has championed a new data base that compares operative outcomes by surgeon and procedure. The methodology of data collection and analysis are exemplary. The director of information technology has just completed the initial analysis and the data clearly show that several of the older surgical attendings have higher than average mortality rates for specific procedures. The vascular surgeon's patients in particular have a statistically significant higher stroke rate following carotid artery procedures, but his other vascular work is satisfactory. He is not scheduled to be recredentialed for 10 months. What should be done?

(A) The vascular surgeon has outstanding credentials, and several times has been selected as a "Best Doctor." Collect more data.

(B) Don't worry. Referring physicians will stop sending him cases because of his outcomes.

(C) Recredential those with poor records by procedure.

(D) The data may not be properly adjusted. Wait until you have more data.

(E) Monitor any surgeon with questionable results for a specific procedure.

Wherever there are some who are the best at something, there must, by definition, be someone who is the worst. As betterment is the goal of all applied science, clinical medicine seeks to improve its performance by finding better ways to reestablish health in patients. A mainstay of clinical studies over the last century has been to divide treatment experiences of a specific disease entity into those patients who did well and those who died or had complications. Standard variables included preoperative, mainly demographic or disease-related, and intraoperative, mainly operative technique used, operative efficiency, and blood loss. Although a hierarchy of surgical talent by institution and individual surgeon has been widely acknowledged, surgical technique was considered uniformly good throughout the profession. After all, the influence of quality of surgical technique influencing both sides of the equation should cancel out in comparative studies.

Each practicing surgeon who performs highly technical procedures, from the first day of residency, harbors no doubt that the outcomes are linked to the exposure, intraoperative judgment, exactitude, efficiency, and hemostasis of their performance. Surely, surgery is a concerted performance, but the surgeon remains the virtuoso. It is frustrating for an accomplished surgeon to operate with a suboptimal surgical team, but an outstanding team cannot make up for a surgeon's suboptimal performance.

The vascular system is most unforgiving of technical errors. By divine providence, perhaps, the busiest and most experienced surgeons at any institution are usually the most respected. They may simply have developed better rapport with referring physicians but, although no sane surgeon fails to court referral sources, the elite are often more rushed and less humble.

More than two decades ago, surgeons began to acknowledge that, unlike the manufacture of luxury automobiles and other high-end merchandise, surgical operative results might depend on the volume of certain procedures in hospitals.[1] The key insight was that low-risk patients had poorer outcomes in low-volume hospitals. After hundreds of articles subsequently examining almost every surgical specialty, especially orthopedic and vascular cases, the overwhelming consensus has emerged that there is a caseload threshold in hospitals below which outcomes worsen significantly.[1-6]

The problem is that surgeons, not hospitals, perform surgery. Results of a high-volume cardiovascular surgical group were no different whether their cases were done at a high or low volume hospital.[6] Birkmeyer and associates examined data from over 474,000 patients undergoing eight different surgical procedures and found that the proportion of beneficial effects of individual surgeons' volume in relation to the hospital volume varied from 100% down to 24%, depending on the procedure.[7] Major vascular procedures were more dependent on the surgeon's experience than nonvascular procedures. Lung resection and cystectomy operations benefited least from more experienced surgeons, which is a reasonable statement to surgeons performing both major vascular and lung procedures; the precision and efficiency required differ. Patients undergoing carotid endarterectomy (CEA) by surgeons doing less than one procedure per month (18% of 35,821 or 6,448 patients) had approximately twice the stroke and mortality rates of busier surgeons.[8] Poor outcomes tripled when performed by dabblers doing a case a year.[9] Dr. Oscar Creech, a vascular surgical pioneer with superb technical talent, summed up the importance of OR performance: "Most postoperative care takes place in the operating room."

These data relate directly to the ethical concept of the physician as fiduciary of the patient, which is the core concept of surgical ethics. Conceptualized at the end of the 18th century by the physician-ethicists John Gregory and Thomas Percival, this formulation has three components. First, the physician commits to becoming scientifically and clinically competent, which includes continuous improvement of knowledge and skills. Second, the physician commits to protecting and promoting the patient's health-related interests as the physician's primary concern and motivation, keeping self-interest systematically secondary. Third, the physician maintains, strengthens, and passes on medicine as a public trust, for the benefit of future physicians and patients. The ethics of scientific and clinical competence, the first component of fiduciary responsibility, restrain surgeons from undertaking procedures for which they are not competent or are no longer competent, perhaps because of atrophy of fine motor skills, or not had occasion to perform the particular procedure in a long time. In the era of evidence-based surgery, competence is now defined in terms of an experienced volume of procedures with acceptable outcomes. Given the well established connection between threshold workloads and acceptable outcomes, a surgeon whose outcomes are no longer acceptable, as in this case, has a strict ethical obligation to stop performing the procedure as soon as the problem is recognized. His surgical processes should be carefully analyzed in a disciplined, professional peer-review. If this review results in a judgment that the surgeon's deficiencies are irremediable, then he should not be permitted to perform the procedure, consistent with his fiduciary responsibility to protect the health and lives of patients. Percival captures what is at stake here, when he addresses the ethical obligations of the aging surgeon: "As age advances, therefore, a physician should, from time to time, scrutinize impartially, the state of his faculties; that he may determine, *bona fide,* the precise degree in which he is qualified to execute the active and multifarious offices of his profession."[10]

Percival's point can be generalized to cover reasons other than age resulting in subpar surgical performance. Percival entrusted this task of self-assessment to the court of individual conscience, a slender reed upon which to hang a weighty responsibility. We should not, opting instead for peer-review through existing quality improvement processes.

Option (A) proposes that a prestigious education and professional accolades are reliable markers for good outcomes. Cardiovascular surgical outcomes are not related to prestige indicators such as medical education at a top rated school or training at an institution renowned for surgical care.[11] Foreign medical graduates' outcomes were no different than those of surgeons with diplomas originating in the United States. Likewise, the professional honor of being elected or selected to a "Best Doctors" publication does not guarantee better results.[12]

Available data suggest that reliance upon the referral process to redirect patients away from surgeons with poor results and toward surgeons achieving higher quality outcomes is not realistic. The accessibility of surgeon-specific risk-adjusted mortality data in the "Consumer Guide to Coronary Artery Bypass Graft (CABG) Surgery of Pennsylvania" is known to 82% of referring cardiologists, but 87% of cardiologists reported that it had "minimal influence on their referrals."[13] In New York, we find similar disinterest among referring physicians. Though risk-adjusted surgeon specific CABG mortality rates are published in the news media, two thirds of referring cardiologists think that the data is accurate and two thirds state that the data does not influence their referral decisions.[14] More surprising, a survey of patients undergoing cardiovascular operations in a geographic area where surgeons' outcomes are readily available found that less than one percent knew the published record of their surgeon.[15] Option (B) is not viable.

Option (D) is a common depreciatory courtroom tactic, attacking the validity of the source. If one does not like what the data say, complain that the data are flawed and, therefore, unworthy of belief. Death is an absolute endpoint, and statistics are as objective a method as science has available. It is, however, hoped that the surgeons were kept informed and had input while the data program was being developed.

Monitoring surgeons with procedural results that are statistically inferior to those of other surgeons, option (E), is an often used practical alternative, but it is not the best ethical answer. Using scientific methodology, the data confirm that the surgeon in question is performing substandard carotid surgery. Monitoring is a qualitative surveillance measure designed only to confirm what is already known. In this case, rehabilitation from formation of new synapses and practice development is highly unlikely. A decision to monitor would allow additional patients to bear the outcome shortfall to extend unwarranted compassion to a fellow surgeon.

Our choice is option (C), because procedural credentialing is a privilege, not a right, which rightly serves a single purpose, to protect patients from practitioners whose skills are less than is otherwise available.

There is a particular red flag in regard to this specific case of a surgeon at career's end who may need to slow down a busy practice because of decreasing stamina and motor skills. The decreasing volume of cases, combined with the ravages of time, can irreversibly reduce the effectiveness of previously highly qualified surgeons.[9,16] This phenomenon is seen in procedures requiring proficient hand-eye coordination, as in CEA. In the same study, the problem was not found in aortic aneurysm procedures.[16] The investigators noted that "For most procedures...surgeon age is not an important predictor of operative risk," implying that recredentialling should be procedure specific, and aging surgeons may continue to be credentialed in procedures they can still do well. Operative experience is more than a surrogate marker for quality, it is the mostly unappreciated mainspring of a surgeon's technical skills. Procedural specialties are separated epistemologically by the difference in knowing something and knowing how to do something. Surgeons must know how to do something. Memorizing and mastering the textbook concepts of surgery do not make a surgeon. A surgeon's essence results from the focusing of acquired motor skills to provide operative therapy. Idle motor skills wane, just like other memories, perhaps even faster.

References

1. Flood AB, Scott WR, Ewy W. Does practice make perfect? Part I: The relation between hospital volume and outcomes for selected diagnostic categories. *Med Care.* 1984;22:98–114.

2. Hannan EL, Wu C, Ryan TJ, Bennett E, Culliford AT, Gold JP, et al. Do hospitals and surgeons with higher coronary artery bypass graft surgery volumes still have lower risk-adjusted mortality rates? *Circulation*. 2003; 108:795–801.

3. Peterson ED, Coombs LP, DeLong ER, Haan CK, Ferguson TB. Procedural volume as a marker of quality for CABG surgery. *JAMA*. 2004; 291:195–201.

4. Wen HC, Tang CH, Lin HC, Tsai CS, Chen CS, Li CY. Association between surgeon and hospital volume in coronary artery bypass graft surgery outcomes: a population-based study. *Ann Thorac Surg*. 2006; 81:835–842.

5. Westvik HH, Westvik TS, Maloney SP, Kudo FA, Muto A, Leite JO, et al. Hospital-based factors predict outcome after carotid endarterectomy. *J Surg Res*. 2006; 134: 74–80.

6. Zacharias A, Schwann TA, Riordan CJ, Durham SJ, Shah A, Papadimos TJ, et al. Is hospital procedure volume a reliable marker of quality for coronary artery bypass surgery? A comparison of risk and propensity adjusted operative and midterm outcomes. *Ann Thorac Surg*. 2005; 79:1961–1969.

7. Birkmeyer JD, Stukel TA, Siewers AE, Goodney PP, Wennberg DE, Lucas FL. Surgeon volume and operative mortality in the United States. *N Engl J Med*. 2003; 349:2117–2127.

8. Cowan JA, Jr, Dimick JB, Thompson BG, Stanley JC, Upchurch GR, Jr. Surgeon volume as an indicator of outcomes after carotid endarterectomy: An effect independent of specialty practice and hospital volume. *J Am Coll Surg*. 2002; 195: 814–821.

9. O'Neill L, Lanska DJ, Hartz A. Surgeon characteristics associated with mortality and morbidity following carotid endarterectomy. *Neurology*. 2000; 55:773–781.

10. Percival T. *Medical Ethics, or a Code of Institutes and Precepts, Adapted to the Professional Conduct of Physicians and Surgeons*. London: Johnson & Bickerstaff, 1803.

11. Hartz AJ, Kuhn EM, Pulido J. Prestige of training programs and experience of bypass surgeons as factors in adjusted patient mortality rates. *Med Care*. 1999; 37:93–103.

12. Hartz AJ, Pulido JS, Kuhn EM. Are the best coronary artery bypass surgeons identified by physician surveys? *Am J Public Health*. 1997; 87:1645–1648.

13. Schneider EC, Epstein AM. Influence of cardiac-surgery performance reports on referral practices and access to care: A survey of cardiovascular specialists. *N Engl J Med*. 1996; 335:251–256.

14. Hannan EL, Stone CC, Biddle TL, DeBuono BA. Public release of cardiac surgery outcomes data in New York: What do New York state cardiologists think of it? *Am Heart J*. 1997; 134:1120–1128.

15. Schneider EC, Epstein AM. Use of public performance reports: A survey of patients undergoing cardiac surgery. *JAMA*. 1998; 279:1638–1642.

16. Waljee JF, Greenfield LJ, Dimick JB, Birkmeyer JD. Surgeon age and operative mortality in the United States. *Ann Surg*. 2006; 244:353–362.

• CASE 61 •

Fiduciary Economization: Your Wealth or Your Health

When are you going to realize that if it doesn't apply to me it doesn't matter?
Murphy Brown

A 64-year-old man is referred to clinic with an asymptomatic 5.0-cm.-abdominal aortic aneurysm (AAA) found by ultrasound screening at the local shopping mall. He is otherwise in good health, with no risk factors for accelerated rupture. The patient's father died from a ruptured AAA and he is quite fretful, requesting repair as soon as possible. He lost his job months ago and allowed his medical insurance to lapse, but he has some savings, owns his home outright, and, as expected, is willing to forfeit everything to be rid of this threat. In 6 months he will be able to scrimp by on Social Security and a modest pension. You offer the option of nonoperative surveillance, which is summarily dismissed. Because you and the hospital where your practice is located attract many international patients, you are aware of the enormity of charges imposed on those without insurance. What should you do?

(A) Explain the economics of waiting until he can enroll in Medicare.
(B) Go ahead and operate. The hospital will write it off as a bad debt.
(C) Call the hospital administrator and negotiate his price downward.
(D) Go ahead and operate. If you don't and the aneurysm ruptures, you could be sued.
(E) Operate. He will just get someone else and you will lose the case.

Calling medicine a business knocks off the top hat of its professional image. Yet surgeons make good livings exchanging restorative, sometimes even curative, services for greenbacks. And medical institutions, hospitals, practice groups, and our billing operations are in every sense complex businesses. The principal driver of physicians' recent reaffirmations of professionalism is concern that overcommercialization has swayed physicians from their ancient ethos.[1,2]

As in few other major purchases, even though the cost may be high enough to negatively affect future lifestyle, one of the rarest questions from patients involves the cost of treatment.[3] When McKneally interviewed patients having major surgery about their process of deciding, he found that the idealistic shared-decision-making model of lawyers and bio-ethicists was better described as an entrustment process, because the patient had already resolved to defer to the surgeon's expertise prior to even meeting him.[4] Since the entrustment process sweeps aside matters of life and limb, cost is but a trifle; the treatment's necessity takes priority in the patient's thinking. One's life, health, or even the outside chance to temporarily avoid death is, as MasterCard ads stress, "priceless."

When the patient does not bring up costs, it is unlikely that the physician will initiate the discussion. The patient's financial status can sometimes be estimated by appearances, but clerks in the hospital business office are the only ones who know accurately. Physicians may be aware of their customary charges for a procedure, but excepting the most common insurers, most physicians are unaware of what the patient's share of their bill will be and are certainly unschooled in ranges of hospital charges or the host of supportive physicians' charges.[5]

Recommendations for operations are based firmly on the criteria we've called "indications" since medical antiquity. Stedman defines indications as, "The basis for initiation of a treatment for a disease or of a diagnostic test; [they] may be furnished by a knowledge of the cause, by the symptoms present, or by the nature of the disease." Indications in the case of aneurysms, as in most diseases with minimal symptoms, derive from favorable risk/benefit ratios. Since in our present state of knowledge abdominal aneurysm repairs have associated mortality, and aneurysms vary in their risk of rupture, the risk-benefit ratio is quite important.

Our patient's disease is less severe than the vascular society's threshold for repair, but the recommended guidelines include taking account of the patient's preference in the decision about surgical management versus watchful waiting.[6] One might rationalize that endovascular repair obsolesces those recommendations, but the available evidence is not yet there,[7] and, in this era of evidence-based practice, collective expert practice recommendations should not be altered by unsubstantiated opinions. In this marginal but acceptable situation, operative therapy would otherwise be indicated. Should the patient's financial situation make a difference? Should those people without funds be treated differently? If so, would that result in an ethically unacceptable, two-tiered medical system?

A two-tiered medical system is obviously ethically unacceptable, if that means that those with a source of payment receive the accepted standard of care and those without do not.[8] From the beginning of recorded history, societies have always victimized their politically weak, particularly the poor, and evidence still exists that there are differences in care of the poor in America.[8] Great strides toward elimination of these differences have been registered, but 45 million uninsured Americans face a crisis every time they need health care.

The ethical objection to such a two-tiered system applies to necessary treatment, not to discretionary treatment, based on the ability to pay. The ethical challenges concerning cost to the patient in this case therefore differ and are more subtle. Cost should not be the sole or even the primary determinant of medical therapy, but physicians' favored economic status should not blind them to the financial hardship major surgical therapy can have on less affluent patients. "[Surgery in] fully insured middle-class people who become ill with critical or life-threatening illnesses can completely ruin their financial health," says Beth Darnley, chief program officer for the Patient Advocate Foundation. "Bankruptcy is just the tip of the iceberg: 29 million Americans are in medical debt," says Jennifer Edwards of the Commonwealth Fund, a private foundation that supports research on health and social issues."[9]

Holden made the case that cost should be a part of the informed consent process, and concluded that, "If we are proposing a treatment that provides a slight improvement in outcome, compared with the second choice treatment, at an added cost equal to an around-the-world luxury vacation or a new luxury car, it is incumbent on us to tell our patients about the less expensive treatment and let them decide how they want to spend their money. I suspect more than a few will opt for the more economical treatment."[10]

This final comment should be taken with a note of caution. In this case, the fiduciary responsibility of the surgeon to this patient includes consideration of the impact that discretionary, clinically unwarranted, expedited surgery will have on the patient's future lifestyle, and therefore his health and well being. The best predictor of health status in our society is socioeconomic status; having surgery now, rather than waiting until he is Medicare-eligible, will drastically reduce this patient's socioeconomic status. The likely impact that long-term increased anxiety and stress, which his suddenly reduced economic circumstances will almost certainly produce, is an ethically significant consideration for the surgeon, and is therefore within the realm of his fiduciary responsibility to the patient.

Should he procede with the surgery, our patient will encounter an unyielding reality. In times of scarcity, many hospitals have developed strategies for vigorously, even harshly, pursuing outstanding debtors.[11] That pursuit, and the likelihood that payment would be demanded on admission or shortly thereafter, exclude option (B), because it assumes that the cost-components of this case are not of economic significance. But they are.

Option (D) suggests that the surgeon is violating the fiduciary role in decision making. The evidence base for (D) is weak: Selecting a therapeutic modality based on medico-legal risks frequently misidentifies those who are likely to sue.[12] Moreover, this option makes self-interest the overriding consideration, which threatens to distort, if not undermine, professional expert judgment about whether surgery is indeed indicated at this time. The legitimate goal of reducing unnecessary liability should never be achieved by putting patients at unnecessary increased clinical risk.

Option (E) is a universal excuse that all of us should have discarded during childhood. Should it be adopted in the legal code, every drug dealer and child pornographer would be released with remuneration for false imprisonment. It also violates the physician's fiduciary duty by dislocating decision making from the patient.

Option (C) is a thoughtful action but should not be the first step taken; it should follow the careful explanation suggested by option (A). The sequelae of surgery in this case are not simply anatomic. Those economic sequelae have clinical consequences, and the patient should be informed about them and factor them into his decision. There is a strict legal obligation, called informed refusal, for a physician to explain the risks that the patient takes when refusing recommended clinical management. That management usually involves intervention, but in this case involves close observation and considered judgments in the future. The physician should take advantage of the legal obligation of fulfilling the requirements of informed refusal—explaining to the patient the risks he is taking by electing surgery at this time—to engage in the ethically significant task of persuading the patient to reconsider. Apprising him of the psychosocial risks he is taking by assuming the enormous financial burdens, and the clinical risks of electing immediate surgery become key educational components in persuading him to reconsider.

Decisions about clinical management should not only be informed, but voluntary. Faden and Beauchamp explain that this means the decision-making process and its outcome should be free of substantially controlling influences, including such substantially controlling emotional influences as unreasoning fear.[13] Part of implementing option A should therefore be a careful exploration with the patient of his attitudes and feelings toward this father's death, and educating him about the fact that the current size of his AAA should not be interpreted to mean that he is at high risk of death within the next year. The goal of this conversation with the patient should be to mitigate the potentially distorting influence of an unreasoning fear on his decision-making processes.

Option A is the best course. Ethical surgeons should invite their patients to consider the attendant biopsychosocial consequences of unnecessary major ethically financial outlays, especially when treatment can be safely enough postponed. Somewhere back in folklore there was a belief that if you saved someone's life, you became responsible for them forever. Thank goodness, it was a myth.

References

1. Professionalism ATFo. Code of professional conduct. *J Am Coll Surg*. 2003; 197: 603–604.
2. Medical professionalism in the new millennium: A physician charter. *Ann Intern Med*. 2002; 136:243–246.
3. McCullough LB, Jones JW, Brody BA. Informed consent: Autonomous decision making of the surgical patient. In: McCullough LB, Jones JW, Brody BA, eds. *Surgical Ethics*. New York: Oxford University Press, 1998:15–37.
4. McKneally MF, Martin DK. An entrustment model of consent for surgical treatment of life-threatening illness: Perspective of patients requiring esophagectomy. *J Thorac Cardiovasc Surg*. 2000; 120:264–269.
5. Jones JW, McCullough LB, Richman BW. Other people's money: Ethics, finances, and bad outcomes. *J Vasc Surg*. 2006; 43:863–865.
6. Brewster DC, Cronenwett JL, Hallett JW, Jr., Johnston KW, Krupski WC, Matsumura JS. Guidelines for the treatment of abdominal aortic aneurysms: Report of a

subcommittee of the Joint Council of the American Association for Vascular Surgery and Society for Vascular Surgery. *J Vasc Surg.* 2003; 37:1106–1117.

7. Schermerhorn M. Should usual criteria for intervention in abdominal aortic aneurysms be "downsized," considering reported risk reduction with endovascular repair? *Ann NY Acad Sci.* 2006; 1085:47–58.

8. Jones JW, McCullough LB, Richman BW. Ethics of boutique medical practice. *J Vasc Surg.* 2004; 39:1354–1355.

9. Appleby J. Medical costs prove a burden even for some with insurance. *USA Today.* 2005.

10. Holden JL. Shouldn't cost be considered a significant issue in medical care? *Am J Surg.* 2002; 183:4–6.

11. Weissman JS. The trouble with uncompensated hospital care. *N Engl J Med.* 2005; 352:1171–1173.

12. Jones JW, McCullough LB, Richman BW. A helping hand bitten: An ethical response to medical malpractice suits. *J Vasc Surg.* 2006; 43:422–425.

13. Faden RR, Beauchamp TL. *A History and Theory of Informed Consent.* New York: Oxford University Press, 1986.

• CASE 62 •

What to Do When a Patient's International Medical Care Goes South

There's nothing that cleanses your soul like getting the hell kicked out of you.
Woody Hayes, Former Ohio State Football Coach

A former patient who traveled to a clinic in India for placement of an aortic endograft several months ago has returned to your clinic with general malaise and as having experienced a low grade an intermittent fever for several weeks. The physical examination was unremarkable but laboratory tests showed substantial evidence of low-grade infection that cannot be isolated to an organ system. MRSA grew on cultures from the groin and blood. The patient traveled abroad for therapy when you diagnosed the aneurysm because she was underinsured and remains so. You are considered one of the foremost authorities on graft infections. What should you do?

(A) Tell her to return from whence she came.
(B) Alert the news media to the problem of cheap international medical care.
(C) Advise the patient to sue in international court.
(D) Provide care for the patient as you would any other.
(E) Advise the patient that once patients leave your care; they leave permanently. Tell her, "It is not my problem."

Globalization is an inevitable modern reality as the economy stretches worldwide, travel cheapens, and all earthlings share common problems such as global warming. Who has not called computer support or other technical assistance to discover they are speaking to someone halfway around the world? One will search long and hard for a pair of athletic shoes or leisure clothing manufactured in the United States.

"Medical Tourism" is international economics in action as patients seeking cheaper medical care have funded a growing multibillion dollar enterprise. For many years medical care in the United States was technologically unsurpassed and the wealthy from around the world flocked here when ill. Many still do, but several decades ago medical centers in Europe began to take more of the international healthcare market share, especially from the Middle East, as their global reputations for excellence blossomed. Currently, the numbers of foreign medical graduates trained in the United States and the worldwide availability of technology has made American-quality care available in many other countries. As implementation of new therapies are delayed by thriving American bureaucratism, cutting-edge technologies are becoming available sooner outside the United States, including some that shouldn't be, to draw the desperate. Although mainland Europeans can freely cross borders to other member countries of the European Union, they rarely do so, even if they live on the border of another country with shorter waits for therapy.[1] The Canadians and British, on the other hand, do participate somewhat in medical tourism because of lengthy delays in certain high-tech procedures. But incredibly, Americans are the largest group of medical tourists from the West with a half-million opting to leave what is assumed to be the best place for medical care in the world.[2] Americans have the problem of almost 50 million uninsured, lack of coverage for cosmetic, preexisting, and unproven "research" therapies, and ever-increasing copays, but one of the biggest problems is the priceyness of American medical care. Far Eastern countries including Malaysia, India, and Singapore offer procedures at 10% to 20% of the cost in the US including air fare and hotel.[3,4] Singapore has opened a second medical school to supply enough future physicians to treat the growing number of foreign patients.[5]

This alarming trend is reminiscent, but unlikely to be of the same magnitude, as the beating that the United States auto industry suffered when car manufacturers mistakenly considered their products' marketability invincible several decades ago. Remember how they had to radically change their business plans in order to survive the competition in price and quality of foreign manufacturers? Much of the American industrial noncompetitiveness still is blamed on the cost of medical care. Whether one manufactures cars or treats patients, volume eventually translates into quality.

Citizens in the United States spend almost double the percentage of the gross national product as other industrialized nations without national health statistics being as good.[6] Comparing the costs by procedure between the United States and other countries can be an eye opener. For example, with respect to inguinal hernias, "it is less expensive to fly someone roundtrip from Boston to the Shouldice Hospital for three days and pay the entire bill than to have the procedure done locally.[2]

The American Medical Association (AMA) considered the developing crisis of medical travel outside the United States serious enough to study the problem this year and produced a report generally critical of the U.S. healthcare system. The AMA concluded that, "currently, competition in American health care is focused not on patient outcomes but rather on shifting costs, restricting access, and supporting bloated administrative expenses."[2] In an article on international health care, Wikipedia considers the U.S. medical economic system to suffer from adverse selection to the extent that it is a market failure.[6] This economic aberration results in the unhealthy being more likely to seek health insurance (raising costs), the healthy to feel it costs too much and choosing to be inadequately insured (raising costs), and insurers expending considerable resources "weeding out" bad risks (raising costs). The only reasonable solution to systemic adverse selection appears to be a solution similar to the Massachusetts compulsory health insurance plan.[7] Consider what would happen if property taxes were optional. Those starting families whose incomes were growing would opt in, those who likely would be in a position to pay the most could opt out, raising the cost alarmingly to those trapped by the system.

Government regulation, managed care contracts, expansion of less invasive therapies, and bundling of payment for operative services have drastically reduced surgeon's fees to a relatively small percentage of the cost of medical care while overall medical care costs continually outstrip the economy.

The surgical mindset resolutely assigns responsibilities of medical care specifically to the attending surgeon—not the assistant, resident, nurses, or anesthesiologist—only to the surgeon of record. This responsibility is independent of whether other participants in care may have been causal. The natural implication is that when complications result from another surgeon's procedure, the operating surgeon alone bears full responsibility. An infected graft is a problem no vascular surgeon wants. Why can't the surgeon in this case simply say, "It's not my problem"? After all, the surgeon is not causally responsible for this patient's complication from previous treatment.

The AMA Ethics Principle VI defends the physician's right, "except in emergencies, [to] be free to choose whom to serve, with whom to associate, and the environment in which to provide medical care."[8] Denial of treatment on the basis of HIV seropositivity is the AMA's sole stated objection to the physician's ethical entitlement to select the patients he or she accepts for nonemergent treatment. There is no evidence in the document that a physician's personal prejudices may be considered as a basis for or against patient exclusion.

The fourth edition of the American College of Physicians' (ACP) Ethics Manual reaffirms the right to refuse non–emergent care to an individual patient when treatment is otherwise available.[9] However, the manual states that "a physician may not discriminate against a class or category of patients." We assume that medical tourism fails to achieve category status; the ACP has in mind race, gender, sexual orientation, and other personal characteristics of patients that, if selected against, result in invidious discrimination.

Declining to treat is valid and ethically necessary when the therapy sought is unnecessary, futile, or contraindicated,[10] when poor patient compliance will severely limit therapeutic effectiveness,[11] or when another available physician can provide better care.[12] Refusing a consultation request may also be ethically acceptable when there is a history of personal animus or other conflict of interest sufficiently negative to harm the physician's relationship with a patient.

Rejecting a patient with an urgent need for care that one is highly qualified to provide because she had sought affordable medical care elsewhere is ethically questionable. Such a decision by the surgeon unwarrantably concludes the causality of a disease determines a physician's professional responsibility to the patient. How the disease process came to be is irrelevant. If it were, most of us would be guilty of bringing maladies upon ourselves by our lifestyles and thus deserving our illnesses, would not deserve optimal therapy. What is relevant is that (1) the patient presented herself to the surgeon, (2) the surgeon is competent to diagnose and manage the patient's problem, and (3) there exist in the surgeon's hospital the human and technical resources necessary to provide the requisite clinical management of her problem.

Options (A) and (E) are ethically unacceptable, representing a fit of pique and not the exercise of professional or individual conscience. Refusing to treat this patient furthermore violates the professional virtue of self-effacement, which obligates the surgeon to set aside factors irrelevant to the care of the patient, especially personal ones. Where the patient received prior surgery is ethically irrelevant; she is in need of the expert clinical judgment and skills the surgeon has to offer. Options (A) and (E) also fail the Kantian criteria of universality of ethical behavior; it would not be proper for every physician to refuse to provide the best therapy because of a perceived personal insult, a trivial self-interest, at best, not valid justification for limiting professional responsibility.

Option (B) assumes that the patient's infection was caused by suboptimal medical care without proof. There is some evidence that patients having transplant surgery at international medical centers do reasonably well.[13] Current newspaper articles are appearing that are quite complementary and one of the larger healthcare networks in Malaysia treats complications from their therapies without added charges. Is there an American hospital willing to take up that gauntlet?

Option (C) is a risk of having a patient's medical or surgical care bungled in a foreign country where their malpractice tort systems are practically nonexistent; don't expect to sue and get compensated even when compensation is deserved.[3] But even with the high-powered legal system developed in the United States, less than 3% of those experiencing malpractice sue and less than half of those suing receive compensation.[14] However, the difference in cost between the two is billions.

Option (D) is the professional choice. Grumble, if needed, as you drive home, about life's injustices but taking care of patients by self-effacing will make one a better surgeon and a better person.

Also, let's hope that changes needed in the medical establishment come about before medicine's economic soul, like Detroit's, is forced to improve by "getting the hell kicked out of it."

References

1. Brouwer W, van Exel J, Hermans B, Stoop A. Should I stay or should I go? Waiting lists and cross-border care in the Netherlands. Health Policy 2003; 63:289–298.
2. AMA OMSS. Medical Travel Outside the U.S. Report B, 2007:1–20.
3. Chinai R, Goswami R. Medical visas mark growth of Indian medical tourism. *Bull World Health Organ* 2007; 85:164–165.
4. Burkett L. Medical tourism. Concerns, benefits, and the American legal perspective. *J Leg Med* 2007; 28:223–245.
5. Soo KC. Singapore's proposed graduate medical school: An expensive medical tutorial college or an opportunity for transforming Singapore medicine? *Ann Acad Med Singapore* 2005; 34:176C–181C.

6. Wikipedia. Medical care, 2007.

7. Steinbrook R. Health care reform in Massachusetts: A work in progress. *N Engl J Med* 2006; 354:2095–2098.

8. Association AM. Code of medical ethics: Current opinions with annotations. The Association, Chicago, 1996.

9. Ethics manual. Fourth edition. American College of Physicians. *Ann Intern Med* 1998; 128:576–94.

10. McCullough LB, Jones JW. Postoperative futility: A clinical algorithm for setting limits. *Br J Surg* 2001; 88:1153–1154.

11. Jones JW, McCullough LB, Richman BW. The surgeon's obligations to the non-compliant patient. *J Vasc Surg* 2003; 38:626–627.

12. Jones JW, McCullough LB. When to refer to another surgeon. *J Vasc Surg* 2002; 35:192.

13. Canales MT, Kasiske BL, Rosenberg ME. Transplant tourism: Outcomes of United States residents who undergo kidney transplantation overseas. *Transplantation* 2006; 82:1658–1661.

14. Jones JW, McCullough LB, Richman BW. From premiums to payouts: Who's behind the malpractice crisis, anyway? *J Vasc Surg* 2006; 43:635–638.

· 8 ·

END-OF-LIFE ISSUES

"End-of-life" euphemizes the beginning of death. Knowledge stops at the end-of-life, death being our universal material finality. Francis Bacon (1561–1626) characterized the human emotions associated with death as, "Fear such as a small child has of the darkness."[1] Death motivates the existence of religion, the medical profession...and gravediggers. Many of the world's great monuments, including the Great Pyramids, the Taj Mahal, the Mausoleum at Halicarnassus, Saint Peter's Basilica, and the dynastic tombs of the Shang and the Han, are representations not only of the awe with which we confront death, but of our efforts to magically project life into death and so withstand it. Because we fear death's ubiquity and the finality it imposes, many of ethics' knottiest challenges are associated with end-of-life issues.

For most of the history of Western medicine, the standard of care was for physicians to shun desperate cases in which the physician could reliably predict a high likelihood of mortality. The correlate of this standard of care was that physicians should stop treating patients who became so desperately ill while in their care that they were likely to die.

These standards date from the time of the Hippocratic texts, and two important concerns supported them. The first was the physician's self-interest. In a crowded, competitive, completely unregulated market place for medical and surgical services, practitioners who became known for losing their patients would not succeed. High mortality rates were not good for a practitioner's reputation and therefore for economic success. Only a practitioner reckless of legitimate self-interest in earning a living—not at all guaranteed in those days—would fail to heed to demands of prudence.

The second standard arose from a keen appreciation for the moment when medicine reaches the limits of its ability to alter the course of disease. The author of the Hippocratic text, *The Art*, argues that,

> For if a man demand from an art a power over what does not belong to the art, or from nature a power over what does not belong to nature, his ignorance is more allied to madness than to lack of knowledge. For in cases where we may have mastery through the means afforded by a natural constitution or by an art, there we may be craftsmen, but nowhere else. Whenever therefore a man suffers from an ill which is too strong for the means at the disposal of medicine, he surely must not even expect that it can be overcome by medicine.[2]

For the ancient Greeks, moral failure resulted from ignorance of intellectual and moral standards of judgment and behavior. A physician who takes on a dying patient, thinking falsely that medicine has at its disposal the power to alter the course of disease and save the patient, is worse than ignorant; that physician has gone mad. That is, to willfully and knowingly violate well founded intellectual and moral standards of clinical judgment and behavior was worthy of even less respect than moral failure. Such hubris was abject intellectual and moral failure.

The Hippocratic texts on the ethics of end-of-life care are therefore marked by a deep tension between self-interest and the moral virtue of prudence, on the one hand, and, on the other, a nascent concept of the intellectual and moral integrity of medicine that requires physicians to acknowledge and observe the limitations of medicine or nature to self-correct injury and disease. In the subsequent history of medicine, this tension was usually resolved, as a matter of practice, in favor of self-interest. Prudence requires that the physician not accept dying patients and stop treating patients who become gravely ill in their care and enter the end-stages of disease or injury; the physician who follows this standard ensures that the disease or injury, and not the physician's ministrations, will be recognized as the cause of the patient's death.

This prudence-based approach to the ethics of end-of-life decision making and medical care was codified in the early 18th century by the German physician and medical educator, Friedrich Hoffmann (1660–1742). His ethics lectures were published under the title, *Medicus Politicus*,[3] meaning "the politic physician," the physician who was wise in the ways of the rational protection and pursuit of self-interest. Hoffmann made the virtue of prudence one of the foundations in his book. Prudence is a virtue that trains us to identify our legitimate self-interests and then act rationally to protect and promote them. It is wise self-governance. Hoffmann's account is distinctive because his concept of the physician's self-interest is enlightened: it incorporates the interests of the patient.

With respect to "malignant and acute," or life-taking, disease, Hoffmann urges physicians to "speak circumspectly" but never to be dishonest with the dying patient. He understood well the *ars moriendi*, the art of dying, and the need of his patients to prepare themselves for their deaths. Patients cannot undertake such preparation if they are buoyed up by false hope engendered by dishonest or misleading statements about the state of their health by the physician. It was also suggested that physicians avoid "heroic medication," such as emetics and surgery, in the management of dying patient. There were two reasons for this approach. Heroic measures carry significant iatrogenic burden (indeed, this was part of the clinical concept of "heroic" medicine), with little expectation of a compensating clinical benefit. Moreover, the administration of heroic medicines or surgery could then be considered the cause of the patient's death, imperiling the physician's reputation and his associated economic interests. The marketplace of medicine in Hoffmann's 18th-century Germany was as unforgiving in its punishment of high mortality rates as it was in Hippocrates' Greece.

Later in the 18th century, Dr. John Gregory argued for a different standard: physicians should not abandon the dying, but continue to provide care for them:

Let me here exhort you against the custom of some physicians, who leave their patients when their life is despaired of, and when it is no longer decent to put them to farther expence. It is as much the business of a physician to alleviate pain, and to smooth the avenues of death, when unavoidable, as to cure diseases. Even in cases where his skill as a physician can be of no further avail, his presence and assistance as a friend may be agreeable and useful, both to the patient and to his nearest relations.[4]

"Smoothing" the "avenues of death" included aggressive pain management with such drugs as laudanum, which was then readily available over the counter. As a result of Gregory's ethics, the standard of care for dying patients began to change and attending to the dying became a commonplace obligation of physicians and surgeons.

With the introduction of the mechanical ventilator and the invention of modern critical care units in the mid-20th century, the technical capacities of medicine and surgery dramatically increased. Mortality rates from acute disease and injury began to come down. With the introduction of anesthesia and asepsis, surgery became a reasonable alternative therapy in cases that previously had meant certain death. The concept of unacceptably high surgical risk became elastic, as surgeons and physicians pushed against old limits and sought to expand their capacities to extend life.

During the 1960s and early 1970s, advanced technology and high-risk surgery was used for sicker and sicker patients in American hospitals, but without much attention to outcomes. As a consequence, physicians and surgeons were slow to appreciate that, despite the dramatically expanded "powers" of surgery and medicine, "nature" still imposed limits on those powers. Powerful drugs such as steroids and antibiotics became available and were tried without hesitation in every conceivable situation. In the early days of high-dose steroid therapy, many patients died with smiling blue lips. A challenge was mounted to the traditional moral logic of high-risk surgery and critical-care medicine that every life extended was worth whatever morbidity and lost functional status that might result. Patients, especially women with breast cancer whose only option was total radical mastectomy, began to complain that the cure was worse than the disease. By the middle of the 1970s, a vigorous debate began about the limits of high-risk surgery and critical care medicine.

It was in this context that the landmark case of Karen Ann Quinlan occurred. She suffered anoxic brain injury of uncertain origin and progressed to what was then called a "chronic, persistent vegetative state." Life-sustaining treatment included mechanical ventilation, antibiotics, and artificial nutrition and hydration. Her father, acting as her surrogate decision maker (before the phrase had been in general usage), requested that mechanical ventilation be discontinued, but her physicians refused his request. The matter was litigated to the New Jersey Supreme Court and decided in 1976.[5]

The Court first took up the question of whether the state had a compelling interest in preserving Ms. Quinlan's life, and whether it should invoke its police powers to compel continuation of mechanical ventilation. The Court found that no such compelling interest existed, because when the invasiveness of treatment is high and the prognosis of recovery to a cognitive, sapient existence very low, the state has no compelling interest to intervene. Ms. Quinlan had a right to refuse treatment, a right that would not be meaningful if her father could not exercise it for her. Turning to the history of medical ethics and practice, the Court next found that discontinuing mechanical ventilation would not violate the integrity of medicine, because that history showed acceptance of limits on medicine in the face of overwhelming injury or disease. The Court also found that discontinuing mechanical ventilation would not constitute homicide or suicide, since the cause of death would be her underlying incurable brain injury. Finally, the Court urged that its views be codified into statute, to keep future such cases from requiring litigation.

The *Quinlan* opinion helped to forge a consensus that patients have the right to refuse even life-sustaining treatment, that others can exercise this right for them when the patient cannot, and when the patient is in the end-stages of disease or terminally ill and the state has no compelling interest in preserving the patient's life. Spurred by *Quinlan*, all states have enacted advance directive legislation.[6]

The basic idea of an advance directive is that a patient, when autonomous, can make decisions regarding his medical management in advance of a time during which he or she becomes incapable of making health care decisions. The relevant ethical dimensions of autonomy in these cases include:

1. A patient may exercise his autonomy now in the form of a request for or refusal of life-prolonging interventions.
2. Autonomy-based request or refusal, expressed in the past and left unchanged, remains in effect for any future time when the patient becomes nonautonomous.
3. Past autonomy-based requests or refusals should translate into physician obligations at the time the patient becomes unable to participate in the informed consent process.
4. In particular, refusal of life-prolonging medical intervention should translate into the withholding or withdrawal of such interventions, including artificial nutrition and hydration.

The living will or directive to physicians is an instrument that permits the patient to make a direct decision, usually to refuse life-prolonging medical intervention in the future. The living will becomes effective when the patient is a "qualified patient," that is, terminally or irreversibly ill, and the attending physician judges that the patient is no longer able to participate in the informed consent process. In keeping with the urging of the Quinlan opinion, court review is not required. Obviously, terminally or irreversibly ill patients who are able to participate in the informed consent process retain autonomy to make their own decisions. Some states prescribe the wording of the living will and some do not. Each individual should become familiar with the legal requirements in his or her own jurisdiction, well in advance of the moment of critical need. A living will, to be useful and effective, should be as explicit as possible. Readers should familiarize themselves with hospital policies on advance directives, which should reflect applicable law. Copies of the living will should be placed in the personal physician's office and in the medical record with each admission.

The concept of a durable power of attorney or medical power of attorney is that any autonomous adult, who later becomes unable to participate in the informed consent process, can assign decision-making authority to another person. The advantage of the durable power of attorney for health care is that it applies only when the patient has lost decision-making capacity, as judged by his or her physician. Court review is not required. It does not, as does the living will, also require that the patient be terminally or irreversibly ill. However, unlike the living will, the durable power of attorney does not necessarily provide explicit direction, only the explicit assignment of decision-making authority to an identified individual or "agent." Obviously, any patient who assigns durable power of attorney for health care to someone else has an interest in communicating her values, beliefs, and preferences to that person. The physician can play a facilitating role in this process. Indeed, in order to protect the patient's autonomy, the physician should play an active role in encouraging this communication process so that there will be minimal doubt about whether the person holding durable power of attorney is faithfully representing the wishes of the patient.

The main clinical advantages of these two forms of advance directives are that they encourage patients to think carefully in advance about their request for or refusal of medical intervention, and that these directives, therefore, help to prevent ethical conflicts and crises in the management, especially, of terminally or irreversibly ill patients who have decision-making capacity. Unfortunately, the use of advance directives is not as widespread as it should be.[17] The reader is encouraged to think of advance directives as powerful, practical strategies for preventive ethics for end-of-life care, and to encourage patients to consider them seriously, especially high-risk surgical patients. The use of advance directives prevents the experience of increased burden of decision making in the absence of reliable information about the patient's values and beliefs.[18]

Except in the Netherlands, there is no acceptance of euthanasia, direct killing of the patient by medical means. In addition, Belgium and Switzerland allow physician-assisted suicide. In the United States, only Oregon allows for physician-assisted suicide. This is understood to mean that the patient must be terminally ill, must be capable of informed consent for the prescription and use of medication to end his life, and must administer the medication himself. The physician is involved only in counseling the patient, obtaining informed consent, and writing the prescription. There is no ethical consensus about the permissibility of physician-assisted suicide managed in this way. Physician-assisted suicide in which the physician, not the patient, administers the lethal medication is illegal in all other jurisdictions in the United States and most other countries. It is ethically very controversial.

In fact, most all the urgent topics we consider in this chapter are intensely controversial, examining as they do the one subject that still abrades the sensitivities of every individual: human death. Not only will we look at clinical situations at the core of futility, advanced directives, and euthanasia, but whether a surgeon should provide life-saving therapy to a death row inmate, what should be done when the most dreaded complications happen in the postoperative period, and even whether dead patients retain their rights. Recalling Bacon, these are areas which men "fear such as a small child in the darkness." Let us shed some light.

References

1. Bacon F. *Essays and New Atlantis.* Walter J. Black, Roslyn, New York, 1923.
2. Hippocrates (attributed to). "The Art." Translated by W. H. S. Jones. In W. H. S. Jones, trans., *Hippocrates, Volume II.* Cambridge, Mass: Harvard University Press, Loeb Classical Library, 1992.
3. Hoffmann F. *Medicus Politicus, sive Regulae Prudentiae secundum quas Medicus Juvenis Studia sue et Vitae Rationem Dirigere Debet. In F. Hoffmanni, Opera Omnium Physico-Medicorum Supplementum in Duas Partes Distributum.* Genevae: Apud Fratres de Tournes, 1749.
4. Gregory J. Lectures on the Duties and Qualifications of a Physician. In McCullough LB, ed. *John Gregory's Writings on Medical Ethics and Philosophy of Medicine.* Dordrecht, The Netherlands: Kluwer Academic Publishers, 1998: 161–248.
5. In re Quinlan, 70 N.J. 10, 355 A.2d 647 (1976), cert. denied, 429 U.S. 92 (1976).
6. Meisel L. *The Right to Die.* 2nd ed. New York: John Wiley & Sons, 1995.

• CASE 63 •

Futility and Surgical Intervention

*If you live to be one hundred, you've got it made. Very few people
die past that age.*
George Burns (1896–1996)

An 86-year-old man presents with a history of multiple endarterectomies, coronary grafting, and severe heart failure. He is now diagnosed with a non-obstructing pancreatic carcinoma and emphysema with an FEV1 of 0.5 liters. Patient and family insist on surgical intervention. The best response is:

(A) Refer the request to the hospital ethics committee.
(B) Refuse the request as inappropriate.
(C) Refer them to another surgeon because you are uncomfortable operating on this patient.
(D) Explain why surgery is likely to be futile in this case, and recommend palliative care.
(E) Involve your hospital's risk management division in subsequent discussions with the patient and his family.

Limits on the obligation to preserve life have been understood in medicine throughout history. The dramatic success of high-technology surgery and critical care since World War II has sometimes made medicine's ability to extend life seem boundless, but of course it is not. Cardiopulmonary resuscitation and advanced surgical procedures have often been implemented with insufficient attention to associated morbidity and lost functional status, as many patients, families, and even some physicians have refused to acknowledge boundaries to medicine's obligation to preserve life.

Despite recent skepticism,[1] clinical assessments of futility can be made and reliably implemented. "Futility" means that the therapeutic goal of a clinical intervention is unlikely to be achieved. The key clinical issues in assessing futility therefore become the specified goal and the evidence that it is unlikely to be reached. Four senses of futility are relevant to the specification of goals:

1. "Physiologic futility" applies when the intervention is reliably expected not to produce its desired physiologic outcome. CPR is routinely discontinued when it can no longer be expected to restore spontaneous circulation and respiration, even though it may produce the transient physiologic effect of an occasional heart beat.

2. "Overall futility" reflects a reliable expectation that the intervention will not restore the patient's capacity to interact with the environment and continue human development. Antibiotics for management of opportunistic

infections can justifiably be withheld from patients in a persistent vegetative state.

3. "Imminent demise futility" characterizes a reliable expectation that the
patient will die before discharge and not recover interactive capacity
before death, as may be the case with our elderly patient.

4. "Quality of life futility" applies when the patient's current or projected
condition will result in an intolerable inability to engage in or derive
pleasure from life, as judged from the patient's perspective, not that of
others.

In this case, there are two likely outcomes of surgical intervention: first, that
the patient will die during or shortly after surgery, or will survive but not be
weanable from ventilation, thereby losing any remaining interactive capacity.
Blackhall[3] set the standard for physiologic futility at a 98–100% expectation
of failure to achieve the desired clinical outcome. This case may not meet that
standard, but can be seen as exemplifying either imminent demise futility or
overall futility.

The surgeon should meet with the patient and his family to discuss the
prognosis of overall or imminent demise futility. The surgeon should explain
that surgery would not be in the patient's best interest, and that a comfortable
and dignified death is the most appropriate available goal. The surgeon should
make a referral to hospice care. If the patient continues to insist on surgery, the
surgeon should consider referral to the hospital Ethics Committee, option (A).

The problem with refusing to perform inappropriate surgery, option (B),
resides in the term's vagueness when clinically applied. The four concepts of
futility can help to clarify the surgeon's reluctance to operate when the outcome will be poor. "Uncomfortable" is an even fuzzier term in clinical discourse and so, until an attempt has been made to reason with this patient and
his family, option (C) is premature. Finally, surgeons should not rely upon
risk managers for clinical guidance in potentially conflictual situations like
option (E). Surgeons should instead form clinical ethical judgments carefully
as patient fiduciaries and guide themselves and their patients accordingly. The
best clinical and ethical response is option (D).

References

1. Helft PR, Siegler M, Lantos J. The rise and fall of the futility movement. *N Engl
J Med*. 2000; 343:293–296.
2. Rabeneck L, McCullough LB, Wray NP. Ethically justified clinical comprehensive guidelines for percutaneous endoscopic gastrectomy (PEG). *Lancet*. 1997; 349:
496–498.
3. Blackhall L. Must we always use CPR? *N Engl J Med*. 1987; 317:1281–1285.

• CASE 64 •

Complying with Advance Directives in the Operating Room

I must die. Must I die moaning?
Epictetus (c. 55–c. 135)

An ambulance brings an unconscious 41-year-old man to the ER following an automobile accident. Emergency CT shows rupture of the liver, spleen, and superior mesenteric artery. He is being prepared for surgery when his business partner arrives with what he claims is the patient's signed advance directive, specifying that in the event of cardiac arrest the patient wishes no resuscitative measures. During surgery the patient suffers an acute hypotensive episode and arrests. Your proper response is:

(A) Do not resuscitate
(B) Resuscitate and continue the operation
(C) Limit your resuscitative efforts to closed chest massage
(D) Consult the business partner
(E) Ignore the advance directive

The "living will" advance directive is defined by most statutes and hospital policies as the medical instructions of a terminally ill or injured patient who can no longer communicate his immediate wishes.[1] Living wills typically concentrate upon end-of-life issues, particularly withdrawing or withholding efforts to sustain a life that cannot be saved or restored to a functional level acceptable to the patient. They may conversely express the wish that all available life-sustaining efforts be fully implemented until death is spontaneous. A "terminal illness or injury" is understood to mean that death is inevitable within a short time regardless of medical intervention. The application of a living will also requires that, in the reasonable clinical judgment of the attending physician, the patient currently lacks the decision-making capacity he had at the time the living will was written. The absence of current decision-making capacity may be the result of traumatic brain injury, dementia, psychosis, or persistent vegetative states. The living will provisions of advance directives should not govern physicians' clinical responses when the patient's clinical status does not meet these criteria. Transient cognitive disturbances, like drunkenness, drug intoxication, panic, delirium, acute unconsciousness secondary to illness or trauma, or induction of general anesthesia, do not activate a living will. The right to informed consent remains intact in these cases, and should be applied when the patient's mental status stabilizes.

Though grievously injured, this patient can recover with timely and competent surgical care. His intraoperative arrest is a correctable complication of fluid management and shock, likely not the culminating event of an inevitably terminal illness or injury. Intraoperative resuscitation maintains homeostatis, and patient recovery in such cases is routine, as opposed to the overall 15% success rate of CPR.[2] The patient's refusal of CPR in the advance directive may ethically be understood to apply in the context of these poor success rates, which include not just death but survival with a greatly diminished quality of life. The advance directive's election of option (A), no resuscitation, was very likely formulated without consideration of functional conditions in the operating room, and would furthermore deny the patient the benefits for which he was originally brought to the OR. Option (B) is fully consistent with the goals of surgery, and is a necessary and proper response for a patient whose condition does not activate the authority of a living will.

Some ethicists argue that advance directives containing do-not-resuscitate (DNR) instructions should be as applicable inside the operating room as in the ICU.[3] Others have argued that the conditions of surgery blur the distinctions between resuscitation and maintenance of homeostasis,[2] or that many physicians routinely dismiss advance directives, or that patients seldom understand the processes of surgical care. Attempting to straddle these issues by limiting the procedural options of the resuscitation efforts, option (C), strengthens neither the physician's ethical posture nor his clinical effectiveness, and is inconsistent with the goals of surgery and conditions under which the advance directive has clinical authority.

The business partner is not the next-of-kin, and has no legal standing as a surrogate decision maker unless he has been named as an agent in a durable medical power of attorney for health care. Furthermore, the patient's own views have been articulated in the advance directive, which would stand as the last available expression of his wishes if it otherwise qualified. Option (D) is therefore not available.

Ignoring the advance directive, option (E), which legend holds is a common tactic among physicians who find such instructions odious, is not acceptable. Notwithstanding, the surgeon is obligated to evaluate the directive in light of the patient's clinical condition to establish its pertinence. As noted, the clinical diagnosis necessary to establish the clinical application of an advance directive, i.e. a terminal condition not susceptible to reversal with medical care, are not present, and the physician is not governed by the terms of the document. In such cases the medical record should reflect why the surgeon is not implementing the directive.

References

1. Youngner SJ, Shuck JM. Advance directives and the determination of death in surgical ethics. In: McCullough LB, Jones JW, Brody BA, eds. *Surgical Ethics*. Oxford 1998:57–77.
2. Cohen CB, Cohen PJ. Do-not-resuscitate orders in the OR. *NEJM*. 1991; 325: 1879–1882.
3. Walker RM. DNR in the OR. *JAMA*. 1991; 266:2407–2412.

• CASE 65 •

Abdominal Aortic Aneurysm in a Death Row Inmate

As men, we are all equal in the presence of death.
Publius Syrus (fl. 1st century BCE)

You are consulted about a 47-year-old male with complaints of abdominal pain. Workup revealed large gastric carcinoma. The patient exercises daily and appears to be in excellent physical condition. Laboratory studies are normal except for a positive HIV test. The patient has resided on the state prison's death row since his conviction and sentencing 3 years ago for multiple aggravated murders in your home-town. His sentence has been under lengthy appeal, and no execution date has been set. You have enjoyed a lucrative capitated contract providing exclusive surgical services for the main prison system for many years. The prison warden has denied the prisoner's request to be transferred to a major medical center in the state's capital city for surgery. What is your most ethical course of action?

(A) Petition the governor for funds to have the procedure done out of state.

(B) Perform the operation to the best of your ability.

(C) Since the patient will be executed anyway, recommend that surgery represents a poor utilization of the prison system's healthcare budget and is therefore not indicated.

(D) Elect to follow the cancer until you know how long the death sentence appeals process will continue.

(E) Heinous crimes of this nature do not deserve civility or professionalism. Tell the patient what you think and decline to operate.

As the designated surgeon for this patient population, you are clearly in a fiduciary relationship with the patient. The most basic ethical component of this fiduciary role is the surgeon's obligation to make the protection and promotion of the patient's health a primary ethical concern.[1] This patient has an urgent need for surgical management, and there are no medical contra-indications to performing the surgery. The risk-benefit ratio, divested of his social status, unequivocally supports surgical intervention.

The fiduciary must place the patient's best interests above his or her own. The patient's HIV-positive status does not pose an unreasonable or unacceptable threat to the surgeon or surgical team if standard infection-control procedures are observed. Any negative personal attitudes you might hold toward prisoners are irrelevant to the determination of your ethical obligations in this case. By signing the contract with the Department of Corrections, you have implicitly confirmed that you will provide high quality medical care to incarcerated patients, without regard to your personal feelings about individual criminals or crimes.

The surgeon's clear duty here is not to act as an agent of the criminal justice system, but as a physician whose social contract obligates him to treat his patients' ailments. The professional virtue of self-effacement requires the surgeon to sublimate his personal repugnance at the patient's crimes, remain silent about them during the course of treatment, and prevent them from adversely affecting the clinical management of the patient's condition. Our culture grants physicians wide latitude in determining the best course for their patients. Determination of legal penalties, assessment of whether the criminal appeals process is too lengthy or stultifying, and implementation of death sentences before the judicially appointed hour are not among the privileges granted within that latitude.

Because gastrectomy is well within the capacity of any certified surgeon, option (A), a petition to the governor to have the surgery performed out-of-state, is based upon no compelling need for locally unavailable specialized services. Instead, it is likely a reflection of your personal distaste at caring for a patient who has committed terrible crimes. This argument lacks ethical justification and must be rejected. Furthermore, this choice would violate your contract to provide the Department of Corrections with any indicated vascular surgical services you are capable of performing.

Option (C), evaluating the cost-benefit ratio of surgery in view of the patient's death sentence, displaces the surgeon from his proper role as professional caregiver. The distribution of the prison's medical budget is the responsibility of administrators within the Department of Corrections, and legislators, not contract surgeons. When and whether this patient will in fact die as punishment for his crimes is still to be determined by an active appeals process and execution certainly should not be presumed by the surgeon. The certainty of death if the cancer is not surgically treated has been fully established. The certainty of death by judicial execution has yet to be fully determined and the surgeon has no proper role in this process.

Electing to follow the patient, option (D), is inconsistent with the standard of care for the clinical management of his disease. This is either a gross medical error, or, as with option (C), an attempt to disguise the surgeon's ill-intent in a medical rationalization. The course and duration of the appeals process is irrelevant to the patient's care.

Option (B), performing the indicated operation to the best of your ability, recognizes that your ethical obligations to all patients needing your care do not vary with their character, social histories, belief systems, or other features unrelated to their medical condition. Furthermore, option (B) properly leaves the prisoner's punishment to those legally empowered to determine and administer it.

Option (E) reflects the perils of physicians and surgeons acting on judgments about the social worth of their patients. Nazi physicians were tried and convicted, largely because they accepted cultural judgments that some people had no social worth, when their professional integrity should have rejected this notion.[2] The health care professionals involved in the Tuskegee Syphilis Experiment from the 1930s to the 1970s acted on the basis of racial bias in the design and conduct of their research.[3] More recently, the "God Committee" at the University of Washington, in making decisions about who should have access to renal dialysis when it first became available and before Medicare funded it, made allocation decisions that were biased by unwarranted judgments of their patients' social value.[4] The physician's clear obligation during treatment is to relieve his patient's ailments rather than society's.

References

1. McCullough LB, Jones JW, Brody BA. Principles and practice of surgical ethics. In: McCullough LB, Jones JW, Brody BA, eds. *Surgical Ethics*. New York: Oxford University Press, 1998:3–14.
2. Grodin M, Annas GJ, eds. *The Nazi Doctors and the Nuremberg Code: Human Rights in Human Experiments*. New York: Oxford University Press, 1992.
3. Jones JH. *Bad Blood: The Tuskegee Syphilis Experiment*. New York: The Free Press, 1981.
4. Jonsen AR. *The Birth of Bioethics*. New York: Oxford University Press, 1998.

• CASE 66 •

Telling the Truth About Terminal Diseases

After the game, the king and the pawn go into the same box.
Italian Proverb

You have excised a pancreatic adenocarcinoma from your respected college biology professor, who is now retired and widowed at age 85. He returns for follow-up examination after 9 months. Laboratory tests and imaging confirm recurrence of the tumor, with widespread metastases. He is being treated by a psychiatrist for depression and mild dementia, but remains legally competent and maintains his own home. His three adult children, two sons and a daughter, are ardent in their request that you withhold the bad news from the patient. Radiation and chemotherapy are marginally indicated for palliation, but he will probably consent to the therapy if you refer him. The patient hasn't asked you for results of the diagnostic tests. What should you do?

(A) Respect the family's request. Don't volunteer the information about prognosis, and refer for palliation.

(B) Ignore the family's request. Tactfully tell the patient that his cancer has recurred, and seek his consent for aggressive treatment.

(C) Tell the patient only if he specifically asks about his prognosis and recommend palliative therapy.

(D) Dissemble and minimize the seriousness, even if he asks. Tell him that some other doctors are going to mop up the remaining cancer cells.

(E) Tell the patient the truth. Provide him with appropriate referrals.

Informing a patient when surgical therapy has failed and the prognosis has changed from good to terminal is an unpleasant and even painful responsibility of surgical practice. Dr. John Gregory (1724–1773), in the first medical ethics book written in the English language, noted that a "Physician is often at a loss in speaking to his patients of their real situation when it is dangerous."[1] Indeed, being frank with seriously ill patients and their families, Gregory added, is one of the "most disagreeable duties" and a "painful office" of the physician. The task becomes all the more emotionally distressing when bad news must be conveyed to younger patients or patients for whom the surgeon has developed a special regard and affection, as in this case. Family members, believing that they are emotionally protecting the patient but acting in their own interests as well, may want the physician to conceal from the patient knowledge that the battle with disease has been lost. In our capacities as healers, our own instincts are to protect our patients from whatever will cause them pain, and our professional nature makes us loath to concede that our therapy has failed. Why not euphemize the message as this family requests?

Option (D) certainly appears at first to be an attractive and sensitive choice, but it is not ethically acceptable. Dissembling and obfuscating are ultimately self-protective mechanisms, intended here to save the family from having to confront an anticipated emotional storm. Sometimes physicians mask this reality when they assume without basis that a terminal patient will not want to know the truth about his condition and prognosis. Not coincidentally, this approach saves the surgeon the torment of breaking the news, supporting the patient through an intensely difficult time, and perhaps even accepting an angry, accusatory response for having failed to arrest the disease. Though advertised as sparing the patient an intolerable insight into his limited future, the real motivation for such a deception is often the self-interest of the family and physician in sparing themselves an emotional storm.

The issue is particularly sharp on the surgical specialties, because when our treatment fails there is usually no saving alternative; we are the doctors of last resort. For many diseases, surgical therapy is the "gold standard" which, when it fails, dashes hope and heralds terminal illness. We cannot truthfully soften the blow by dangling the hope that other specialties will have the answer that we could not find. Once surgical therapy has failed, the surgeon's role is reduced to nibbling around the edges—two-thirds of surgeons readily admit they are not trained in competencies for nonsurgical care such as pain management, care coordination, and nutrition.[2] The surgeon's last important duty is to fully inform the patient and the family of how well or poorly surgical therapy has turned out and what they can expect, not just immediately post-op, but at every stage of follow-up until indicated referrals have been made to specialists in end-of-life and/or palliative care. In this case, the surgeon's duty attaches directly to this patient, who remains competent to make his own decisions about accepting palliative care.[3] Wear considers informed consent for terminally ill patients different from the standard informed consent, and calls for "a candid, to the point of bluntness, explanation of the patients' basic situation and prospects, with and without treatment, and a clear sense of the potential downsides and limitations of the course of therapy being proposed."[4] Option (E) therefore emerges as ethically mandated, out of respect for this patient's autonomy.

Honesty also helps to protect the patient from overtreatment, which is neither benign nor beneficial. The availability of technologically advanced therapies has particularly increased utilization of medical resources in terminally ill cancer patients without necessarily lengthening their lives or improving their comfort. Aggressive chemical and radiation therapy after recurrence in advanced pancreatic cancer metastases typically buys the patient little or no extension of life, but in this case assures additional suffering.[5-7]

The survival of patients with unresectable pancreatic cancer is measured in months regardless of medical therapy. Earle examined Medicare claims of 28,777 patients 65 years and older dying of cancer and found that 15.7% received chemotherapy within the last 2 weeks of their lives.[8] In a study typical of current literature on patients with advanced pancreatic cancer, after 45 cycles of chemotherapy the median survival was a paltry 6.8 months.[6] The authors' Panglossian conclusions were, "Treatment with NFL is well-tolerated in patients with advanced pancreatic cancer...survival in these patients with poor prognoses compares favorably with other treatment options." There are aggressive oncologists who administer therapy costing 100% more than those less aggressive measures. Despite the increased cost and higher morbidity, survival is the same.[9]

By not informing patients of the natural course of their chronic or recurrent diseases, or by mis-characterizing a terminal reality and handing the case off to an aggressive oncologist, the surgeon may be depriving his patient of what end-of-life specialists call "a good death," an opportunity to come to terms with unresolved emotional, interpersonal, and spiritual issues. These intensely private concerns are within everyone's personal experience, and cannot rightfully be denied a dying patient by well-meaning spouses, adult children, or compassionate physicians. The considerable majority of patients want their physicians to tell them if they have a terminal illness,[10] and elderly patients, oblivious to the physician's feelings of helplessness and frustration in this regard, typically expect the discussion in terminal illness to be initiated by their doctor.[11] There are many obvious problems in confronting the termination of life, and patients need genuine direction and useful consultations. What they often get is a baffling shift of responsibility to another specialist who may address the wrong issues. The surgeon now assumes the same ethical obligations as the physicians who referred the patient for surgery: a comprehensive objective description of the disease and prognosis, and referral to the specialist who can best care for the patient. This does not necessarily mean the physician who can briefly extend the patient's life, but the one who best understands how the patient wants to die. We will therefore rule out option (A), because it deprives this intelligent and competent patient of information he is entitled to have and initiates the process of palliative care without his informed consent, thus doubly violating his right to autonomy in the control of his care. Option (B) gets it half right by informing the patient, but ignores overwhelming evidence that aggressive treatment will mean additional avoidable morbidity without significantly improving outcome. Option (C) relieves the physician of the painful burden of breaking terrible news to the patient, and usually leads to a protracted evasion of professional responsibility.

Telling terminally ill patients the truth about their diagnosis and prognosis is probably the most painful of all physicianly responsibilities to fulfill. This seems particularly true for surgeons, who intend to deliver definitive cures. When the patient is personally dear to the surgeon, as in our case, or is young with an entire life to forfeit the reluctance to bear the bad news is naturally that much greater; our professional training gives us no special insight into the mysteries and terrors of death, and we hate and fear it as all humans do. Nonetheless, sparing the patient with false hope betrays the surgeon's important role as a trusted authority figure, and thinking that oncological therapy is a recommended continuation of therapy is likely to encourage patient demands for overtreatment, with all the useless suffering it may bear. The moral obligation is to give the patient information and offer several directions depending on the clinical situation and the patient's desires. Using a surgeon's practical knowledge to educate and properly direct such a patient is your last and perhaps most meaningful duty.

References

1. McCullough LB. *John Gregory and the Invention of Professional Medical Ethics and the Profession of Medicine*. Dordrecht, the Netherlands: Klwuer Academic Publishers, 1998.
2. Darer JD, Hwang W, Pham HH, Bass EB, Anderson G. More training needed in chronic care: A survey of US physicians. *Acad Med*. 2004; 79:541–548.
3. McCullough LB, Jones JW, Brody BA. Informed consent: Autonomous decision making of the surgical patient. In McCullough LB, Jones JW, Brody BA, eds. *Surgical Ethics*. New York: Oxford University Press, 1998:15–37.
4. Wear S, Milch R, Weaver W. Care of dying patients. In McCullough LB, Jones JW, Brody BA, eds. *Surgical Ethics*. New York: Oxford University Press, 1998:171–197.
5. Rocha Lima CM, Green MR, Rotche R, Miller WH, Jr., Jeffrey GM, Cisar LA, et al. Irinotecan plus gemcitabine results in no survival advantage compared with gemcitabine monotherapy in patients with locally advanced or metastatic pancreatic cancer despite increased tumor response rate. *J Clin Oncol.* 2004; 22:3776–3783.
6. Garcia AA, Leichman L, Baranda J, Pandit L, Lenz HJ, Leichman CG. Phase II clinical trial of 5-fluorouracil, trimetrexate, and leucovorin (NFL) in patients with advanced pancreatic cancer. *Int J Gastrointest Cancer*. 2003; 34:79–86.
7. Emanuel EJ, Young-Xu Y, Levinsky NG, Gazelle G, Saynina O, Ash AS. Chemotherapy use among Medicare beneficiaries at the end of life. *Ann Intern Med*. 2003; 138:639–643.
8. Earle CC, Neville BA, Landrum MB, Ayanian JZ, Block SD, Weeks JC. Trends in the aggressiveness of cancer care near the end of life. *J Clin Oncol*. 2004; 22:315–321.
9. Hoverman JR, Robertson SM. Lung cancer: A cost and outcome study based on physician practice patterns. *Dis Manag*. 2004; 7:112–123.
10. Fernandez D, Perez Suarez M, Cossio Rodriguez I, Martinez Gonzalez P. [Attitude to incurable disease]. *Aten Primaria*. 1996; 17:389–393.
11. Carmel S, Lazar A. [Telling the bad news: Do the elderly want to know their diagnoses and participate in medical decision making?]. *Harefuah*. 1997; 133:505–509, 592.

• CASE 67 •

Arsenic and Old Lace: End-of-Life Care in the Postoperative Period

Death, the undiscover'd country, from whose bourn no traveler returns.
Shakespeare (1564–1616), Hamlet, Act III, Sc. 1

The patient's family and the institution's ethics committee agree with your recommendation to discontinue mechanical ventilation of a postoperative patient in a persistent vegetative state. The family wishes to be present when ventilation is discontinued, and you want the event to proceed as comfortably as possible for all involved. Which of these measures would be most ethically satisfactory in these circumstances?

(A) Morphine drip at 0.3 mg/ minute.
(B) Morphine drip titrated to provide sedation.
(C) Injection of curare.
(D) Injection of potassium chloride.
(E) Morphine drip wide open

Medical ethics and the law recognize that critical and other life-prolonging care may be withheld or withdrawn from patients in terminal (death expected in the near future despite maximal medical intervention) or irreversible conditions (susceptible to palliation but permanently incapacitating to mind and body, and ultimately fatal).[1,2] The ethical justification for this consensus is based on an understanding that the physician's obligation to delay death is neither absolute nor unconditional. In the landmark 1976 case of Karen Ann Quinlan, the New Jersey Supreme Court recognized such limits when it held, consistent with the long history of medical ethics, that the obligation to preserve life is predicated upon the patient's prognosis and the extent of invasive therapy necessary to delay death. The Court held in *Quinlan* that when there is no realistic expectation for a return to cognitive, sentient existence, particularly the ability to interact with one's surroundings and continue human development, and when measures necessary to maintain survival are so invasive that they risk increasing the patient's pain and suffering, the physician's duty to preserve life approaches its limits. The Court also acknowledged the ethical and compassionate principle of proportionality. When the iatrogenic and disease-related discomfort of ongoing clinical management outweigh the clinical benefits *for the patient*, it becomes conscionable to withhold or withdraw such medical interventions and permit the disease process to complete its course.[3] Furthermore, competent adult patients and the surrogates of patients with significantly impaired decision-making capacity are entitled to refuse treatment when the patient's condition is terminal, irreversible, and intolerable. This right has been legislatively sanctioned in all states by recognition of advance directives as legally binding.

Both the ethics and law of end-of-life care recognize the importance of palliation as one of its essential components. Palliative care, including analgesia and sedation, is grounded in the ethical principle of "double effect." Double effect refers to a single action, like analgesia or sedative administration, which has two causally independent effects, one of which is ethically and legally acceptable (relief of pain and agitation), and the other contrary to law and ethics (directly causing the patient's death). It is crucial to clinical application of the double effect principle that the acceptable outcome not be dependent upon occurrence of the unacceptable. When the two are causally independent, it is reasonable to assume that the physician intends palliation, while understanding the risk of, but not intending, the patient's death.[4] The principle of double effect recognizes a distinction between killing and permitting death, which has been endorsed in recent United States Supreme Court decisions affecting physician-assisted suicide.[5]

In our hypothetical situation, clinical administration of morphine titrated to provide sedation and relieve suffering, option (B), is supported by the principle of double effect. Effective relief of pain and suffering can be achieved without administration of lethal doses—eliminating pain and suffering by causing the patient's death—which would violate the principle of double effect.

Option (A) is not acceptable because the dosage level of morphine is too low to result in sedation and pain relief, thereby failing to meet the standard of care for palliation. The bedrock professional virtue of integrity requires that the physician always act in a clinically competent fashion.

Option (C), curare injection, will prevent the family from recognizing suffering, but without actually relieving the suffering, and likely causing death. Intellectual honesty compels the reasonable physician to recognize options (C), (D), and (E) as methods of directly and intentionally causing the patient's death. These three options clearly violate the principle of double effect. Each introduces a new, life-threatening change in the treatment regimen; option (B) does not. Moreover, option (B) provides a gradual trial of palliation that is consistent with the principle of double effect.

Some have argued that the physician is ethically justified in causing the patient's death to prevent pain and suffering when further care will restore neither consciousness nor function. This is of course an ethically controversial view. Except in the state of Oregon, and there only under strict conditions, killing patients, even with their consent, is illegal.

References

1. Wear S, Milch R. Weaver LW. Care of dying patients. In: McCullough LB, Jones JW, Brody BA, eds. *Surgical Ethics*. New York: Oxford University Press, 1998:171–197.
2. Texas Advance Directive Act, Texas Health and Safety Code. Chapter 166 (Vernon 1999).

3. In re Quinlan, 70 N.J. 10, 355 A.2d 647 (1976), cert. denied, 429 U.S. 92 (1976).

4. Garcia JLA. Double effect. In Reich WT, ed. *Encyclopedia of Bioethics.* 2nd ed. New York: Macmillan, 1995:636–641.

5. Annas GJ. The bell tolls for a constitutional right to physician-assisted suicide. *N Engl J Med.* 1997; 337:1098–1103.

6. Battin MP, Rhodes R, Silver A, eds. *Physician-Assisted Suicide: Expanding the Debate.* New York: Routledge, 1998.

· CASE 68 ·

Training on Newly Deceased Patients

Where is there dignity unless there is honesty?
Cicero (106–43 BCE)

You are the attending surgeon of a patient who has just expired. It is late in the evening; both a junior resident and a medical student have been helping with the attempted resuscitation. The ICU is almost empty. A central line kit lies on the bed, opened but not used. The junior resident asks your permission for herself and the student to practice the technique of subclavian catherization and tracheal intubation on the fresh cadaver to get a "feel" for the procedures. What is your most ethical response?

(A) Tell them to go ahead and practice.
(B) They can only practice intubation, which leaves no external wounds.
(C) You should supervise them yourself to assure their educational benefit.
(D) They should wait until you speak to the family.
(E) Tell them to practice on live patients.

A tradition in medical education allows physicians in training or medical students to "rehearse" technical procedures without consent on patients who are recently dead or near death. The rationale that no further harm can result to the patient, and improving the trainee's education will benefit future patients, seems to be *en passant* defensible, utilitarian, justification. In addition, it is often thought that explicit permission to use the newly dead will be refused by family members, thereby impairing the teaching mission.

Utilitarian philosophical arguments such as this generally ignore individual rights, and from this perspective are often found inadequate in medical ethics. Most surgeons intuit benefit from procedures on the dead, although there is no hard evidence confirming that the custom as it is currently practiced is a worthwhile educational experience.[1]

It would be difficult to argue against the practice on the basis of the rights of the newly dead patient, inasmuch as the rights of patients expire when they expire. Autonomy attaches to living persons, not cadavers. Physicians, however, are not exempt from societal customs of respect for the dead. As in requirements for permission to autopsy, harvest organs for transplantation, and use donated cadavers for teaching purposes, there is an obligation to demonstrate rituals of respect for the cadaver and to honor the preferences and decisions of those who survive deceased patients. Legally, permission is required for possession of human remains and their transportation. From the mid-19th century, every medical school must obtain the permission of a legally empowered donor before using a cadaver for teaching or research. Status as the deceased's attending physician does to invest one with the right to decide disposition of the remains. The traditional custom of using the recently deceased as teaching material without explicit family authorization assumes a highly suspect moral authority for faculty physicians.

Berger et al. have recently advanced a powerful criticism of the tradition of training on the newly dead. They argue that the contemporary norms of informed consent and of respect for the family of dead patients create an obligation to obtain informed consent for this important training experience. They conclude that "current ethical norms do not support the practice of using newly and nearly dead patients for training in invasive medical procedures absent prior consent by the patient or contemporaneous surrogate consent."[1]

The Council on Ethics Judicial Affairs (CEJA) of the American Medical Association has emphasized the importance of maintaining the trust of patients' families and the public in medical education. That trust is nurtured by an explicit consent process and threatened by its absence.[2] CEJA has further expanded the argument to include assessing the impact of this traditional teaching method on the "sentiments of the health care team and trainees," which relates directly to the importance of maintaining the integrity of the educational enterprise. CEJA notes that the normal apprehension of trainees in the presence of patients who have just died can be "intensified when the newly deceased are used in clinical training without consent." Such a practice invites trainees to put their own self-interest first, rather than their obligations to patients, thus undermining proper professional formation as fiduciaries of the patient. Because medical education should be committed to such professional formation, lack of consent for training on the newly dead does indeed threaten its moral integrity.

CEJA also notes that there are data to support a practice of explicit consent. The concern that not enough families would consent is not supported by the evidence.[3] Several prospective studies on obtaining consent for postmortem training found that medical staff received consent in from 50% to 70% of cases, when it was solicited, and very rarely noted any related emotional anxiety of family members.

Clearly a moral consensus has recently formed that training on the newly dead should be brought up to standards of moral and intellectual excellence. To achieve this goal, CEJA calls for reform of medical education regarding this practice. First, teaching crucial skills should not be episodic or happenstance, but carefully planned and supervised, so that the experience of learning on the newly dead is indeed a valid learning experience. Second, training on the newly dead "should not be undertaken without reasonable efforts to obtain informed consent, as would be done for other medical decisions." We would add that having a well thought-out and carefully designed educational plan would make consent more likely to occur, because formalization will promote trust by families in the integrity of both educators and trainees.

Option (A) is not acceptable, though we suspect it is the common practice, because the learning experience is unstructured. It is also not clear when in the educational process a student should be taught, and can retain the skills of, placing a central line. Moreover, consent has not been obtained and its absence should not be assumed to be benign in terms of impact on professional formation of the resident and student.

Option (B) is inadequate because it focuses on external appearances, perhaps even intended for deception, rather than fundamental ethical considerations. The difference in whether or not the procedure leaves external marks has no ethical relevance; requirements for permission are essentially the same whether or not epithelial surfaces are penetrated. Thus, there is good ethical reasoning for prohibiting the practice of endotracheal intubation without consent. A number of European medical societies have forbidden the practice.[4]

Option (E) assumes that there is no possible ethical rationale for training on the newly dead, which is not the case.

Options (C) and (D) together best represent the ethical rationale described by CEJA and the emerging moral consensus. Their combined effect, which respects others and structures a better learning experience, should be established as surgical academic policy in the management of this issue. In effect, CEJA has proposed a careful and respectful ethical approach to enable this traditional practice. Training programs should abandon the custom of forgoing consent in favor of policies and practices that respect the newly dead and their families, are designed to achieve relevant educational goals, and contribute to the professional development of fellows, residents, and students.

It has been suggested that implicit permission has been given for cadaver procedures in organ donors. The surgeon must decide whether the professional fiduciary obligation to the patient terminates at death or impending death, and when the professional obligation to the patient's family ends. This is an area in which a preventive ethics approach would favor obtaining permission from patients or their families before death. A failure to obtain permission displays disrespect for the deceased and the family and is consequently inconsistent with ethical practice.

References

1. Berger JT, Rosner F, Cassell EJ. Ethics of practicing medical procedures on newly dead and nearly dead patients. *J Gen Intern Med.* 2002; 17:774–778.
2. The Council on Ethics Judicial Affairs of the American Medical Association. Performing procedures on the newly deceased. *Acad Med.* 2002; 77:1212–1216.
3. McNamara RM, Monti S, Kelly JJ. Requesting consent for an invasive procedure in newly deceased adults. *JAMA.* 1995; 273:310–312.
4. Ardagh M. May we practice endotracheal inntubation on the newly dead? *J Med Eth.* 1997; 23:289–294.

• CASE 69 •

Advanced Age, Dementia, and an Abdominal Aneurysm: Intervene?

I prefer to die by the hand of God.

Ambrose Paré, a father of surgery (1510–1590), to a colleague who proposed amputating his gangrenous toes.

A 79-year-old female with advanced Alzheimer's disease is brought to the ER with increasing back pain from a 10 cm infrarenal abdominal aneurysm. The aneurysm is not suitable for endovascular repair. She is incontinent, bedridden, and unable to provide a history, her name, or respond appropriately to questions. There is no advance directive, but an accompanying elderly woman who identified the patient as "my best friend" states that, "she would not want to live this way." The friend reports that the patient has a son living in another city with whom she has not had contact for many years. The hospital has been unsuccessful in efforts to locate him. Your most ethical action is:

(A) Get a CT scan and determine whether the aneurysm is leaking to decide whether to operate or not.

(B) Do a standard open repair.

(C) Admit her, make her comfortable with analgesia, and do not intervene further.

(D) Send her back to the nursing home with orders for oral analgesia.

(E) Meet with the friend to discuss the patient's values, beliefs, and preferences, and select your clinical intervention accordingly.

Surgeons are ethically obligated to protect the health-related interests of their patients, the foremost of which is the preservation of life. Nevertheless, for as long as the practice of medicine has been associated with ethical behavior, limitations on the physician's obligation to preserve a patient's life have been acknowledged not only on the basis of his finite ability, but as an ethical obligation to contain pain and suffering. In *The Art,* the Hippocratic writers noted that medicine is sometimes powerless to alter the course of fatal disease, and that struggling against nature's boundaries represents hubris, and therefore a kind of madness.[1] Recognition of our limited ability to challenge the borders of life, and the ethical implications of doing so, have not been confined to medicine's prescientific era, and ethicists are to this moment embroiled in white-hot debate about our right to engage ourselves in the earliest and latest stages of human existence.[2] Fiduciary responsibility to patients includes the obligation to recognize the limits of medicine and surgery; responsibility to society includes recognition of finitude. Engelhardt believes that medicine's failure in this regard has allowed managed care to "redefine the character of the encounter between physicians and patients...because of a reluctance [of physicians] to accept medicine's finite abilities in postponing death and curing disease."[3]

Physiologic futility remains the most clearly defined limitation on medicine's capacity to extend life. Physiologic futility applies in clinical situations in which no surgeon can reasonably expect that the usual physiologic therapeutic outcome will result from a specified surgical procedure or intervention, however well performed.[4] This limitation does not apply in the present case because timely surgery can repair the aneurysm that is the immediate threat to our elderly patient's life.

Iatrogenic burdens of surgical or medical intervention can be so great that they become disproportionate to the expected benefits of the planned intervention and constitute a second limitation upon the surgeon's ability to intervene successfully. When a frail elderly patient's capacity to withstand the physiologic and emotional stresses of a major open surgical procedure are so severely compromised that a satisfactory outcome cannot be confidently predicted, the risk of serious harm is substantially greater than the likelihood of clinical benefits. In this case, the severity of the patient's brittle physiological reserves and the advanced state of her dementia are likely to profoundly affect her ability to cooperate in critical postoperative care, in even such basic procedures as clearing her lungs in preparation for weaning from the ventilator, and her condition is likely to deteriorate to the extent that she is unable to respond to loved ones or care givers, or interact with other elements of her environment. The reliable expectation of such an outcome is the *overall futility* described in the last case discussed in the last chapter and elsewhere.[3] If the patient has no other major medical deficits, however, she could conceivably recover to her preoperative baseline, suggesting that prediction of an inevitable unacceptable iatrogenic burden is insufficient ethical justification to withhold surgery in this case. If the patient is unable to recover interactive capacity postoperatively, then clinical or overall futility should be recognized, and discontinuation of life-sustaining interventions considered as an ethically sound course of action at that time.

The burden of disease itself constitutes yet a third major limitation upon the physician's ethical obligation to extend the life of an elderly debilitated patient. Competent adult patients are the most authoritative judges of the quality of their lives and their capacity to either derive satisfaction from or endure the hardships of their place in the world. When disease and its attendant pain and disability irrevocably overwhelm the capacity to experience pleasure in any of its manifestations or withstand misery, then the concept of *quality of life futility* applies.[4] This is likely what our patient's friend is trying to communicate in her report that the patient "would not want to live this way," bereft of the capacity to function, to sense pleasure or satisfaction, or to further experience personhood because of her disease-ravaged condition.

The surgeon does not bear unmitigated responsibility for this life-ending decision, and should take care to determine that the situation is as it appears to be by further exploring with the friend the patient's past expressions of feeling in this regard, and specifically what the patient may have intimated about her own attitudes toward profound disability and dependence. The surgeon might ask the friend about the patient's premorbid revelations of individual values, religious convictions, or personal philosophy that could provide guidance into how she would prefer to be helped through her current predicament. From this information the surgeon might infer the equivalent of an advance directive that could best characterize the patient's wishes for management of her present illness and provide some degree of authoritative guidance about the appropriate level of intervention, with options ranging from palliative care to open surgery. The dominant consideration in this case is that the iatrogenic burdens of aggressive surgical management, overlaid upon the suffering and disability of the underlying dementing process and the inevitable institutional life to follow, may not be worth enduring, but the decision must reflect as much as possible the patient's value system and not the surgeon's. The goal is to meet the substituted judgment standard for surrogate decision making, and option (E) most nearly answers that need.

It has been argued that when the patient finds the quality of life unendurable, limits on the physician's obligation to preserve life are ethically justified.[5] Option (B), simply operating, or option (D), returning the patient to the nursing home with palliative care only, are precipitous. The first of these choices presumes that surgery is unequivocally indicated, and all other values irrelevant; the second presumes just as narrowly that surgery has no meaningful role in this patient's treatment plan, and that the time has come for her life to be surrendered. Neither choice is acceptable without first consideration of a wider context. Option (A) is merely a temporizing measure; whether or not this large tender aneurysm is leaking has no real bearing upon a decision to operate. Option (C) provides more effective and carefully titrated palliative care than if the patient was returned to the nursing home, but at a vastly inflated cost for a small clinical return, and a markedly increased risk of additional major iatrogenic disease.

The surgeon is the final decision maker in such cases. Sixty-five percent of English surgeons would not operate to relieve bowel obstruction from volvulus in a demented 70-year-old patient.[2] In addition, 26% would not even perform a sigmoidoscopy.

A considerable portion of our massive national expenditures on health care is spent on end-of-life interventions, much of which may be wasted because of misdirected surgical beneficence. The decision to limit care is properly placed at the bedside, not at a bureaucratic desk. However, just as professional excellence requires reasonable certainty of the clinical diagnosis, ethics requires reasonable certainty of the status and will of the patient. One cannot summarily assume patients with diminished mental capacity lack value systems. Under the stress of acute illness, the capacity and quality of life may be obscured, and therefore, needs defining. Once the futile state is realized, it is unethical to apply surgical skills uselessly.

References

1. Jones WHS, ed. *Hippocrates.* Cambridge, Mass: Harvard University Press, Loeb Classical Library, 1923.
2. Gallagher P, Clark K. The ethics of surgery in the elderly demented with bowel obstruction. *J Med Ethics.* 2002; 28:105–108.
3. Engelhardt HT. The deprofessionalization of medicine. In: Bondeson WB, Jones JW, ed. *The Ethics of Managed Care: Professional Integrity and Patient Rights.* Boston: Kluwer Academic Publishers, 2002:93–107.
4. McCullough LB, Jones JW. Postoperative futility: A clinical algorithm for setting limits. *Brit J Surg.* 2001; 88:1153–1154.
5. Rhymes JA, McCullough LB, Luchi RJ, Teasdale TA, Wilson NL. Withdrawing very low-burden interventions in chronically ill patients. *JAMA.* 2000; 283:1061–1063.

• CASE 70 •

Withdrawal of Life-Sustaining Low-Burden Care

Technology is a way of organizing the universe so that man doesn't have to experience it.
Max Frisch (1911–1991), Homo Faber, 1957

A 90-year-old diabetic man with unresectable esophageal cancer, end-stage COPD, relentless arthritic pain, and severe disability, returns to your clinic asking you to deactivate his implanted pacemaker. To do so would likely precipitate his demise, and you ask him if he is aware of this. He tells you that he is, and that he has been considering this request since he last saw you 3 months ago. He has been evaluated by a psychiatrist and found to be mentally competent. His treatment by a pain specialist, who utilized his full armamentarium of high-dose narcotics, electronic devices, nerves blocks, and psychological techniques, has been unsuccessful. You do not reside in Oregon. What is your most ethical course of action?

(A) Comply with his request.
(B) Inform him that barbiturates are the preferred drugs for suicide, and give him a prescription.
(C) Refer him to a physician practicing in Oregon who will comply.
(D) Seek emergency commitment to a psychiatric inpatient unit, with suicide precautions.
(E) Tell him that you cannot violate good medical practice by an action that would be harmful.

Advances in medical technology often have replaced a "natural death" in the United States with various life-prolonging therapies. The artificial extension of life against disease or injury during the last century was not only approved legally and ethically, it became mandatory medical practice. Prolonging life was the supreme measure of success. For the last two decades and still in evolution, consideration of when to use life support technologies, when to discontinue them, and who should make those decisions have become potential questions.

It is well established in both law and the medical ethics of informed consent that a competent adult patient is entitled to accept or refuse a proposed medical therapy. It is similarly well accepted in law and ethics that a competent adult patient has the right to decline continued administration of an ongoing treatment modality. Most often, patients exercise this right by discontinuing their own medications or no longer appearing for scheduled follow-up visits. When patients elect to discontinue treatment without further notifying their physician, the physician has no ethical basis for intruding upon the decision. Medical paternalism has been out of favor for at least half a century.

Competent adult patients likewise have the right to refuse intensive treatment requiring the close involvement of their physicians. A competent patient hospitalized in a surgical intensive care unit, intubated and on a ventilator, is entitled to refuse further mechanical ventilator support. The surgeon in such cases is ethically and legally obligated to ensure the patient understands that imminent death will be the likely, if not certain, consequence if that decision is implemented. The patient should also be advised of any pain and discomfort associated with discontinuation of therapy, and the physician should offer help in reducing these undesired side effects. Should the competent adult patient remain committed to withdrawal of care, even life-sustaining care, the physician should promptly order palliation and extubation as requested. Patients also have the right to make and record such decisions in advance directives, before they contract terminal or irreversible conditions and can no longer make decisions for themselves. Nevertheless, our patient's pacemaker is neither the source of his intolerable discomfort, a cause of additional pathology, nor in and of itself burdensome for him to endure.[1,2] His pacemaker is physiologically effective in maintaining normal heart function.[3] Should this affect his right to insist that his physician discontinue the treatment?

This patient's current quality of life is not acceptable to him and cannot be significantly improved by medical treatment. He is continually miserable and in the terminology of our psychiatric colleagues, anhedonic—he is no longer able to experience happiness. His pain can be mitigated only by sedating him into unconsciousness, eliminating as well his ability to act and interact within his environment. Quality of life is a subjective measure of an individual's ability to engage in chosen activities and to derive satisfaction from them.[4] The determination of an individual's quality of life is not an expert judgment; indeed, external observers tend to underestimate quality of life when compared to patient self-evaluations.[5] This patient's ability to engage in valued activities and emotions has been thoroughly nullified by the severity and persistence of his pain and disability. While physiologically successful in extending his life, ongoing pacemaker management is qualitatively futile for this patient.[6] Is it ethically defensible, or desirable, to permit a patient to lapse into death by meeting his request to terminate a life-sustaining treatment which causes him no pain, inconvenience, or dangerous side effects, because, in his estimation, his chronic disease processes have utterly and irremediably destroyed the quality of his life?[7]

Option (B) is not an appropriate response to this question, constituting as it does a physician-assisted suicide, which is illegal in all states but Oregon. Violating the law by writing an intentionally lethal prescription constitutes neither principled civil disobedience nor an expression of moral purpose, and no moral authority attaches to it. The State of Oregon limits access to the provisions of its Death With Dignity Act to bona fide residents of the state.

Out-of-state referrals cannot call upon Oregon physicians to assist them in ending their lives, even when other criteria are met. Option (C) is therefore not available as a remedy for the patient.

The patient has been evaluated psychiatrically and found to be mentally competent, and as such is not a legitimate candidate for involuntary commitment to inpatient care and the highly restrictive measures associated with suicide precautions. Clearly these steps will do nothing to relieve his intolerable chronic pain or his progressive physiological disease processes. They would actually say more about your attitude toward patients' deaths and your morbidity/mortality statistics than about your concern for patients' suffering. They would represent a misuse of the psychiatric commitment process, which in most states permits involuntary hospitalization only when a patient is dangerous to himself or others *by virtue of mental illness*. Despite his very advanced age, the patient has shown no evidence on formal examination, or in his interactions with you, of cognitive or affective deficit. Although his conclusions may be debated, and indeed are the subject of the present debate, this patient has made a rational decision to end his suffering by ending his life. Option (D) is therefore not an ethically acceptable selection.

Many physicians would elect option (E), explaining to the patient that you cannot ethically perform a medical procedure which would be harmful to a patient. Modern medicine challenges the concept of natural death. In considering requests for hastened death by terminally ill patients with overwhelming suffering despite excellent palliative care, the End-of-Life Care Consensus Panel of the American College of Physicians and the American Society of Internal Medicine concluded, "In legal application, the biggest stumbling block is the physician's intention: whether it is the relief of suffering (legal) or the active hastening of death (illegal)."[7] It is becoming generally accepted that when a physician extubates a terminally ill patient in irreversible respiratory failure by request, the physician is not introducing a new pathology as a cause of death; that pathology is already present, and is then permitted to run its natural course without further intervention. We argue that in de-activating the pacemaker, the surgeon is not introducing a new pathology; the patient's existing heart disease is being allowed to run its natural course.[8] Our patient's response to the physician who says he cannot consent to a harmful procedure will likely be that the greater harm is done by facilitating his continued pain and suffering, the lesser by relieving it. Nevertheless, no turn of logic can escape the fact that de-activating this patient's pacemaker will very likely result in his death within 48 hours. If a physician's conscience simply cannot accept that relief of even the most intense and intractable suffering can be ethically purchased at such a price, then an impasse has been reached between the patient's understanding of his needs and best interests and the physician's. Referral to another physician better prepared to work with this patient should then be considered.[9]

In the tightly circumscribed conditions described, we recommend option (A) over option (E) as the most ethically sound course. This competent adult patient autonomously requests de-activation of the pacemaker after long consideration and thoughtful judgment about his negative quality of life in full awareness of the consequences of doing so. The surgeon's responsibility to preserve life then becomes properly secondary to respect for the patient's autonomy, concern for the magnitude of his suffering, and empathy for the qualitative futility of continuing to support his life with medical technology.

References

1. Paola FA, Walker RM. Deactivating the implantable cardioverter-defibrillator: A biofixture analysis. *South Med J.* 2000; 93:20–23.
2. Paola F, Walker RM. Is it ethical to withdraw low-burden interventions in chronically ill patients? *JAMA.* 2000; 284:1380.
3. Lane DJ. Is it ethical to withdraw low-burden interventions in chronically ill patients? *JAMA.* 2000; 284:1380–1381.
4. Walker LJ. Quality of life in clinical decisions. In: Reich WT, ed. *Encyclopedia of Bioethics.* 2nd ed. New York: Macmillan, 1995:1353–1358.
5. Leplège A, Hunt S. The problem of quality of life in medicine. *JAMA.* 1997; 278: 47–50.
6. Tomlinson T, Brody H. Ethics and communication in do-not-resuscitate orders. *N Engl J Med.* 1988; 318:43–46.
7. Meisel A, Snyder L, Quill T. Seven legal barriers to end-of-life care: Myths, realities, and grains of truth. *JAMA.* 2000; 284:2495–2501.
8. Rhymes JA, McCullough LB, Luchi RJ, Teasdale TA, Wilson N. Is It ethical to withdraw low-burden interventions in chronically ill patients? *JAMA.* 2000; 284: 1380–1382.
9. Jones JW, McCullough LB. Stem cell research: Obligations when religious values conflict with professional values. *J Vasc Surg.* 2004; 40:589–591.

• CASE 71 •

Physician-Assisted Suicide: Has It Come of Age?

I have learned from my life in medicine that death is not always an enemy.
Often it is good medical treatment. Often it achieves what medicine cannot
achieve—it stops suffering.
Christiaan Barnard (1922–2001), *Good Life, Good Death*

A 90-year-old diabetic man with unresectable recurrent cancer, severe disability, and unremitting pain returns to your clinic, repeatedly requesting that
you help him end his life. He explains to you that his recent life experience has been only agony, and that he derives neither satisfaction nor pleasure
from extending his painful journey to a certain death from his disease. He
has refused hospice care because he is annoyed by the hospice's emphasis on
spirituality. You have tried trans-cutaneous electrical nerve stimulation, spi-
nal cord stimulation, anticonvulsants, and antidepressants, all without success
in relieving the patient's torment. You have increased his narcotic analgesia
beyond the highest recommended doses, but still without significant effect
upon his intractable pain. He has been evaluated by a psychiatrist, who found
his affect somewhat blunted by severe chronic pain, but saw no evidence of
major depression or psychosis. You do not reside in Oregon. Today he insists
that the prescription be increased to provide a lethal dosage. What is your most
ethical course of action?

(A) Tell him that you will comply and write the prescription he requests.
(B) Seek involuntary hospital commitment with suicide precautions.
(C) Refer him to a physician practicing in Oregon, where physician-
assisted suicide is legal.
(D) Go to his home and provide assistance.
(E) Explain that what he's requesting is against the law, but incrementally
increase his dosage for pain and caution him about dangerous levels.

In the finale of 2004's Academy Award–winning best film, a fatherly friend
euthanizes a quadriplegic heroine who has pleaded for death. After discon-
necting her ventilator, the friend administers a dose of epinephrine "four times
what would kill you" (a regimen unlikely to be chosen for the purpose by a
knowledgeable physician). Without an agonal gasp or a facial grimace, the
young woman instantly goes into ventricular fibrillation and dies painlessly. It
was a movie.

Million Dollar Baby and the Schiavo case in 2005, which stimulated extraordinary interventions by the U.S. Congress and president have concentrated the
nation's attention on end-of-life issues and the role of well-intentioned help-
ers. Our most ardent advocate and practitioner of physician-assisted suicide

and euthanasia, Dr. Jack Kevorkian, was paroled in 2007 after serving 8 years in a Michigan prison for actively aiding seriously ill patients who wished to die, an occasion that fanned the flames of public opinion for and against the practice. Many people find their deeply held religious sensibilities stirred by these issues, and many link them to the nation's furious ongoing abortion debate. For physicians, including those who count themselves among one or both of these groups, these current events have necessarily reminded us of a question both ancient and basic to our art and science. Is our most important role to preserve life, or to relieve suffering?

Usually the question demands no answer: to do one is to do both. The astonishing advances in clinical medicine during the last half century have nevertheless have increased our ability to extend life, perhaps farther than our ability to prevent or relieve suffering. The roars of medicine's self-congratulations at postponing a family's pain at the pronouncement of death have sometimes made us deaf to the patient's wails. What is our responsibility when the patient tells us that enough is enough?

Suicide has been condemned as a violation of the sanctity of life. Institutional censure emerges from Church and State, which have claimed that one's life is the property of either God or the King, and therefore not the individual's to take. The Bible includes the stories of five suicides, but, despite many modern assumptions, registers neither clear approbation nor clear condemnation of the act. In Plato's Phaedo, the condemned Socrates asks, "Why, when a man is better dead, is he not permitted to be his own benefactor, but must wait for the hand of another?" Socrates concludes that the gods are ultimately the owners of men, and characterizes the suicide's offense with the question, "If one of your own possessions, an ox or an ass, took the liberty of putting himself out of the way... would you not be angry with it?" A similar position was subsequently adopted by the Christian Church. Aristotle called suicide "a denial of one's civic responsibility," and St. Thomas Aquinas said it was indicative of "a negative attitude toward God as the giver of life." Dante condemned the suicides in an even deeper pit of the Inferno than the murderers, for the sin of "denying one's own life". In the 16th and 17th centuries, English Common Law considered suicide a criminal act which deprived the king of his rightful subjects and therefore his source of homage, income, and military service. The suicide's property was seized by the King in England and by the authorities in the Colonies, leaving his family destitute. The harsh punishment was nevertheless much reduced when illness and pain were the motivating factors. The consideration that suicide is a selfish act provides most of the stigma that is removed in the suicides of martyrs who are "not merely praised but justified—- indeed, highly praised—for their deed."[1] Almost every organized religion still condemns suicide in all contexts except martyrdom, acts of valor, or most incredibly, war. Only in the last century were legal penalties for suicide lifted.

Among the 44 countries of Europe, just Belgium, the Netherlands, and Switzerland permit physician-assisted suicide, and only Oregon within the

United States. The Oregon Death With Dignity Act authorizes physician-assisted suicide. Through 2004, 208 terminally ill patients have elected to end their lives with the assistance of their physicians, or about 30 a year since the Death With Dignity Act was passed.[2] Under provisions of the law, physicians may prescribe medications for patient self-administration to end the life of a terminally ill patient, with no further involvement by the physician. Malignant neoplasms (79%) and amyotrophic lateral sclerosis (8%) have thus far been the most prominent conditions prompting Oregon patients to seek this service from physicians.[3] A rather elaborate series of conditions designed to protect patients and avoid tragic misunderstandings must be observed before the lethal prescription can be written. Monitoring by the state has shown that no more than 5% of participating physicians have been surgeons.[3] A federal court has certified the Oregon state law as constitutional, but the U.S. Department of Justice has repeatedly appealed the ruling to the U.S. Supreme Court. In earlier rulings, the high court held that there is neither a constitutional right nor a constitutional prohibition in assisted suicide. In 2006 the Supreme Court held that the U.S. Attorney General could not prohibit the use of prescribed medication in physician-assisted suicide.[4] No state, including Oregon, has legalized euthanasia, that is, direct physician administration of medication or any other procedure for the immediate purpose of causing death, even at a patient's request. No professional medical organization endorses euthanasia by doctors as ethically permissible.

John Schwartz's 2005 article in the *New York Times* cited a 2004 Gallup poll finding that 65% of respondents "agreed that a doctor should be allowed to assist a suicide when a person has a disease that cannot be cured and is living in pain." 52% of the people agreed with the principle when asked a similar survey question in 1996.[5] Many physicians nevertheless remain thoroughly uncomfortable with the idea of assisting a suicide, no matter the degree of suffering the patient must endure on the path to an otherwise certain death. The "Goldilocks Principle" is prominent among these practitioners, holding that "death by assisted suicide is too soon, death after high-tech life-prolonging treatment is too late, and natural death is just right."[6] In the discussion, Rogatz points out that a "natural death" assumes that God has an interest in the time we die. The prohibition of interference with a "natural death" apparently applies only to a "death too soon." Between "death too soon" and "death too late" is in fact the passive version of physician-assisted suicide, the withdrawal of care, nowadays a regular occurrence. Pellegrino writes that the morality of withdrawing care should be measured by whether the value of life is absolute, relative, or instrumental.[7] The balanced, or "relative" value of life suggests a rational assessment based in standards of quality and medical possibility. Does an elderly, pain-wracked terminal cancer patient's life have the same value to him and society as a healthy child's? The growing prominence of the advance directives suggests that, for almost everyone, it is not.

Option (A) requires your absolute commitment to assisting the patient in his suicide, regardless of local legal prohibitions or the availability of yet-unexplored medical measures which might afford relief without death. Physicians, like any other citizen, have ethical obligations to obey the law or oppose it through political action, which may even include civil disobedience. Moral authority does not attach to simply violating the law. In doing so one becomes a common criminal. Option (A) is not the best ethical choice.

Option (B), seeking involuntary hospital commitment and suicide precautions, may, as noted in the previous case, be more reflective of a physician's horror at the idea of a patient suicide than of his desire to actually help the patient. This patient has been psychiatrically examined and found to be psychologically clear. His suicidal thoughts have the rational intent of relieving intolerable suffering, which he's been given no reason to believe can be otherwise stopped. Involuntary hospitalization and the intensely restrictive conditions of suicide precautions violate this patient's personal autonomy and abuse the process of court commitment for treatment of mental illness. The choice should be rejected.

Patients availing themselves of the Oregon Death With Dignity Act must have been residents of the state of Oregon for at least 6 months. Out-of-state referrals for physician-assisted suicide are not accepted, eliminating option (C) as a practical choice. As an ethical consideration, even if assistance were available in Oregon, a death far from family, friends, and familiar surroundings could only add to your fragile patient's emotional trauma, and should not be recommended.

Visiting the patient's home to assist him in his suicide suggests that you are intending to administer the fatal dose of medication yourself. This would constitute euthanasia, not assisted suicide. Even if you did not plan to personally administer or even deliver the drug, your visit to the home could realistically make the patient feel obligated to go through with the suicide, even if he had begun to feel reservations. Option (D) must therefore be rejected.

Undermedication of chronic pain patients has been confirmed in numerous studies over the last decade,[8] but physicians continue to prescribe the most powerful narcotics gingerly for even the most severely afflicted terminal patients, fearing acute overdosage, legal sanctions, and, puzzlingly, dependency. Many patients in the terminal stages of cancer require analgesic dosages well beyond limits described in the pharmaceutical textbooks. If pain relief is actually achieved at these high doses, patient function and quality of life can be expected to improve rather than further deteriorate in a narcotic haze, and the motivation for suicide might actually be eliminated or reduced to tolerable levels. The continually refractive patient may of course elect to misuse this same prescription to pursue his initial plan after being advised comprehensively about critically dangerous dosages. A suicide in this manner cannot be said to be physician-assisted since the medicine was not intended for that purpose. (E) is the best option at this stage in the still developing history of ideas about physician-assisted suicide.

Unassisted suicide in terminally ill patients is higher than most would suspect. The overall suicide rate among men in general over 65 years is 0.55% yearly.[9] In a study of over 7500 young adults followed for 8 years with serious medical illnesses, 35% had suicidal ideation and 16.2% attempted suicide.[10] The suicide attempts rose to about 20% when subjects had cancer, not necessarily in the terminal phase.

So, the time has not quite come, but it appears to be approaching. Most people quietly accept the concept of physician-assisted suicide when disease-related death is certain and the intervening misery unbearable. Their acceptance has nonetheless not yet matured to the degree that they are challenging their legislators to legalize physician-assisted suicide in their states. The durability of the Oregon experiment and its ability to withstand any renewed federal pressures will be influential in determining whether other states will follow its example. The well-contained utilization of the law in Oregon suggests that it has been judiciously applied, by patients and physicians, and has thus far not created the slippery slope that opponents of anything so often invoke when neither evidence nor reason supports their views. Ultimately, it must be up to each individual patient and his physician to decide whether a higher premium should be placed on maintaining life or relieving suffering when a choice must be made. If we continue to make sure it's done that way, we will be certain to have performed ethically.

References

1. Zohar N. Jewish deliberations on suicide. In: Battin M, Rhodes R, Silvers A, eds. Physician Assisted Suicide, New York: Routledge, 1998.
2. Okie S. Physician-assisted suicide—Oregon and beyond. *N Engl J Med.* 2005; 352:1627–1630.
3. Annan GJ. Congress, controlled substances, and physician-assisted suicide— elephants in mouseholes. *N Engl J Med.* 2006; 354:1079–1084.
4. Leman R. *Sixth Annual Report on Oregon's Death with Dignity Act.* Portland, Ore: Department of Human Services, Health Services, Office of Disease Prevention and Epidemiology, 2004.
5. Schwartz J. New openness in deciding when and how to die. *New York Times.* 3/21/2005:A1.
6. Rogatz P. Physician assisted suicide should be legalized. In: Haley J, ed. *Death and Dying: Opposing Viewpoints.* Farmington Hills, Mich: Greenhaven Press, 2003.
7. Pellegrino ED. Decisions to withdraw life-sustaining treatment: A moral algorithm. *JAMA.* 2000; 283:1065–1067.
8. Addington-Hall J, McCarthy M. Dying from cancer: Results of a national population-based investigation. *Palliat Med.* 1995; 9:295–305.
9. Llorente, MSD, Burke M, Gregory GR, Bosworth HB, Grambow SC, Horner RD, Golden A, Olsen EJ. Prostate cancer: A significant risk factor for late-life suicide. *Am J Geriatr Psychiat.* 2005; 13:195–201.
10. Druss B, Pincus H. Suicidal ideation and suicide attempts in general medical illnesses. *Arch Intern Med.* 2000; 160:1522–1526.

· Index ·